T5-DGR-019

IMAGING HANDBOOK
FOR HOUSE OFFICERS

IMAGING HANDBOOK FOR HOUSE OFFICERS

Edited by

Paul M. Silverman, MD
Professor of Radiology and Medical Oncology
Director of Computed Tomography
Co-Director of Abdominal Imaging Division
Georgetown University Medical Center

Douglas J. Quint, MD
Associate Professor of Neuroradiology
and Magnetic Resonance Imaging
University of Michigan Medical Center

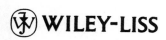 **WILEY-LISS**

A John Wiley & Sons, Inc., Publication
New York · Chichester · Brisbane · Toronto · Singapore · Weinheim

This text is printed on acid-free paper.

Copyright © 1997 by John Wiley & Sons, Inc.

All rights reserved. Published simultaneously in Canada.

Reproduction or translation of any part of this work beyond that permitted by Section 107 or 108 of the 1976 United States Copyright Act without the permission of the copyright owner is unlawful. Requests for permission or further information should be addressed to the Permissions Department, John Wiley & Sons, Inc., 605 Third Avenue, New York, NY 10158-0012.

While the authors, editors, and publisher believe that drug selection and dosage and the specification and usage of equipment and devices, as set forth in this book, are in accord with current recommendations and practice at the time of publication, they accept no legal responsibility for any errors or omissions, and make no warranty, express or implied, with respect to material contained herein. In view of ongoing research, equipment modifications, changes in government regulations, and the constant flow of information relating to drug therapy, drug reactions, and the use of equipment and devices, the reader is urged to review and evaluate the information provided in the package insert or instructions for each drug, piece of equipment, or device for, among other things, any changes in the instructions for indication of dosage or usage and for added warnings and precautions.

Library of Congress Cataloging-in-Publication Data:

Imaging handbook for house officers / edited by Paul M. Silverman, Douglas J. Quint.

    p.   cm.

    Includes index.

    ISBN 0-471-13767-7 (pbk. : alk. paper)

    1. Diagnostic imaging—Handbooks, manuals, etc. 2. Diagnosis, Radioscopic—Handbooks, manuals, etc. I. Silverman, Paul M. II. Quint, Douglas J.

    [DNLM: 1. Diagnostic Imaging—handbooks. WN 39 I31 1997]

RC78.7.D53I4415   1997

616.07′54—dc20

DNLM/DLC

for Library of Congress   96-20853

Printed in the United States of America

10 9 8 7 6 5 4 3 2 1

To

My wife, Amy, and children, Zachary and Rebecca
PAUL M. SILVERMAN, MD

My wife, Leslie, and sons, Jason and Mark
DOUGLAS J. QUINT, MD

▶ Contents

▶ Contributors

Marie D. Acierno, MD
Director, Department of Ophthalmology, University of Mississippi
Medical Center, Jackson, Mississippi

Mohamed Mohamed Amin, MD
Lecturer, Department of Radiology, University of Michigan Medical
Center, Ann Arbor, Michigan

Bernard A. Birnbaum, MD
Associate Professor of Radiology, Hospital of the University of
Pennsylvania, Philadelphia, Pennsylvania

Harry Cloft, MD
Fellow, Department of Radiology, University of Virginia Medical Center,
Charlottesville, Virginia

Richard H. Cohan, MD
Associate Professor of Radiology, University of Michigan Medical
Center, Ann Arbor, Michigan

Wayne Cornblath, MD
Assistant Professor, Departments of Neurology and Ophthalmology,
University of Michigan Medical Center, Ann Arbor, Michigan

Deborah J. Crowe, MD
Senior Staff Radiologist, Henry Ford Hospital, Detroit, Michigan

Michael DiPietro, MD
Professor of Radiology, University of Michigan Medical Center, Ann
Arbor, Michigan

O. Petter Eldevik, MD
Associate Professor of Radiology, University of Michigan Medical
Center, Ann Arbor, Michigan

James H. Ellis, MD
Associate Professor of Radiology, University of Michigan Medical Center, Ann Arbor, Michigan

Stephen S. Gebarski, MD
Associate Professor of Radiology, University of Michigan Medical Center, Ann Arbor, Michigan

Barry H. Gross, MD
Professor of Radiology, University of Michigan Medical Center, Ann Arbor, Michigan

Katrina Gwinn, MD
Fellow, Department of Neurology, Mayo Clinic, Scottsdale, Arizona

Barbara Hertzberg, MD
Associate Professor of Radiology and Assistant Professor of Obstetrics and Gynecology, Duke University Medical Center, Durham, North Carolina

Jacquelyn P. Hogge, MD
Assistant Professor of Radiology, Georgetown University Medical Center, Washington, DC

David Jamadar, MB, BS, FRCS, FRCR
Lecturer, Department of Radiology, University of Michigan Medical Center, Ann Arbor, Michigan

Ella Kazerooni, MD
Assistant Professor of Radiology, University of Michigan Medical Center, Ann Arbor, Michigan

Thomas Kim, MD
Fellow, Department of Radiology, University of Michigan Medical Center, Ann Arbor, Michigan

Nirish R. Lal, MD
Radiology Resident, University of Michigan Medical Center, Ann Arbor, Michigan

Laurie Loevner, MD
Assistant Professor of Radiology, University of Pennsylvania Medical Center, Philadelphia, Pennsylvania

James Meaney, MRCPI, FRCR
Lecturer, University of Michigan Medical Center, Ann Arbor, Michigan

Douglas J. Quint, MD
Associate Professor of Neuroradiology and Magnetic Resonance Imaging,
University of Michigan Medical Center, Ann Arbor, Michigan

Stephen E. Rubesin, MD
Associate Professor of Radiology, Hospital of the University of
Pennsylvania, Philadelphia, Pennsylvania

Allen E. Schlesinger, MD
Associate Professor of Radiology, Baylor University, Houston, Texas

William W. Scott, Jr., MD
Associate Professor of Radiology and Orthopaedic Surgery, Johns
Hopkins Medical Center, Baltimore, Maryland

Marilyn J. Siegel, MD
Professor of Radiology and Pediatrics, Mallinckrodt Institute of
Radiology, Washington University School of Medicine, St. Louis,
Missouri

Paul M. Silverman, MD
Professor of Radiology and Medical Oncology, Director of Computed
Tomography, and Co-Director of Abdominal Imaging Division,
Georgetown University Medical Center, Washington, DC

Duc Tran, MD
Lecturer, Department of Radiology, University of Michigan Medical
Center, Ann Arbor, Michigan

Todd E. Wilson, MD
Assistant Professor of Radiology, University of Michigan Medical Center,
Ann Arbor, Michigan

Rebecca A. Zuurbier, MD
Director of Breast Imaging, Georgetown University Medical Center,
Washington, DC

▶ Preface

The subspecialty of radiology and, more specifically, diagnostic imaging has undergone extremely rapid growth over the past few decades. It now occupies a pivotal position in the triage, diagnosis, and subsequent treatment of most patients with significant medical or surgical abnormalities. Prior to the ready availability of even basic radiologic imaging, the diagnosis of the vast array of medical and surgical illnesses literally fell upon the eyes, hands, and experience of the examining physician. Skills in taking an accurate clinical history and integrating it with the findings on physical examination were paramount. Despite the high level of acumen many of these physicians developed over a long course of training, apprenticeship, and personal practice, arriving at a correct diagnosis remained a great challenge. Misdiagnosis often resulted in delays of treatment or even unnecessary surgical exploration.

In more modern years, the development of a vast array of laboratory tests and radiologic studies has dramatically changed the ability and approach of physicians to diagnose complex disease processes. Early on, radiologic studies were basically limited to plain films, barium studies of the gastrointestinal tract, and use of iodinated contrast material to perform intravenous pyelograms for displaying the genitourinary tract. Radioisotopes were employed to evaluate the bony skeleton, liver, spleen, kidneys, and other organs such as the thyroid gland. These studies served to benefit both patients and physicians by yielding important clinical information that complimented the history and physical examination. Over the past two decades there has been a dramatic increase in the number of diagnostic radiologic procedures available. Much of this has been technology-driven. These studies include sophisticated nuclear medicine studies, computed tomography (CT), and magnetic resonance imaging (MRI), as well as various functional studies. The dramatic explosion in the number and types of diagnostic procedures available has become a "two-edged sword." In many cases these studies are both highly sensitive and highly specific, allowing one to expeditiously make a correct diagnosis and implement appropriate therapy. On the other hand, incorrect usage of many of these studies has added significant costs to the health care system and has occasionally contributed to patient morbidity.

In the present climate of significant concerns over the cost of providing universal health care and the widespread takeover by managed care operations (MCOs) wishing to cut medical costs severely, it has become evident that there will be significant limitations imposed on the total expenditure of funds allocated for medical care. This begs the question, "How are we to utilize our medical resources efficiently and appropriately to optimize patient care?" For many years I have struggled in my role as a radiologist to deal more effectively with this issue. I am fortunate to have gained experience at a number of excellent medical centers—Stanford University, Duke University, and Georgetown University—teaching medical students, training house officers, and being involved on a daily basis as part of a consultative service in trying to plan an appropriate radiologic workup of various symptom complexes. It is through this experience of working with house officers, general practitioners, internists, and subspecialists that I began to appreciate the complexities these physicians face daily when confronted with the vast array of radiologic imaging studies that are available. My daily clinical experience provided an impetus to design a book that was symptom-complex oriented as an approach to guiding *nonradiologists* to the appropriate radiologic workup for their patients. Although it would be valuable to be able to have radiologists involved in the workup of each patient from the earliest point of presentation, this is not the reality of the present state of medical care. In fact, many if not most radiologic studies are ordered by physicians prior to consultation with the radiologist based on their knowledge and perception of what these tests can offer. As one can imagine, there is variability between physicians as a result of their knowledge, areas of expertise, and length of experience.

The goal of this handbook is to provide nonradiologists with a succinct guide for organizing the radiologic workup of patients suffering from certain basic symptom complexes. The handbook is divided into the following organ-based subspecialties: *Musculoskeletal Disease and Trauma, Gastrointestinal Disease, Genitourinary Disease, Obstetrics and Gynecology, Pediatrics, Breast Disease, Chest and Cardiac Disease,* and *Central Ner-*

vous System and Head and Neck Disease. Within each major section there are a number of major subheadings representing a wide variety of common clinical symptoms or patient presentations. After considerable personal reflection and consultation with my clinical colleagues, I decided a valuable and consistent organization under each symptom complex would be (1) *Clinical Findings,* (2) *Imaging Modalities,* (3) *Recommended Imaging Approach,* and (4) *Differential Diagnostic Considerations.* The first section, *Clinical Findings,* is a review of the clinical findings most commonly found to be associated with the patient's chief complaint or clinical presentation. Contained within this section are also important associated clinical or laboratory findings. In some cases additional information is provided related to the necessity of any imaging tests or the most likely etiology based on certain aspects of the clinical presentation. In the second section, *Imaging Modalities,* various radiologic imaging modalities are listed and the expected findings from each of these studies are presented as they relate to the patient's principal clinical presentation. The pros and cons as well as the strengths and limitations of the different studies are discussed. This assists the clinician in anticipating the radiologic findings associated with various clinical presentation or disease entities. The third and perhaps most important section is *Recommended Imaging Approach.* This was the most difficult section to organize. In some cases the least expensive test was applied as a screening test with more expensive examinations performed only as necessary later in the workup. In certain workups it was found to be important to relay to the clinician which radiologic tests were of minimal or no added value, providing only an additional cost to the patient. In some cases we found that an expensive test such as an MRI study is actually more cost-effective and definitive than a battery of less expensive but less specific studies. Within this section the reader will note that each of the radiologist's contributions provide a "roadmap" for what is perceived as the optimal radiologic workup for a given clinical presentation. In some cases certain radiologic tests are mentioned as an alternative examination if other tests are not available, as in the case of CT being a substitute for MRI.

This section also includes details of particular value to the referring physicians on more sophisticated radiologic studies such as the value of

contrast enhancement in CT and MRI, which may lead to increased specificity or to the use of noninvasive studies such as sonography of the lower
extremities for deep venous thrombosis. For example, in the latter case, patients clinically suspected to have pulmonary embolism may benefit from
lower extremity Doppler sonography to demonstrate deep venous thrombosis to increase the diagnostic certainty when the ventilation perfusion
nuclear medicine lung scan is interpreted as "indeterminant." A positive
Doppler sonogram can potentially obviate the necessity of expensive, invasive, and potentially dangerous pulmonary angiography, allowing the
prompt institution of anticoagulant therapy.

Perhaps most enlightening is the fourth section, *Differential Diagnostic Considerations.* In this section, the contributors had the freedom to describe various notable aspects of the radiologic imaging workup, providing
the reader with clinical, pathophysiologic, and imaging information about
a wide spectrum of clinical diseases. If specific clinical entities could be
confused with the primary diagnosis, these are described. The radiologic
workup is placed in the context of the clinical disease with differential diagnostic possibilities. Included in this section are facts related to the radiologic findings of specific diseases and the relative value and reliability of
positive or negative findings. Limitations of certain examinations are described, and, importantly, certain radiologic findings are not just described
but placed in the appropriate clinical context to assist the clinician in arriving at a confident final diagnosis. A limited number of references are also
included for the reader to pursue more in-depth study.

As you will note, the book is soft-covered rather than hard-covered
and has been specifically designed to fit in the pocket of a laboratory coat.
The aim of the contributors was to provide portability so that the book
could function as a guide or "handbook" for the practical ordering of radiologic examinations and appreciation of the significance of the results.
The organization in an outline form was thought to be the easiest way to
provide readability and easy access to the material. Although some algorithms were used, it was not thought during the design of the book that a
rigid algorithmic approach would be the most effective one. As one of the
contributors related to me, "the proper algorithm path is often only obvious
once the diagnosis is known" (M.DiP.). There is much truth to this state-

ment. Algorithms, which in retrospect appear to be wonderful guides, are often much more difficult to follow in the prospective evaluation of patients since our patients do not always read the textbooks.

It is my hope, along with that of my co-editor Douglas Quint and all my colleagues who worked so diligently on this project, that this handbook will provide a valuable manual for navigating the increasingly complex array of radiologic imaging studies now available.

PAUL M. SILVERMAN, MD

► CHAPTER 1

Musculoskeletal Disease and Trauma

William W. Scott, Jr., MD
Johns Hopkins Medical Center

Imaging Handbook for House Officers, Edited by Paul M. Silverman and Douglas J. Quint.
ISBN 0-471-13767-7 © 1997 Wiley-Liss, Inc.

CERVICAL SPINE FRACTURE OR DISLOCATION

A. Clinical Findings

1. History of motor vehicle accident, fall (often down stairs), or other trauma.
2. Pain in neck.
3. Neurologic signs referable to the C-spine.
4. The above are unreliable if the patient is intoxicated, has a decreased level of consciousness, or has multisystem injury.

B. Imaging Modalities

1. Plain radiography with lateral, AP, and AP open-mouth odontoid views has a sensitivity of over 90% for cervical spine fractures. The lateral view alone has a sensitivity of about 80%. Some authorities advise also obtaining supine oblique views of the injury victim. All of these initial studies are obtained with the patient supine in a neck collar. In patients with short necks and thick shoulders, downward traction on the arms aids in visualization of the lower C-spine on the lateral view. If this fails, the swimmers view is an alternative. Flexion-extension lateral views, in the alert cooperative patient with the patient actively doing the flexing and extending, are useful in diagnosis of hyperflexion sprain.

2. Conventional tomography is useful in suspected odontoid fracture, because the fracture is in the axial plane. Many prefer conventional tomography to CT in this situation, although CT reconstructions, especially from spiral CT, may provide the same information.

3. CT provides greater detail of fractures identified on conventional radiographs and not infrequently demonstrates additional fractures, although usually not major ones. CT can "clear" the lower C-spine when all pain film maneuvers have proven unsuccessful.

4. MRI has not been extensively used in the trauma setting because of difficulty with life support equipment in the scanner and surrounding area. Where this limitation has been overcome, MRI has proven quite useful. It provides unique information about the spinal cord

that has prognostic value. It can diagnose hyperextension injuries in which the anterior column is disrupted, but the plain radiographs are normal or near normal. Bone, however, is not as well seen as on CT so that there is a danger of missing posterior element fractures unless some other imaging modality is also used.

C. Recommended Imaging Approach

1. Lateral, AP, and open-mouth odontoid views of C-spine.
2. Supplement above with swimmers view of lower C-spine if C7 not initially visualized.
3. In alert patient with question of hyperflexion sprain after initial exam, obtain active flexion-extension lateral views.
4. If any portion of the C-spine remains nonvisualized, do CT of that portion.
5. If any fracture is identified or any area is suspicious, do CT of that level and the level above and below.
6. If subtle odontoid fracture is suspected, obtain AP and lateral conventional tomography. If not available, use CT with reconstructions.
7. Obtain MRI in patients with normal plain radiographs and neurologic deficit.

D. Differential Diagnostic Considerations

1. History and physical examination are very reliable in alert individuals and may allow one not to obtain an imaging study of the C-spine.
2. In patients with altered consciousness and history and/or other injuries to suggest C-spine injury, a full evaluation must be done.
3. Lack of prevertebral soft tissue swelling does not exclude fracture—do not let this finding lessen your suspicion.
4. The open-mouth odontoid view is not only good for visualization of odontoid fractures but is also the best view to detect the burst fracture of C1 (Jefferson fracture).

References

Orrison WW Jr, Benzel EC, Willis BK, Hart BL, Espinosa MC (1995). Magnetic resonance imaging evaluation of acute spine trauma. Emerg Radiol 2:120–128.

Pathria MN, Petersilge CA (1991). Spinal trauma. Radiol Clin North Am 29:847–865.

DIAPHYSEAL LONG BONE FRACTURE

A. Clinical Findings

1. History of trauma.
2. Pain.
3. Deformity.
4. Abnormal motion.
5. Crepitus.
6. Local tenderness to palpation.

B. Imaging Modalities

1. Plain radiography of suspected fracture site. Two views in orthogonal projections must be obtained.
2. Computed radiography (CR) would be comparable where available.
3. CT, MRI not indicated.
4. Angiography may be needed to evaluate arterial injuries in cases of severe trauma with pulse deficit or penetrating injury.

C. Recommended Imaging Approach

1. Plain radiographs in orthogonal projections.
2. Include adjacent joints on radiographs, especially in tibia–fibula and radius–ulna examinations.
3. Additional views of suspicious areas where initial radiographs are not conclusive.
4. If there is a pulse deficit, gunshot wound, or penetrating injury with suspected arterial injury, perform arteriogram.

D. Differential Diagnostic Considerations

1. Check for additional fractures or dislocations where there are paired bones as in the radius–ulna and tibia–fibula.
2. Consider age-related fracture types in guiding your search. Torus fractures and bowing deformities occur in young, more deformable bones. Salter-Harris type injuries must be considered near growth plate in immature skeletons.
3. Transverse fractures of long bones are very unusual in normal bone and suggest an underlying pathologic condition such as Paget's disease of bone, metastasis, myeloma, or other lytic lesion of bone. Fractures with little or no trauma and ill-defined fracture margins should suggest the possibility of preexistent bone abnormality.

References

Kerr R (1989). Diagnostic imaging of upper extremity trauma. Radiol Clin North Am 27:891–908.

Mitchell MJ, Ho C, Resnick D, Sartoris DJ (1989). Diagnostic imaging of lower extremity trauma. Radiol Clin North Am 27:909–928.

FRACTURE INVOLVING A JOINT

A. Clinical Findings

1. History of trauma.
2. Joint effusion.
3. Swelling, discoloration, local tenderness near joint.
4. Loss of joint function.

B. Imaging Modalities

1. Plain radiographs, often with three views, are diagnostic in most cases. Additional radiographic projections are more likely to be useful than for fractures of the diaphyses of long bones.
2. CT is frequently useful to measure displacement of articular frag-

ments, detect additional fractures, and define the relationship of the fragments to one another in complex comminuted fractures.

3. MRI is very sensitive to subtle fractures such as "bone bruises," which are often seen in conjunction with ligamentous injuries. The utility of demonstrating these is as yet unclear. MRI can be used in the knee to evaluate tibial plateau fractures and accompanying ligamentous injuries simultaneously. Not infrequently, when MRI is used to evaluate the soft tissues, an unsuspected fracture is discovered. One example of this is the finding of a nondisplaced fracture of the greater tuberosity of the humerus while investigating suspected rotator cuff injury. MRI is good for further evaluation of osteochondral fractures as to degree of attachment and displacement of the fragment. MRI can demonstrate growth plate fractures that may only be inferred from plain film examination or cannot be detected.

4. ^{99m}Tc bone scan is useful to diagnose or exclude radiographically occult fractures of the scaphoid or radial head in situations where the patient's occupation makes a trial of immobilization difficult.

C. Recommended Imaging Approach

1. Plain radiographs in at least two perpendicular projections. Often an oblique view is useful.
2. Additional views in suspicious cases for scaphoid, radial head, tibial plateau, patella, calcaneus, and shoulder.
3. For suspected, initially nonvisualized fractures, one option is to treat for 10–14 days and then reexamine and reradiograph. This is used most often for suspected scaphoid and radial head fractures.
4. CT can be employed for displaced tibial plateau fractures and comminuted calcaneal fractures to plan surgery. It also permits evaluation of the distal radioulnar joint, even through a cast.
5. ^{99m}Tc bone scan or MRI can be used to detect or exclude fracture in important weight-bearing areas such as the hip and also in the scaphoid and radial head where radiographically occult fractures are not uncommon.
6. MRI is useful to characterize Salter type fractures of the elbow in very young children where most of the elbow is cartilaginous.

D. Differential Diagnostic Considerations

1. A trial of therapy followed by reexamination may be a safe and economical way to deal with a suspected occult fracture of the scaphoid or radial head if acceptable to the patient.

2. In obtaining follow-up radiographs to detect initially occult fractures, wait at least 10–14 days to permit radiographically visible healing to occur.

3. Oblique views are often useful to detect nondisplaced tibial plateau fractures.

4. The axillary view of the shoulder is useful for dislocations and for fractures of the coracoid process and acromion.

5. The sunrise view demonstrates sagittal patellar fractures.

6. A fluid–fluid level in a joint may be a lipohemarthrosis and should stimulate an exhaustive search for a fracture.

7. Fat pad displacement in the elbow is a reliable sign of joint effusion and strong predictor of fracture, more so in adults than in children.

References

Newberg, AH (1990). Computed tomography of joint injuries. Radiol Clin North Am 28:445–460.

Rubin DA, Dalinka MK, Kneeland JB (1994). Magnetic resonance imaging of lower extremity injuries. Semin Roentgenol 29:194–222.

HIP FRACTURE

A. Clinical Findings

1. History of a fall on the hip with inability or great difficulty bearing weight on the involved lower extremity.

2. Pain in the region of the hip, groin, and/or thigh.

3. Bruising in the hip region.

4. Excessive external rotation or other unusual positioning of the femur.

B. Imaging Modalities

1. AP and lateral radiographs of the involved hip. These will be diagnostic in the vast majority of cases.
2. ^{99m}Tc-MDP radionuclide bone scan to detect or exclude occult fractures in radiographically negative cases where there is still a reasonable clinical suspicion of fracture. In a small fraction of patients, especially the elderly, this study may give false-negative results during the first 72 hours after fracture. In highly suspicious cases, a delayed study will be necessary.
3. MRI, if obtainable on an emergent basis, is very sensitive for radiographically occult fractures. T1-weighted coronal views are suggested. MRI should be positive immediately after the trauma, a potential cost-saving advantage over bone scan.
4. CT may show some radiographically occult fractures but cannot be relied on to "exclude" a fracture. It is more useful to give additional anatomic information about a known fracture when such information is necessary for treatment planning.

C. Recommended Imaging Approach

1. Plain radiographs in AP and lateral projections of the proximal femur. If these demonstrate the fracture, imaging is often complete.
2. In rare cases of comminuted fractures, CT may be necessary for planning of operative treatment.
3. In plain radiograph-negative cases that have a high clinical suspicion of fracture, MRI T1-weighted coronal views should be obtained to detect or exclude nondisplaced fracture. The patient must be kept non-weight bearing until fracture is excluded.
4. If MRI is unavailable, ^{99m}Tc bone scan should be performed. If initially negative in elderly individuals, a repeat scan should be done after 72 hours of the injury to reliably exclude fracture.

D. Differential Diagnostic Considerations

1. Keep the patient non-weight bearing until a fracture has been excluded to prevent displacement of an occult nondisplaced fracture. Displacement could have significant impact on prognosis, increas-

ing the chance of avascular necrosis of the femoral head and making reduction and fixation more difficult.

2. Be certain to obtain two perpendicular views of the proximal femur on the plain radiographs. Often the lateral view obtained initially is poorly positioned due to the patient's condition and inability to cooperate.

3. Remember that, especially in elderly patients, the bone scan may give false-negative results prior to 72 hours after injury.

4. If fracture margins are poorly defined or portions of bone appear to be missing, consider the possibility of pathologic fracture through a lytic lesion.

References

Deutsch AL, Mink JH, Waxman AD (1989). Radiology 170:113–116.

Holder LE, Schwarz C, Wernicke PG, Michael RH (1990). Radionuclide bone imaging in the early detection of fractures of the proximal femur (hip). Radiology 174:509–515.

PELVIC FRACTURE

A. Clinical Findings

1. History of major trauma.
2. Pain to lateral compression of the pelvis.
3. Hematuria.
4. Overlying swelling, discoloration.
5. Possible major internal blood loss.

B. Imaging Modalities

1. Plain radiography: AP view of pelvis. Permits identification of most major fractures without moving patient, who may have multiple injuries.

2. Additional plain radiographs for further classification of major fractures or exclusion or diagnosis of suspected minor fractures. Views

include bilateral "Judet" obliques, inlet view (AP angled caudad), and outlet view or tangential view (AP angled cephalad).

3. CT provides further analysis of major fractures and detects fractures missed on plain radiographs. About 70% of sacral fractures are initially not recognized on plain radiography. Bone fragments in the hip joint often cannot be identified on plain radiography but are easily seen on CT. CT with 3D reconstructions can entirely replace the additional radiographs in (2) above and does not require rolling the patient for oblique views. CT can thus provide the overview and the details in one exam. CT also identifies major hemorrhage and soft tissue injuries. It often is required to evaluate other injuries in the multiple-injury patient (head, C-spine, thorax, abdomen).

4. Angiography may be useful in cases with associated major pelvic hemorrhage to identify the site of bleeding and to treat it by embolization.

5. Especially in fractures of the anterior pelvis, the posterior urethra or bladder may be injured (7%). Retrograde urethrogram followed by a cystogram are the tests to evaluate these injuries.

6. MRI has been little used in this setting due to difficulties supporting a multiple-injury patient in the MRI environment.

C. Recommended Imaging Approach

1. AP radiograph of pelvis.
2. To exclude or detect suspected minor fracture, do oblique views.
3. If major fracture (involving the acetabulum or multiple locations in the pelvic ring) is detected and patient's condition permits, do CT for further evaluation. If need is thought for 3D orientation for a major fracture, do 3D reconstructions from the CT; if that is not available, do oblique, inlet, and outlet conventional views.

D. Differential Diagnostic Considerations

1. Pelvic fractures have a high associated mortality (9%–19%) because of frequent multiple associated injuries and hemorrhage. All the injuries must be treated in a prioritized manner.

2. Study the sacral foramina to detect subtle, otherwise overlooked sacral fractures.
3. The pelvis is a ring; always look for the second fracture.

References

Scott WW Jr, Fishman EK, Magid D (1987). Acetabular fractures: optimal imaging. Radiology 165:537–539.

Young JWR, Resnik CS (1990). Fracture of the pelvis: current concepts of classification. AJR 155:1169–1175.

STRESS FRACTURE OR INSUFFICIENCY FRACTURE

A. Clinical Findings

1. History of unaccustomed repetitive activity (or lesser activity in a person with osteoporosis).
2. Development of localized pain and tenderness.
3. Characteristic location of symptomatic area (e.g., tibia, metatarsals, lower back, groin).
4. Pain relieved by rest, aggravated by activity.

B. Imaging Modalities

1. Plain radiography, two orthogonal views, may show healing stress fracture and helps differentiate other etiologies for the pain such as complete fracture, osteoid osteoma, neoplasm, and infection.
2. ^{99m}Tc-MDP bone scan will show focal fusiform increased uptake at site of stress fracture very early in the course of the process. Stress fracture and "shin splints" can be differentiated in most cases. In the presence of known malignancy, one may be unable to differentiate stress fracture (or insufficiency fracture) from metastasis.
3. CT can add specificity. It is especially good for confirmation of sacral insufficiency fractures in osteopenic individuals.
4. MRI is sensitive to stress fractures as well as ordinary fractures. The findings may be nonspecific. The test is expensive.

C. Recommended Imaging Approach

1. Plain radiographs in two orthogonal projections. If stress fracture or other lesion responsible for pain is identified, stop here.
2. If radiographs are negative and the diagnosis must be made immediately, do ^{99m}Tc bone scan. Or, rest, treat, and radiograph again in 10–14 days.
3. CT is quite useful to confirm suspected sacral insufficiency fracture.

D. Differential Diagnostic Considerations

1. Prompt diagnosis of femoral neck stress fractures is important to avoid progression to displaced fracture.
2. Conventional radiographs are negative at initial presentation in over 50% of stress fractures.
3. Tibial stress fracture requires cessation of the inciting activity and often casting, and "shin splints" may be treated with decreased activity. These entities can be differentiated by bone scan.
4. A knowledge of the usual site of stress fractures is important, because the diagnosis depends on a typical history and symptoms at a typical location.

References

Lee JK, Yao I (1988). Stress fractures: MR imaging. Radiology 169:217–220.

Rupani HD, Holder LE, Espinola DA, Engin SI (1985). Three phase radionuclide bone imaging in sports medicine. Radiology 156:187–196.

PAINFUL WRIST

A. Clinical Findings

1. Pain that may be ulnar or radial side predominantly.
2. Limitation of motion.
3. Decreased strength.

4. Jerky motion and "popping" or "clunking" sounds with certain motions.
5. Possible trauma history, recent or remote.

B. Imaging Modalities

1. Plain radiographs: PA, lateral, and oblique. Scaphoid view(s). Carpal tunnel view. Instability series: clenched fist, radial deviation, ulnar deviation, flexion, extension.
2. Arthrography with contrast injection into one or all of three joints: wrist, midcarpal, and distal radioulnar. If several are injected, the procedure takes several hours to permit the contrast to be absorbed from one joint before the next is injected. Arthrography demonstrates tears of the triangular fibrocartilage, the scapholunate ligament, and the lunotriquetral ligament.
3. MRI can demonstrate abnormalities of the intercarpal ligaments similar to arthrography. The contents and abnormalities of the carpal tunnel are demonstrated. Tendons and tendinitis can be diagnosed. Soft tissue masses including ganglion cysts can be evaluated, especially prior to surgery. Subtle scaphoid fractures and early avascular necrosis of the scaphoid or lunate can be diagnosed.
4. CT can provide detailed images of scaphoid and other fractures if needed for surgery and can assess the results of surgery and fracture or fusion healing. It is useful to detect radiographically occult fractures suspected from positive bone scan. It provides the definitive method of investigation of possible subluxation or dislocation of the distal radioulnar joint when conventional radiographs are equivocal. The scan can even be done through a cast.
5. Radionuclide bone scan can identify or exclude subtle fractures such as of the scaphoid under circumstances when a trial of therapy is not satisfactory, as in the case of a professional athlete.

C. Recommended Imaging Approach

1. For arthritis, almost all fractures and dislocations, and possible bony changes associated with a mass, obtain plain radiographs: PA, later-

al, and oblique views. Add scaphoid view if appropriate. Carpal tunnel view good for hook of hamate fracture.

2. Obtain instability series if instability is clinically suspected or suspected from initial radiographs.

3. Obtain bone scan to exclude fracture under special circumstances (professional athlete).

4. Obtain CT scan rarely for distal radioulnar joint subluxation/dislocation.

5. Obtain wrist joint arthrography for suspected tear of triangular fibrocartilage, scapholunate ligament, or lunotriquetral ligament. With a high degree of clinical suspicion, add distal radioulnar injection and midcarpal injection to demonstrate the small percentage of unidirectional communications.

6. Obtain MRI as alternative to arthrography.

7. Use MRI for evaluation of soft tissue masses and their relationship to other structures prior to surgery.

D. Differential Diagnostic Considerations

None.

References

Manaster BJ (1991). The clinical efficacy of triple-injection wrist arthrography. Radiology 178:267–270.

Zlatkin MB, Chao PC, Osterman AL, Schnall MD, Dalinka MK, Kressel HY (1989). Chronic wrist pain: Evaluation with high resolution MR imaging. Radiology 173:723–729.

PAINFUL SHOULDER

A. Clinical Findings

1. Pain.
2. Limitation of motion.

3. Instability.
4. Possible history of previous trauma, dislocation.

B. Imaging Modalities

1. Plain radiography permits detection of soft tissue calcifications in the rotator cuff suggestive of calcific tendinitis. Arthritic changes sufficient to result in osteophytes of the glenohumeral joint or acromioclavicular joint are demonstrated, as is glenohumeral joint narrowing on a Grashey view. Osteophytes from the acromion in the insertion of the coracoacromial ligament, which suggest possible impingement, are demonstrated on an outlet view. Decreased distance between acromion and humeral head and cystic and proliferative changes in the greater tuberosity suggest chronic rotator cuff disease. Hill-Sacks deformity of the humeral head and bony Bankhardt lesions of the glenoid rim may be seen after shoulder dislocation. Late-stage avascular necrosis is easily diagnosed. Erosive changes may be seen in synovial inflammatory processes.

2. Arthrography consists of injection of contrast medium (single contrast) or contrast medium and air (double contrast) into the shoulder joint followed by radiography. It is very accurate for demonstration of full thickness rotator cuff tears and not reliable for partial tears. It cannot demonstrate bursal side partial tears. It must be combined with tomography or CT to study the glenoid labrum (see below). It can confirm a diagnosis of adhesive capsulitis by demonstration of a small capacity joint.

3. MRI permits examination of the rotator cuff for reliable recognition of complete tears and less reliable detection of partial tears. The glenoid labrum can be examined in cases of suspected instability. Joint effusions, ganglion cysts, synovial cysts, and any other fluid collections are demonstrated. Early-stage avascular necrosis can be detected. Calcifications are not particularly well demonstrated. Gadolinium DTPA can be injected into the joint and arthrography performed, which may give improved results in some cases.

4. CT alone is rarely useful in this situation, but CT arthrography provides very reliable detection of full thickness rotator cuff tears and

very accurate examination of the glenoid labrum in cases of suspected instability due to labral tear.

5. Ultrasound has proven useful for detection of rotator cuff tears in some instances.

C. Recommended Imaging Approach

1. Plain radiography: internal and external rotation AP views, axillary view.

2. Single contrast arthrography to confirm suspected full thickness rotator cuff tear.

3. CT arthrography to study the glenoid labrum in cases of instability or MRI—choice may depend on local preferences, availability, and interpretational skills.

4. MRI for the problem shoulder when great clinical uncertainty exists. It permits evaluation of many possible sources of pain with one (expensive) examination.

5. Ultrasound results in the investigation of the rotator cuff have been operator dependent. For this reason it is not widely used. Other methods are generally more reliable and provide a better record of the disease process.

D. Differential Diagnostic Considerations

1. If plain radiographs show features of chronic rotator cuff tear with apposition of humeral head and acromion, no other studies are needed to diagnose rotator cuff tear and to be rather certain that the remaining rotator cuff is atrophic.

2. Patients with claustrophobia and very large patients may prefer arthrography to MRI in cases where it is an appropriate substitute.

References

Kursunoglu-Brahme S, Resnick D (1990). Magnetic resonance imaging of the shoulder. Radiol Clin North Am 28:941–954.

Wilson AJ, Totty WG, Murphy WA, Hardy DC (1989). Shoulder joint: Arthrographic CT and long term follow-up with surgical correlation. Radiology 173:329–333.

PAINFUL HIP

A. Clinical Findings

1. Pain in groin, near greater trochanter of femur, or in thigh.
2. Limp.
3. Limited range of motion.

B. Imaging Modalities

1. Plain radiography: AP view of pelvis and frog-leg lateral view of hip. AP pelvis permits comparison of hips and evaluation of sacroiliac joints. Evaluation of cartilage thickness and surrounding bony and soft tissue changes permits diagnosis of most conditions.
2. ^{99m}Tc bone scan will demonstrate the presence or absence of disease and show its distribution.
3. CT can demonstrate calcifications and ossifications around the hip that may not be well seen on plain radiographs. CT is also available in determining the integrity of the femoral head articular surface in staging of avascular necrosis when joint replacement is contemplated. It is useful to define the nidus of osteoid osteoma when the history and plain radiographic and bone scan findings make this a likely possibility.
4. MRI permits early diagnosis of avascular necrosis of the femoral head, stress fracture, joint effusion, marrow defects due to primary and secondary neoplasm, and the soft tissue extent of tumors. Synovium is imaged with gadolinium-DTPA enhancement. MRI is helpful in diagnosis of transient osteoporosis of the hip and relatively specific in diagnosis of pigmented villonodular synovitis.
5. Arthrography, injection of contrast medium into the hip joint followed by radiography, is primarily useful following joint aspiration in cases of suspected septic hip. Contrast injection and radiography document the source of the fluid.

C. Recommended Imaging Approach

1. Plain radiography: AP pelvis and frog-leg lateral view hip. Most disease will be identified.

2. ^{99m}Tc bone scan. If negative, disease is unlikely. If positive, the diagnosis may be clear from the scan and the history: stress fracture, avascular necrosis. If positive but the diagnosis is unclear, additional studies are indicated.

3. MRI can clarify most of the cases not diagnosed by plain radiography and bone scan.

4. CT is used in limited circumstances to define the nidus of an osteoid osteoma and to stage femoral head avascular necrosis if not adequately done by MRI.

5. Joint aspiration should be performed in cases of suspected septic hip. Source of the fluid obtained is documented by contrast medium injection and radiography.

D. Differential Diagnostic Considerations

1. In children, hip disorders frequently present with knee pain.

2. In suspected infection, always promptly aspirate the joint.

3. In cases of severe hip joint and lumbar spine disease, the contribution of the hip disease to the patient's pain can be assessed by local anesthetic injection into the joint.

References

Beltran J, Knight CT, Zuelzer WA et al (1990). Core decompression for avascular necrosis of the femoral head: Correlation between longterm results and preoperative MR staging. Radiology 175:533–536.

Brower AC, Kransdorf MJ (1990). Imaging of hip disorders. Radiol Clin North Am 28:955–974.

PAINFUL HIP PROSTHESIS

A. Clinical Findings

1. Pain in or around the hip often extending distally in the thigh.

2. Possibly leukocytosis, elevated sedimentation rate, temperature elevation.

B. Imaging Modalities

1. Plain radiography: AP view of pelvis and frog-leg lateral of hip. These views will detect fracture of bone or prosthesis, heterotopic bone formation, lytic lesions due to "particle disease," wear of the acetabular polyethylene liner, dislocation of the prosthesis, some cases of loosening, and rare cases of infection.

2. Arthrography can show additional cases of loosening if the contrast medium, injected under pressure, demonstrates a gap between prosthesis and bone or between cement and bone or between cement and prosthesis. Analysis and culture of fluid obtained at the time of arthrography is the best way to detect or exclude infection.

3. Radionuclide arthrography can also be done and may show cases of loosening not demonstrated by contrast arthrography.

4. ^{99m}Tc bone scan is useful to detect loosening or infection. Increased radionuclide uptake around the prosthesis may be seen in either situation. A negative scan makes infection unlikely.

5. ^{111}In-labeled WBC scan provides more specificity for infection.

C. Recommended Imaging Approach

1. Plain radiography: AP view of pelvis and frog-leg lateral view of hip. Use operating room lateral if acetabular positioning is a question.

2. If no loosening on plain radiography, do ^{99m}Tc bone scan.

3. Aspirate hip to detect suspected infection. Confirm intraarticular needle location with contrast medium injection.

D. Differential Diagnostic Considerations

1. Radiographical detection of loosening does not necessarily mean a poor clinical result. If the prosthesis remains pain free, it will generally not need revision.

2. Due to the danger of pathologic fracture, large lytic lesions around the prosthesis, resulting from histiocytic reaction to particulate material in the joint fluid, may require prosthesis revision even though the patient is pain free.

References

Tigges S, Stiles RG, Meli RJ, Roberson JR (1993). Hip aspiration: a cost-effective and accurate method of evaluating the potentially infected hip prosthesis. Radiology 189:485–488.

Weissman BN (1990). Current topics in the radiology of joint replacement surgery. Radiol Clin North Am 28:1111–1134.

PAINFUL KNEE

A. Clinical Findings

1. Pain: localization may be useful in diagnosis.
2. Locking: suggests portion of meniscus or loose body being trapped in joint.
3. Instability, giving way.
4. Swelling, joint effusion.
5. Previous injury.

B. Imaging Modalities

1. Plain radiographs: lateral view, AP standing view, and PA flexed standing views to evaluate cartilage thickness; sunrise view of patella to evaluate patellofemoral joint and patellar position. Tunnel view to evaluate intercondylar notch, tibial spines, and possible loose bodies in this area. In acute post-trauma situations, the cross-table lateral view is useful to demonstrate lipohemarthrosis. Oblique views are also useful in suspected tibial plateau fracture cases.
2. CT is useful in evaluation of acute complex fractures of the tibial plateau.
3. Ultrasound is useful for demonstration of suspected popliteal cyst. It can also diagnose popliteal artery aneurysm.
4. Arthrography is useful for demonstration of meniscal tears and popliteal cysts if MRI is not available or cannot be performed, for example, because of claustrophobia or patient size. Steroid injection for treatment can be carried out at time of popliteal cyst demonstration in patients with rheumatoid arthritis.

5. MRI provides comprehensive evaluation of the knee with very accurate detection of meniscal, cruciate ligament, and collateral ligament tears. Joint effusions, popliteal and meniscal cysts, and other fluid collections are demonstrated well. MRI demonstrates occult fractures and osteonecrosis. MRI is good for evaluation of osteochondritis dissecans, showing if the fragment is free and needs to be removed.

6. ^{99m}Tc bone scan can show stress fractures and osteonecrosis but is less specific than MRI and generally less useful. It also cannot demonstrate all the other abnormalities demonstrable by MRI.

C. Recommended Imaging Approach

1. In the post-trauma situation, start with AP and cross-table lateral radiographs. Add oblique views in cases suspicious for tibial plateau fracture. Add sunrise view patella in suspected patella fracture. Add CT with multiplanar reconstruction to detect occult tibial plateau fracture or to evaluate complex plateau fracture prior to surgery.

2. For suspected arthritis, obtain standing AP view, lateral view, and sunrise view of patella. Add flexed PA standing view if other features cause suspicion that joint narrowing is more severe than demonstrated on AP view.

3. For suspected meniscal or cruciate ligament tear and/or popliteal or meniscal cyst or generally puzzling situation, obtain MRI.

4. For popliteal cyst and pseudothrombophlebitis versus deep venous thrombosis, obtain ultrasound.

5. Arthrography is second choice study for meniscal tear.

D. Differential Diagnostic Considerations

1. A fat-fluid level in the knee joint on the cross-table lateral view post-trauma is very suggestive of intraarticular fracture and should be followed by oblique views and CT if necessary to demonstrate a subtle fracture.

2. The patellofemoral joint is a common source of knee pain and is not imaged on the AP view of the knee. For radiographic evaluation, the

lateral and sunrise views are required. Dynamic CT and MRI have been used to study patellar tracking.

3. Deep venous thrombosis and pseudothrombophlebitis due to rupture of a popliteal cyst or pressure on the calf veins by a popliteal cyst can be confused clinically. Ultrasound is the study of choice for diagnosis of deep venous thrombosis and can also demonstrate a popliteal cyst. It is effective in this situation.

4. MRI shows potential for the demonstration of early cartilage abnormalities in arthritis. However, clinical decisions can generally be made on the basis of plain radiographs. Early and moderate degenerative arthritis are usually treated with nonsteroidal antiinflammatory drugs. Joint replacement is considered when end-stage disease is reached—"bone on bone" narrowing on the plain radiograph.

References

De Smet AA, Fisher DR, Graf BK, Lange RH (1990). Osteochondritis dissecans of the knee: Value of MR imaging in determining lesion stability and the presence of articular cartilage defects. Am J Roentgenol 155:549–553.

Ruwe PA, Wright J, Randall RL, Lynch JK, Jokl P, McCarthy S (1992). Can MRI imaging effectively replace diagnostic arthroscopy? Radiology 183:335–339.

PAINFUL LOWER BACK

A. Clinical Findings

1. Pain in lower back and/or near sacroiliac joints.
2. Pain may radiate down lower extremities.
3. Variable response of pain to activity—standing, lying down, and straight leg raising, depending on etiology.
4. Variable change in lower extremity reflexes depending on etiology.

B. Imaging Modalities

1. Plain radiographs: AP and lateral and oblique views and coned lateral L-5 view. The oblique views aid in evaluation of spondyloly-

sis and facet joint arthritis. The lateral L-5 spot view provides better detail of the lower lumbar disc changes. Plain radiographs potentially diagnose spondylolysis, chronic degenerative disc disease, ankylosing spondylitis, pathologic fracture, aortic aneurysm, and kidney and gallbladder calculi if these are sufficiently calcified. Radiography is not useful for diagnosis of acute herniated disc.

2. Myelography permits diagnosis of herniated disc if the disc distorts the contrast column. Myelography was formerly the method for making this diagnosis. It cannot demonstrate lateral or foraminal discs and has decreased sensitivity at L-5–S-1 due to the large canal at that level. Today, this study, using water-soluble contrast medium, is usually performed in conjunction with CT and usually in complex postoperative cases. CT myelography is invasive and expensive.

3. CT without contrast is very satisfactory for diagnosis of acute disc disease in the unoperated spine. Postoperatively it may be difficult to differentiate scar from residual or new disc herniation. CT is preferred by some for the imaging of bony hypertrophic changes in older patients with symptoms of spinal stenosis. CT is considerably less expensive than MRI.

4. MRI has become the study of choice for most spinal disease because it images all the tissues of the entire lumbar and lower thoracic spine in one study and thereby can detect the rare unsuspected tumor or other process mimicking disc disease. Contrast enhancement with gadolinium-DTPA makes possible differentiation of scar (enhances) and residual or recurrent disc herniation (no enhancement). Metallic surgical devices cause a local signal void that makes the MRI examination useless in close proximity to the device. The lack of ionizing radiation is a significant benefit in younger patients.

C. Recommended Imaging Approach

1. AP and lateral radiographs to detect the occasional disorder for which they are useful (see above).

2. MRI for its accurate diagnostic ability in many different conditions and lack of ionizing radiation.
3. CT if MRI is not available.
4. CT myelography and/or gadolinium-enhanced MRI for recurrent pain and disability following surgery (if metal is not present in the region of interest).

D. Differential Diagnostic Considerations

1. Studies have shown that imaging of asymptomatic individuals will reveal a relatively high percentage of anatomic abnormalities that under some circumstances cause symptoms. Therefore, one should not do any imaging unless there is strong clinical suspicion of disease with neurologic findings present.
2. Any abnormalities found on imaging studies must be carefully correlated with the clinical findings to be certain that the abnormalities found are actually responsible for the clinical problem.

References

Gaskill MF, Lukin R, Wiot JG (1991). Lumbar disk disease and stenosis. Radiol Clin North Am 29:753–764.

Jensen MC, Brant-Zawadski MN, Obuchowski N et al (1994). Magnetic resonance imaging of the lumbar spine in people without back pain. N Engl J Med 331:69–73.

ARTHRITIS

A. Clinical Findings

1. Pain in one or more joints.
2. Systemic complaints.
3. Gel phenomenon.
4. Associated skin lesions.
5. Synovial thickening.
6. Joint effusion.

B. Imaging Modalities

1. Plain radiography of the involved joints in three projections permits evaluation of joint cartilage narrowing, erosions, alignment, and overall bone density.

2. CT can demonstrate arthritic changes in the sacroiliac joints, the sternoclavicular joints, and subtalar joints with greater sensitivity than conventional radiography. It can demonstrate tarsal coalition responsible for rigid, painful flat foot. High-resolution CT may be useful to evaluate pulmonary disease associated with some types of arthritis.

3. MRI permits detection of earlier cartilage change than conventional radiography. Hypertrophic synovium can be imaged, especially with gadolinium contrast enhancement. MRI is the most sensitive means for early diagnosis of avascular necrosis of the femoral head, an important complication of steroid therapy employed in many arthritides. Suspected internal derangements of knee, shoulder, and wrist are well imaged.

4. Radionuclide bone scan demonstrates the distribution of arthritic changes throughout the skeleton.

5. Arthrography can demonstrate cysts communicating with joints, meniscal tears, rotator cuff tears, triangular fibrocartilage tears, and intercarpal ligament tears.

6. CT arthrography and MRI arthrography are excellent for display of the glenoid labrum of the shoulder, which may be injured in cases of shoulder instability.

C. Recommended Imaging Approach

1. Plain radiographs of the affected joints are the first imaging study and usually the only imaging study. They permit diagnosis of type of arthritis and progression of disease since previous examination.

2. To evaluate severity of knee arthritis, obtain standing AP and, if these do not show significant narrowing, standing PA flexed views. Lateral and sunrise views of the patellas are necessary to evaluate the patellofemoral joint.

3. Use CT for evaluation of possible infection in the sacroiliac joint or sternoclavicular joint.
4. Use MRI for suspected internal derangement of the knee.
5. Use single contrast arthrography to confirm full-thickness rotator cuff tear.
6. Use MRI or CT arthrography to evaluate rotator cuff and glenoid labrum simultaneously.

D. Differential Diagnostic Considerations

1. Degenerative arthritis causes asymmetric cartilage narrowing and osteophyte formation. Distal and interphalangeal and first carpometacarpal joints of hand, knees, and hip are affected commonly.
2. Rheumatoid arthritis causes symmetric cartilage narrowing without prominent osteophytes and often with osteopenia. Metacarpophalangeal, intercarpal, wrist, and distal radioulnar joints are commonly affected in the hand. Alignment abnormalities are prominent in more advanced cases. Hips show axial migration of femoral head and symmetric cartilage narrowing. Knees show involvement of medial and lateral compartments, not seen in degenerative arthritis. Remember possibility of C1–C2 subluxation—evaluate with flexion-extension lateral views if necessary.
3. Gout favors the first metatarsophalangeal joint. Requires 6 years to show erosive changes—early diagnosis made by aspiration and history. Any joint can be involved; distribution is asymmetric. Bone density is normal. Erosions with well-defined margins, erosions away from a joint, soft tissue masses near the erosions, erosions with "overhanging margins," and substantial erosions at the margin of a joint with normal cartilage thickness are highly suggestive features, as is olecranon bursitis without a history of trauma.
4. Systemic lupus erythematosus and Jaccoud's arthropathy show alignment abnormalities without significant erosive changes.
5. Psoriatic arthritis has three patterns, one like rheumatoid arthritis, one involving distal and interphalangeal joints, and a mixed pattern. The "sausage digit" and involvement of the joints of one ray are

suggestive. Fingernail changes may be noted on the radiograph. Psoriatic skin changes are present on examination of the vast majority.

6. If a single joint is involved, be sure to consider infection.

References

Kaye JJ (1990). Arthritis: Roles of radiography and other imaging techniques in evaluation. Radiology 177:601–608.

Recht MP, Resnick D (1994).MR imaging of articular cartilage: Current status and future directions. AJR 163:283–290.

CERVICAL DISC HERNIATION

A. Clinical Findings

1. Radiculopathy: pain radiating to shoulder, arm, or hand. Neck stiffness and pain. Interscapular pain. Upper extremity paresis.
2. Myelopathy: broad-based, staggering gait, hand and arm weakness, and interosseous muscle atrophy.
3. Insidious onset of symptoms.

B. Imaging Modalities

1. Plain radiographs show the bony structures relatively well. AP and lateral views demonstrate alignment, disc narrowing, osteophyte formation, and gross facet joint arthritis. Oblique views show encroachment on the neural foramina by osteophytes from the adjacent vertebrae and from the facet joints. Flexion-extension lateral views may demonstrate abnormal motions such as subluxation not visualized on the neutral lateral view and often not visualized by more expensive imaging modalities.
2. Myelography: introduction of intrathecal contrast followed by radiographic examination permits detection of most disc herniations, but not far lateral herniation. It is invasive, uncomfortable, and may be compromised by contrast medium dilution. It does permit evalu-

ation of different spinal positions on the extent of neural compromise.

3. CT myelography: addition of CT examination of selected areas to the conventional myelogram. The study compares well with MRI for evaluation of cervical radiculopathy and is superior to conventional myelography for lateral disc herniation and in the presence of dilute contrast and other technical problems. Spinal cord area can be measured.

4. Plain CT can be diagnostic of disc herniation and can define narrowing of the bony canal and neural foramina. Beam-hardening artifacts related to the shoulders may make the study nondiagnostic in the lower cervical region. The study can be improved by the addition of contrast enhancement with intravenous iodinated contrast medium.

5. MRI images most cord and nerve root disease extremely well and can provide images in any plane. Sagittal images are very convenient for reference and demonstration of many findings. There is no problem with poor images in the lower cervical spine where CT is hampered by beam-hardening artifact. Gadolinium-DTPA contrast medium or equivalent can be used to enhance visualization of tumors and inflammatory tissue and is probably safer than nonionic iodinated contrast medium used with CT. A disadvantage is the relative insensitivity of MRI to small osteophytes, which may be important to foraminal narrowing.

C. Recommended Imaging Approach

1. In patient with clinical myelopathy, use MRI with contrast enhancement if necessary after unenhanced images. CT myelography is an alternative.

2. In patients with radiculopathy not responsive to conservative therapy, plain radiography should be the first study.

3. Following radiography, any patients with short necks and poor visualization of the lower C-spine should get MRI or CT myelography, while in anatomically favorable patients CT with intravenous contrast enhancement is an option.

D. Differential Diagnostic Considerations

1. Disc herniation and spondylosis (vertebral osteophyte formation) cause radiculopathy.
2. Cervical stenosis causes myelopathy.
3. Uncovertebral joint osteophyte formation is a more common cause of cervical radiculopathy than is disc herniation.
4. Disc herniation; 20–40 years of age.
5. Spondylosis: 40–60 years of age.
6. Ninety percent of disc herniations and most spondylosis C4–C7.

References

Jahnke RW, Hart BL (1991). Cervical stenosis, spondylosis and herniated disc disease. Radiol Clin North Am 29:777–791.

Russell EJ (1990). Cervical disk disease. Radiology 177:313–325.

SOFT TISSUE NEOPLASM

A. Clinical Findings

1. Discovery of a mass not previously noted.
2. Variable history of trauma, pain, interference with function of nearby structures.
3. Growth rate may help in differential diagnosis.

B. Imaging Modalities

1. Plain radiographs are poor for the delineation of extent of a mass due to poor contrast resolution in soft tissues. However, they are useful to show bone involvement of benign or aggressive appearance. Grossly fatty lesions and calcifications within the lesion can be identified. Phleboliths may be diagnostic of hemangioma.
2. CT is more useful than plain radiography to define lesion extent and relationship of the lesion to vessels and nerves. However, it has been largely supplanted by MRI.
3. MRI is best to define extent of disease due to the unsurpassed soft

tissue contrast that is possible. The ability to obtain high-resolution images in any plane is advantageous in defining the relationship of a mass to other structures.

4. Angiography may be useful prior to surgical intervention in a mass that is primarily vascular, such as a vascular malformation, aneurysm, or pseudoaneurysm.

C. Recommended Imaging Approach

1. Plain radiographs of the suspected mass in two orthogonal projections to detect bone involvement and calcification.
2. MRI to define lesion extent and relationship to vessels, nerves, bones, fascial planes, and other important structures.
3. Angiography primarily in vascular lesions.

D. Differential Diagnostic Considerations

1. Lipomas can be positively identified by MRI.
2. Multiple lesions should suggest nerve-sheath tumors, lipomas, or metastases.
3. Size less than 3 cm, homogeneous signal intensity, well-defined margin, and lack of encasement of neurovascular structures are typical features of a benign lesion on MRI.

References

Berquist TH, Ehman RL, King BF, Hodgman CG, Ilstrup DM (1990). Value of MR imaging in differentiating benign from malignant soft-tissue masses: Study of 95 lesions. AJR 155:1251–1255.

Totty WG, Murphy WA, Lee JKT (1986). Soft tissue tumors: MR imaging. Radiology 160:135–141.

PRIMARY BONE NEOPLASM

A. Clinical Findings

1. Pain.
2. Swelling.

3. Variable history of trauma.
4. Age usually under 40 years.

B. Imaging Modalities

1. Plain radiographs in two orthogonal planes provide the most accurate imaging prediction of histologic diagnosis but poor estimation of extent of disease.
2. CT can show extent of bone abnormality and matrix calcification better than plain radiographs in some locations, such as the pelvis. CT is much better than plain radiographs for soft tissue extent but is inferior to MRI.
3. ^{99m}Tc bone scan may be useful to identify additional lesions when benign conditions such as fibrous dysplasia are in the differential diagnosis and to identify additional lesions if metastases are a possibility.
4. MRI is the best procedure following plain radiographic examination to determine the extent of an aggressive lesion.

C. Recommended Imaging Approach

1. Plain radiographs in two orthogonal projections is best to predict histologic diagnosis and separate out benign lesions needing no further imaging or treatment, such as fibrous cortical defect. Other lesions, such as enchondroma or exostosis, may need follow-up plain radiographs or surgery depending on the clinical circumstances. Aggressive lesions representing possible primary malignancies or aggressive benign processes require further imaging.
2. In areas not well seen on plain radiographs, such as the pelvis, CT can aid in the histologic diagnosis by demonstration of calcified matrix in lesions and the aggressiveness of their margins.
3. In cases of suspected osteoid osteoma, CT should be used after plain radiographs to define the nidus if not clearly seen on the initial studies.
4. In most cases requiring further imaging, MRI is the best choice to define extent of disease and involvement of important anatomic structures.

5. If the lesion on plain radiographs may be fibrous dysplasia, Paget's disease, or a metastasis, a bone scan is often useful to detect additional lesions. The additional lesions may have characteristic features allowing a more definitive diagnosis.

D. Differential Diagnostic Considerations

1. MRI should be performed prior to any biopsy to avoid confusion between tumor and post-biopsy changes.
2. In older patients, consider metastases and myeloma.
3. In older patients, osteogenic sarcoma is frequently secondary to previous radiation therapy or Paget's disease.
4. Separation of "leave me alone" lesions from others is the most important diagnostic task.

References

Berquist TH (1993). Magnetic resonance imaging of primary skeletal neoplasms. Radiol Clin North Am 31:411–424.

Sundaram M, McLeod RA (1990). MR imaging of tumor and tumorlike lesions of bone and soft tissue. AJR 155:817–824.

SKELETAL METASTASES

A. Clinical Findings

1. Bone pain.
2. Pathologic fracture.

B. Imaging Modalities

1. Plain radiography in two orthogonal projections of the area(s) involved. These will identify pathologic fractures, sizeable blastic lesions, and most lytic lesions that have destroyed the cortex. Even large medullary lesions will go undetected. Lytic lesions likely to undergo pathologic fracture can be detected. A skeletal survey or metastatic survey is a set of radiographs that covers the axial skele-

ton, the skull, the shoulders, and the lower extremities to the knees. This is the red marrow region most likely to be involved by myeloma or metastases.

2. The ^{99m}Tc radionuclide bone scan is the standard method to survey the entire skeleton for potential metastases. It is much more sensitive than radiography. Some patterns are diagnostic of multiple metastases, but in other cases radiographs of areas of increased radionuclide uptake are required for specificity. The bone scan may be falsely negative in myeloma, aggressive lytic metastases, and some blastic metastases of prostatic cancer.

3. CT is very useful to evaluate scan-positive regions that are not explained by plain radiographs.

4. MRI is very sensitive to metastases and myeloma. It can be used to evaluate scan-positive areas of the skeleton. It is not as convenient for initial survey as the bone scan and is expensive.

C. Recommended Imaging Approach

1. Radionuclide bone scan is the screening exam of choice to exclude or detect possible metastases to the skeleton except suspected multiple myeloma for which a radiographic skeletal survey should be obtained. The bone scan should only be done if the detection of metastases will affect management.

2. Obtain radiographs of scan-positive regions if benign lesions such as arthritis or old fractures might be responsible.

3. Obtain CT or MRI to evaluate scan-positive, radiograph-negative regions.

4. In prostate cancer a radiograph of the pelvis is useful to identify those metastases not detected by bone scan.

D. Differential Diagnostic Considerations

1. Destruction of a vertebral pedicle is empirically more likely due to metastasis than myeloma.

2. Obtain orthopaedic consultation for large lytic lesions in weight-bearing bones that might be subject to pathologic fracture. Prophylactic treatment can decrease morbidity.

3. In the older patient, a lytic lesion should be considered metastasis or myeloma until proven otherwise.

4. Common metastases include blastic lesions in older male due to prostate cancer; blastic and/or lytic lesions in a female due to breast cancer; aggressive lytic lesion male or female due to lung cancer; and renal cancer.

5. Paget's disease can sometimes be distinguished from blastic metastasis by its tendency to enlarge the involved bone.

6. A large soft tissue mass is unusual with metastasis, in contrast to primary bone neoplasms.

References

Merrick MV, Beales JSM, Garvie N, Leonard RCO (1992). Evaluation and skeletal metastases. Br J Radiol 65:803–806.

Rougraff BT, Kneisl JS, Simon MA (1993). Skeletal metastases of unknown origin. J Bone Joint Surg 75-A:1276–1281.

SCOLIOSIS

A. Clinical Findings

1. Possible spinal curvature noted by parent, school nurse, or physician or on radiograph taken for some other reason.

2. Typically asymptomatic adolescent female.

3. Pain uncommon with idiopathic scoliosis until secondary degenerative changes develop.

4. Late findings include marked cosmetic deformity and cardiopulmonary compromise due to distortion of the thorax.

B. Imaging Modalities

1. Plain radiography: PA and lateral views of the entire thoracolumbar spine in the upright position. PA view limits breast radiation exposure, and the upright position maximizes the severity of the scoliosis. A supine view is not comparable and generally shows less severe scoliosis. Wedge filtration of the x-ray beam is used to match

exposure to body thickness, and high-speed, high-efficiency, screen–film combinations limit patient radiation exposure. A coned, centered lateral view of the lumbosacral junction is useful if spondylolysis or spondylolisthesis of the lower L-spine is suspected on the full spine views. PA standing views taken with the patient bending first to one side and then to the other demonstrate how much the curves can change and help predict response to treatment.

2. Computed radiography (CR) offers potential for better control over exposure and the possibility of making electronic measurements of the curves on the display screen. Thus far this method has not been widely employed. Problems include the lack of proper sized cassettes and scanners for the long, narrow image format.

3. CT with multiplanar image reconstruction or conventional tomography can be used to evaluate underlying bony anomalies such as hemivertebra and bar formation whose presence can lead to cases of so-called congenital scoliosis. Following fusion procedures for scoliosis, these studies can be used to evaluate possible pseudoarthrosis.

4. MRI can evaluate possible neurologic abnormalities related to impingement on spinal cord or nerve roots by the abnormal spine. Some diseases, such as neurofibromatosis, have other abnormalities well imaged by MRI.

5. Painful scoliosis in a young person suggests an underlying lesion, and the radionuclide bone scan can exclude or localize such a process. This might be an osteoid osteoma or infection.

C. Recommended Imaging Approach

1. Upright PA and lateral thoracolumbar spine.
2. If question of spondylosis or spondylolisthesis, lower L-spine, get lateral L-5 spot view.
3. For painful scoliosis with plain radiographs negative for underlying lesion, obtain radionuclide bone scan.
4. CT to follow up positive findings of bone scan in (3).
5. Conventional tomography or CT with multiplanar reconstruction to evaluate bony congenital anomalies.

6. Upright lateral bending views to evaluate fixed versus flexible nature of curves, usually prior to surgery.
7. MRI to evaluate any suspected neurologic lesions associated with spinal deformity.

D. Differential Diagnostic Considerations

1. Scoliosis can progress 1 degree per month in the child and adolescent and 1 degree per year in the adult. Do not fail to seek appropriate orthopaedic consultation promptly, and do not fail to get regular follow-up radiographs in the skeletally immature individual at 6-month intervals.
2. Idiopathic scoliosis is generally painless in the young person who has not developed secondary degenerative changes. Pain should raise the possibility of an underlying lesion such as osteoid osteoma.
3. Idiopathic scoliosis usually has a right-convex thoracic curve. A left curve is associated with a greater number of other anomalies such as cardiac malformations.
4. Scoliosis is associated with a number of systemic disorders that have other important manifestations to be looked for, including neurofibromatosis, Marfan syndrome, osteogenesis imperfecta, and neuromuscular disorders.
5. Scoliosis may result from radiation therapy during childhood for paraspinal lesions such as Wilm's tumor.
6. Congenital scoliosis (i.e., that due to vertebral anomalies) has an association with other congenital anomalies of the cardiovascular, genitourinary, and gastrointestinal systems.

References

Mehta MH, Murray RO (1977). Scoliosis provoked by painful vertebral lesions. Skeletal Radiol 1:223–230.

Weinstein SL, Zavala DC, Ponseti IV (1981). Idiopathic scoliosis. J Bone Joint Surg 63A:702–712.

OSTEOMYELITIS

A. Clinical Findings

1. Fever.
2. Elevated WBC.
3. Ulcerations and/or cellulitis overlying bone (diabetic foot, decubitus ulcers near ishial tuberosities, greater trochanters, ulcerations of leg and forearm in "skin poppers").
4. Bone pain.

B. Imaging Modalities

1. Plain radiographs of suspected location(s) in two orthogonal projections can show bone destruction and/or periosteal reaction. These changes require 10 days to 2 weeks to develop. When present, they are rather specific in the appropriate clinical setting. Earlier, comparison views of the opposite extremity may show subtle loss of deep soft tissue planes in the involved extremity.

2. The ^{99m}Tc bone scan is much more sensitive than plain radiographs and is positive sooner after infection. It is nonspecific and often requires radiographic correlation. In some instances specificity can be increased by also performing a ^{67}Ga-citrate scan. The sulfur colloid marrow scan is advised by some for examination of the marrow-containing portions of the skeleton. The ^{111}In-labeled WBC scan is very useful to detect acute infection in an area of chronic changes such as posttrauma or postsurgery.

3. Conventional and computed tomography can show destructive changes of osteomyelitis in bone around infected sacroiliac joints and sternoclavicular joints when the plain radiographs are negative or equivocal.

4. MRI is sensitive to osteomyelitis, demonstrating loss of the normal high signal from marrow fat on T1-weighted images and showing high signal on T2-weighted images in involved areas. In the spine, suspected disc infection and adjacent vertebral osteomyelitis are

conveniently evaluated along with the possible complication of paravertebral or epidural abscess.

C. Recommended Imaging Approach

1. Plain radiographs of suspected location(s) in two orthogonal projections. If positive, this may be sufficient.
2. CT of locations that are anatomically difficult to image with plain films: sacroiliac and sternoclavicular joints. CT may be useful to guide diagnostic biopsy.
3. [99mTc] bone scan in plain radiograph-negative cases to show early lesions and screen for other distant unsuspected lesions. If new lesions are found, radiographs of these areas should be obtained. In neonates, follow with [67Ga]-citrate scan if negative.
4. For suspected discitis and osteomyelitis, obtain MRI of spine.
5. For diabetic neuropathic arthropathy of foot with suspected superimposed osteomyelitis, some success reported with the [111In] WBC scan and with MRI.
6. For suspected osteomyelitis superimposed on fracture or surgery, [99mTc] bone scan (or [99mTc] sulfur colloid scan in red marrow areas) and [111In] WBC scan.

D. Differential Diagnostic Considerations

1. Especially in the foot, stress and trauma can lead to periosteal reaction that could be misinterpreted as osteomyelitis.
2. Severe osteoporosis can mimic bone destruction.
3. Osteomyelitis in the long bones can have an aggressive appearance and is in the differential diagnosis of tumors causing "moth eaten" bone destruction such as Ewing's sarcoma in the young and metastases in the older population.
4. In the spine, discitis and osteomyelitis of the adjacent vertebrae can resemble a Charcot joint, arthropathy due to microglobulin amyloid deposition, and crystal-induced arthropathy (CPPD).

References

Erdman WA, Tamburro F, Jayson HT, Weatherall PT, Ferry KB, Peshock RM (1991). Osteomyelitis: characteristics and pitfalls of diagnosis with MR imaging. Radiology 180:533–539.

Schauwecker DS (1992). The scintigraphic diagnosis of osteomyelitis. AJR 158:9–18.

OSTEOPOROSIS

A. Clinical Findings

1. Fractures occurring with little trauma. Typical locations include vertebrae (compression fractures), neck, and intertrochanteric portions of the femur, distal radius, and proximal humerus.

2. Predisposing factors include Caucasian race, female sex, low body weight, family history of osteoporotic fractures, smoking, and alcohol consumption.

3. Loss of height and increasing thoracic kyphosis and back pain may be present.

B. Imaging Modalities

1. Plain radiographs are insensitive. A 40% loss of bone mineral is necessary to make a detectable difference on usual plain radiographs.

2. Despite their insensitivity, plain films do detect the important consequences of osteoporosis—fractures. In many studies of osteoporosis and its therapy, lateral spine radiographs are used to detect and grade compression fractures as the measure of osteoporosis.

3. Dual energy x-ray absorptiometry (DEXA) is a study that uses the amount of x-ray absorption at two different x-ray energies to calculate the amount of bone mineral in the portion of the skeleton examined. It can measure almost any area, including the important femoral neck and vertebral column. Precision and accuracy are high

and radiation dose very low. It is not as sensitive to trabecular bone loss in the spine as in quantitative CT (QCT).

4. QCT measures spinal bone mineral by comparing attenuation values in the spine with those of standard bone mineral equivalent solutions or solids in a phantom. It is very sensitive to loss of trabecular bone in the spine. Radiation dose is higher than for DEXA, and it is not practical to measure the femoral neck with this technique under most clinical conditions. Accuracy and precision of measurement are similar to DEXA. QCT and DEXA are the studies of choice for reliable, practical bone mineral determination in clinical practice and most research at this time.

5. Ultrasound transmission through the calcaneus or patella can be used to provide estimates of bone mineral that correlate well with other measures. There is active research in this area, and it may provide additional structural information leading to better estimation of fracture risk. Currently, it is not widely available and, without standards, not practical for clinical use.

C. Recommended Imaging Approach

1. Fractures due to osteoporosis are detected by the same means as other fractures discussed in sections on trauma. Plain radiographs are always the first step.

2. To quantitate bone mineral and relate it to age-specific standards, DEXA or QCT should be used. If the hip is of particular interest DEXA is preferable. In the spine QCT is more sensitive to trabecular bone loss. Whichever study is chosen must be used for follow-up studies, preferably on the same machine to improve precision.

3. A single study permits comparison with the population and "fracture thresholds."

4. Serial studies are necessary to determine rate of bone loss, such as in the postmenopausal period, and to determine the effects of medications that increase or decrease the rate of bone loss.

D. Differential Diagnostic Considerations

1. A small percentage of persons with "osteopenia" will not have age-related osteoporosis but instead some other condition whose discovery is important. One radiographic presentation of myeloma is diffuse osteopenia, which may be very severe. Hyperthyroidism can lead to increased bone turnover osteoporosis. Osteomalacia results in decreased bone mineral measurements as does osteoporosis.

2. Before measuring bone mineral, decide what will be done differently depending on the results. If the patient requires steroid medications for a serious, life-threatening condition, it will not be possible to stop administration of steroids even if they are causing osteoporosis. Estrogen therapy is the most reliable and effective therapy for postmenopausal osteoporosis. It has other beneficial effects and a few possible ill effects. One can treat without measurement.

References

Guglielmi G, Grimston SK, Fischer KC, Pacifici R (1994). Osteoporosis: diagnosis with lateral and posteroanterior dual x-ray absorptiometry compared with quantitative CT. Radiology 192:845–850.

Herd RJM, Blake GM, Ramalingam T, Miller CG, Ryan PJ, Fogelman I (1993). Measurements of postmenopausal bone loss with a new contact ultrasound system. Calcif Tissue Int 53:153–157.

► CHAPTER *2*

Gastrointestinal Disease

Stephen E. Rubesin, MD
Bernard A. Birnbaum, MD
Hospital of the University of Pennsylvania

Imaging Handbook for House Officers, Edited by Paul M. Silverman and Douglas J. Quint.
ISBN 0-471-13767-7 © 1997 Wiley-Liss, Inc.

OVERVIEW: What Every Clinician Needs To Know About Gastrointestinal Radiology Examinations for Adults

PREPARATION PRIOR TO GASTROINTESTINAL RADIOLOGY EXAMINATION

A. Patient preparation

1. Clinician describes examination to patient before patient goes for radiologic procedure.

2. Clinician provides a written set of instructions specific for each radiologic examination stating the necessary preparation. These should be provided to the clinician by the radiologist.

B. Radiologist preparation: the request slip includes pertinent

1. Clinical history.

2. Physical examination findings.

3. Laboratory data.

4. Medications that may cause complications or alter the study being performed, e.g., opiates will alter intestinal motility.

5. Surgical history: It is crucial for the radiologist to know what the surgical anatomy is beforehand, so the study can be appropriately tailored.

C. Preparation for upper gastrointestinal series, videopharyngoesophagram ("barium swallow"), and small bowel series (without per-oral pneumocolon)

1. Nothing by mouth after 9 PM the evening before the examination.

2. No insulin the day of the examination.

3. Avoid things that stimulate salivary secretion: smoking, chewing gum.

4. No oral medications that coat the gastrointestinal mucosa: antacids.

5. Leave dentures or other oral appliances in place.

D. Preparation for barium enema

Principle: There is no ideal barium enema preparation. Success of preparation relates to the patient's age, intrinsic colonic motility, underlying colonic diseases, and medications. Patients who are "difficult to clean out" include elderly, bedridden, or debilitated patients, patients taking opiates or medications with anticholinergic side effects, patients with hypomotility disorders such as diabetes, scleroderma.

CONSULT YOUR RADIOLOGIST FOR RECOMMENDED PREPARATION

Listed below is a suggested preparation.

1. Clear liquids the entire day before the examination.
2. One bottle (10–12 oz) magnesium citrate 5 PM day before the exam.
3. Several glasses of water throughout the day before exam (hydration).
4. Four 5-mg bisacodyl tablets with one full glass of water 10 PM day before exam.
5. Nothing by mouth after midnight until after the barium enema.
6. Bisacodyl suppository, early on morning of exam.
7. ALTERNATIVES
   a. Two-liter tap water cleansing enema at least 1 hour prior to barium enema in addition to above-stated prep.
   b. Oral colonic lavage agents (e.g., Golytely) not preferred, as they leave excessive fluid and diminish barium coating.
   c. Small-volume enemas are not advised, as these push fecal material in a retrograde fashion into the right colon.

E. Preparation for per-oral pneumocolon or enteroclysis
   1. At minimum, feces should be removed from the cecum and terminal ileum, so administer a colonic (cecal) stimulation agent such as four 5-mg bisacodyl tablets.
   2. Some institutions may prefer a full barium enema preparation.

F. Preparation for ultrasonography
   1. An overnight fast minimizes air and fluid in the intestines and is helpful for most abdominal studies. An overnight fast maximizes gallbladder filling and is required for all but emergent biliary studies.

G. Preparation for angiography
   1. If the angiographic study is elective, standard bowel cleansing improves the interpretation of the study.
   2. Because these are invasive procedures, preoperative clinical history,

physical examination, and pertinent laboratory values should be obtained before angiography. This especially applies to the anesthesia risk of the patient, including respiratory, cardiovascular, and renal status. Pertinent laboratory values including blood coagulation parameters and renal function parameters (e.g., creatinine) should be known.

3. The clinician must alert the radiologist if intravascular iodinated contrast has been used recently.

H. Preparation for computed tomography

1. Because there is a risk of vomiting after injection of iodinated contrast, patients should ideally have nothing by mouth 3–4 hours prior to study.

2. Bowel cleansing with barium enema preparation may be of value in patients with suspected or known carcinoma, unless obstruction is suspected.

3. As with any patient receiving intravascular iodinated material, the patient's renal function should be documented. The clinician should alert the radiologist if intravascular contrast agents have been administered recently.

4. If a CT-guided biopsy or invasive procedure is planned, local anesthesia risk and coagulation parameters should be assessed prior to scheduling the study.

5. Notify radiologist if patient has history of any allergic reaction to contrast, asthma, significant cardiac disease, multiple myeloma, sickle cell disease, or diabetes.

I. Preparation for magnetic resonance imaging

1. Patients with metallic implants, pacemakers, or metallic foreign bodies may not be candidates to undergo MRI. Consult MRI staff to see if patient can be studied.

2. An overnight fast may be helpful.

3. Claustrophobic patients may require premedication.

DESCRIPTION OF EXAMINATIONS

A. Definitions: Double-contrast (air-contrast, biphasic) versus single-contrast (full-column) technique

1. Almost all patients who can stand and turn on a fluoroscopic table,

have normal mental capabilities, are able to communicate, and who are undergoing preoperative examinations should undergo "double-contrast" technique. This is a "biphasic" study combining both air-contrast with single-contrast techniques.

2. Single-contrast techniques are used only when patients cannot stand or turn on a fluoroscopic table, are unable to understand or cooperate with the radiologist, are in the immediate postoperative state, or when the small intestine is to be studied without an intubation technique.

B. Videopharyngoesophagram
   1. Examines oral, pharyngeal, and esophageal motility with dynamic recording (video; true cineradiography; rapid-sequence 105-mm fluorospots or digital images do not suffice).
   2. Examines pharyngeal, esophageal, and gastric cardia morphology with double-contrast and single-contrast techniques. Expect spot films of pharynx in distension by phonation or modified Valsalva; erect double-contrast spot films of esophagus; double-contrast view of gastric cardia; prone drinking views of esophagus. Solid bolus (e.g., barium-impregnated tablet) given if history of solid food dysphagia or with normal study but history of dysphagia.

C. Upper gastrointestinal series (upper GI)
   1. The standard upper GI series combines double-contrast and single-contrast techniques.
   2. Studies the esophagus, stomach, and duodenum to the ligament of Treitz.
   3. Hypotonia induced in all patients (with intravenous glucagon in the United States) except diabetics, patients with vomiting, and patients with contraindications to glucagon (pheochromocytoma, insulinoma).
   4. Except double-contrast views of esophagus, stomach, duodenum; single-contrast views of esophagus, antrum, duodenum using compression or mucosal relief.

D. Dedicated small bowel series
   1. Single-contrast examination relies on frequent compression of each loop of small intestine when the loop is variably filled with barium.

   2. Use "thin" barium appropriate for the small intestine, not high-density barium used during double-contrast upper GI.
   3. This study should not be combined with a double-contrast upper GI series because high-density barium from the double-contrast study may obscure lesions in the small bowel, giving "white out" of pelvic loops.
   4. Expect spot films of at least four quadrants of abdomen, prone compression of pelvic loops, spot film of terminal ileum, and lateral fluoroscopy of abdomen to rule out a hernia.
   5. A per-oral pneumocolon can be combined with this examination if terminal ileal disease is suspected, for example, "rule out Crohn's disease."
E. Enteroclysis (small bowel enema)
   1. Barium examination of choice for malabsorption and unexplained blood loss and if small bowel tumor or Meckel's diverticulum is suspected.
   2. Employs barium designed for small bowel and luminal distension by radiolucent agent (methylcellulose or air).
   3. Expect spot films of all jejunal or ileal loops. Because catheter is placed beyond ligament of Treitz, evaluation of duodenum should either have been previously accomplished by upper endoscopy or upper GI series or is done at end of examination before catheter is pulled out.
F. Barium enema
   1. Expect double-contrast (air-contrast) study unless patient is debilitated, cannot stand or turn on the fluoroscopic table, cannot communicate with the radiologist, or has poor rectal tone. This radiologist even prefers double-contrast exams to rule out diverticulitis or fistula.
   2. Spot films include coned-down views of rectum, sigmoid, flexures, cecum, and terminal ileum if refluxed with barium. Spot films are preferred to wide use of overheads because radiologist can control amount of luminal distension, projection, and barium coating.
   3. Overheads used for projections that radiologist cannot take with

fluoroscopic images: decubitus views, cross-table lateral views, angled views.

4. Single-contrast examination reserved to rule out obstruction.

G. Angiography

1. The clinician should view angiography as a percutaneous surgical procedure. Studies include angiography to evaluate or control a site of gastrointestinal bleeding, to evaluate bowel ischemia, to evaluate tumor resectability (such as carcinoma of the pancreas), to identify tumors (such as islet cell tumors or the pancreas or hypervascular liver lesions), or to deliver chemotherapeutic agents. The clinician must carefully communicate with the angiographer as the order of the vessels to be examined depends on the question to be answered (e.g., what is the source of bleeding?).

2. Patients may be premedicated with agents such as fentanyl and midazolam.

3. Intraprocedural monitoring includes EKG, pulse, blood pressure, and arterial oxygenation with a pulse oximeter.

4. Patients may receive glucagon to reduce bowel motion artifacts.

5. A Foley catheter may be placed to drain the bladder of iodinated contrast material if the study includes vessels overlying the pelvis.

H. Ultrasonography

1. The clinician must choose the most efficacious modality to start a workup utilizing cross-sectional imaging of the gastrointestinal tract. The clinician should not order an ultrasound, followed by a CT, then followed by an MRI or nuclear medicine examination. Choosing the right modality depends on local equipment availability, radiologic expertise, efficacy of the particular modality in diagnosing the suspected clinical disorder, and the ability of study to provide unsuspected information.

2. Ultrasound is the first study to order for suspected disease in the female pelvis, the gallbladder and biliary tree, and in some diseases associated with vascular abnormalities (e.g., portal hypertension evaluation). Ultrasound is of utmost importance in pregnant women and in children. The portable capabilities of ultrasound make its use

invaluable in the evaluation of intensive care unit patients, as well as intraoperative evaluation of liver and pancreas. Ultrasound is extremely valuable at guiding biopsy and percutaneous procedures.

3. Ultrasound should not, however, be used as a replacement for CT or MRI when these modalities are available and for workup of diseases that are more reliably and better demonstrated by CT or MRI. In most places in the United States, there is no dearth of CT scanners or ultrasound equipment. If the clinician has a question of how to image a patient, contact the radiologist.

4. Although ultrasound occasionally identifies gastrointestinal tract lesions (such as appendicitis or terminal ileitis), CT is a better choice, in general, for evaluation of lumenal disorders of the gastrointestinal tract, liver, pancreas, and retroperitoneum. Ultrasound is superior in workup of the gallbladder and proximal biliary tree.

I. Computed tomography

The radiologist must tailor the examination to the clinical problem by varying the use of intravenous and oral contrast and by varying the collimation (slice thickness and site). This requires that the radiologist is provided with adequate clinical history.

1. Collimation

The radiologist will perform routine thickness slices (7–15 mm). When appropriate, thinner slices (3–5 mm) will be employed in specific areas.

2. Oral contrast agents

Complete bowel opacification with contrast agents is essential. Positive contrast agents include 1%–2% barium and 2%–3% water-soluble contrast media. These concentrations are much less than the concentrations used for barium radiography. A sufficient amount of time (30–45 minutes) is necessary for contrast media to reach the colon. The clinician must realize that drinking oral contrast adds time to the overall performance of the study. Water-soluble contrast agents are generally administered if a perforation is suspected, in trauma patients, if the patient is going to the operating room, or to those patients undergoing percutaneous biopsy. For patients with an expected slow intestinal transit time, contrast may be administered before the patients come to the radiology department. If another radiologic study is to follow the CT scan, a bowel preparation similar to a barium enema preparation will be necessary to clear the colon of oral CT contrast agent.

Negative contrast agents such as air may be administered into the colon via rectal catheter or into the stomach by swallowing or nasogastric tube.

Some radiologists use metoclopramide to speed passage of oral contrast. Contraindications include those patients with bowel obstruction or pheochromocytoma.

Oral contrast agents may not be used in patients with suspected choledocholithiasis or intraluminal objects such as calcified enteroliths, foreign bodes, or intraluminal gallstones (gallstone ileus).

3. Intravenous contrast agents
    a. The clinician must alert the radiologist if there has ever been a prior reaction to intravenous contrast agents or if there are any risk factors that may preclude the use of intravenous contrast agents. This clinical information will alert the clinician to use a steroid preparation, arrange anesthesia backup during the procedure, or alert the radiologist to use a nonionic contrast agent.

    Prior contrast reactions include

    - Urticaria
    - Facial or neck edema
    - Shortness of breath
    - Chest pain
    - Laryngospasm or bronchospasm
    - Hypotension or shock
    - Loss of consciousness
    - (a sensation of heat or flushing or a single episode of nausea or vomiting does not constitute a risk factor)

    Risk factors include

    - Previous significant contrast reaction
    - Asthma
    - Severe allergies

- Known cardiac dysfunction including poorly compensated congestive heart failure, severe arhythmias, unstable angina pectoris, recent myocardial infarction, and pulmonary hypertension
- Generalized severe debilitation
- Sickle cell disease or multiple myeloma
- Patients who are unable to communicate to determine the presence or absence of risk factors
- Patients using the oral hypoglycemic agent glucophage should stop taking the drug 48 hours prior to the use of intravenous contrast, according to the package insert

b. Steroid preparation

Each institution has its own indications for the use of a steroid preparation prior to the use of intravenous contrast agents. Consult your radiologist. At the Hospital of the University of Pennsylvania, the steroid premedication is prednisone 50 mg PO 24, 12, and 1 hour before the examination.

c. A scan not employing intravenous contrast should be obtained first if the following disorders are suspected
- Kidney stones, common duct stones
- Calcified mass
- Hepatocellular carcinoma
- Hypervascular liver metastases, e.g., islet cell tumors; melanoma; breast, kidney, or thyroid cancer
- Heavy metal deposits in the liver
- Fatty infiltration of the liver

Nonenhanced scans may also be used for
- Enterovesical fistula
- Abdominal aortic aneurysm

After these scans have been performed, in most cases, intravenous contrast will be administered if intravenous access is available.

4. CT is the best cross-sectional modality for workup of luminal or ex-

traluminal gastrointestinal tract disorders, intraperitoneal processes such as abscess or metastases, and pancreatitis (see below).

J. Magnetic resonance imaging

1. At most institutions, MRI is used as a problem-solving modality after a screening CT has been performed. At other institutions MRI is the primary cross-sectional modality used. MRI may be ordered initially in patients with known or suspected liver lesions, pancreatic carcinoma, renal carcinoma, or adrenal mass lesions. The clinician should consult with the radiologist to help choose the appropriate study.

K. Nuclear medicine

1. Nuclear medicine studies are best when using radioisotopes that emphasize imaging based on physiology rather than anatomy. This may result in information that is different than that obtained by modalities that have superior anatomic definition, such as CT, ultrasound, or MRI.

2. For gastrointestinal disorders nuclear medicine is most valuable for

a. Acute cholecystitis
   - ^{99m}Tc iminodiacetic acid (IDA) agents to rule out cystic duct obstruction by edema or calculus.

b. Characterization of hepatic lesions
   - ^{99m}Tc-labeled red blood cell studies to characterize suspected hemangioma.
   - ^{99m}Tc-labeled sulfur colloid scans to differentiate adenoma from focal nodular hyperplasia (moderately effective).

c. Detection of subtle metastasis with radioisotope-labeled monoclonal antibodies.

References

Gore RM, Levine MS, Laufer, I (1994). Textbook of Gastrointestinal Radiology. Philadelphia: WB Saunders.

Katayama H, Yamaguchi K, Kozuka T et al (1990). Adverse reactions to ionic and nonionic contrast media: A report from the Japanese Committee on the Safety of Contrast Media. Radiology 175:621–628.

Symptom Complexes in Gastroenterology

DYSPHAGIA: GENERAL PRINCIPLES

A. Clinical Findings

1. Oral phase symptoms
   a. Dribbling
   b. Difficulty chewing
   c. Difficulty initiating swallow
2. Pharyngeal, soft palate symptoms
   a. Nasal regurgitation
   b. Referred earache
3. Esophageal phase symptoms
   a. Substernal dysphagia, odynophagia
   b. Chest pain
   c. Heartburn

B. Differential Diagnostic Considerations

1. Patient's subjective assessment site of dysphagia does not always correlate with the site of pathology. Coexistent diseases may involve pharynx and esophagus. Oral phase abnormalities may alter pharyngeal function. Esophageal disorders may alter pharyngeal function. Gastroesophageal reflux or gastric cardia abnormality may alter pharyngeal or esophageal function.
2. When symptoms are referred above the suprasternal notch, start with a videopharyngoesophagram. When symptoms are referred below the suprasternal notch, start with an upper GI tract series.
3. What the clinician should expect from routine videopharyngoesophagram
   a. Videofluoroscopy oral cavity, pharynx, esophagus
   b. Double contrast views the pharynx, esophagus, gastric cardia
   c. Single contrast, mucosal relief views the esophagus

    d. Evaluation esophageal motility, check for gastroesophageal reflux

SUPRASTERNAL DYSPHAGIA

A. Clinical Findings

1. Indications for pharyngography
   a. Choking, coughing during or after swallowing
   b. Respiratory problems: chronic pneumonia or asthma
   c. Cerebrovascular accident
   d. Neuromuscular disease
   e. Pharyngeal tumor
   f. Head or neck surgery or irradiation
2. Definitions
   a. Laryngeal penetration: barium enters laryngeal vestibule during the act of swallowing. Penetration due to
      - Leakage from oral cavity
      - Neuromuscular disease
      - Inflammatory dysmotility: gastroesophageal reflux, pharyngitis
      - Tumors
      - Irradiation
   b. Overflow aspiration: barium enters laryngeal vestibule while patient is breathing. Overflow aspiration due to
      - Stasis of pharyngeal contents: tumors, lateral pharyngeal diverticula, Zenker's diverticulum
      - Reflux of esophageal contents into pharynx from gastroesophageal reflux, achalasia, or obstructing stricture, tumor, or web

B. Imaging Modalities

1. Videopharyngoesophagram
2. Modified barium swallow with speech pathologist/occupational

therapist. Study designed to discover modifications of swallowing to allow patient to swallow some or all of daily fluid and caloric requirements.

3. Nuclear medicine studies. Primarily detect gastroesophageal reflux or gross aspiration in infants or young children.

C. Recommended Imaging Approach

1. Start with videopharyngoesophagram before endoscopy in general workup of dysphagia. Barium study gives information about motility as well as morphology and views the entire swallowing tract. Barium study shows structural abnormalities, e.g., Zenker's diverticulum, which make endoscopy difficult or dangerous.

2. Barium swallow cannot suffice for screening for pharyngeal cancer, but often is the first study to detect cancer.

3. In patients with pharyngeal cancer, barium studies define the anatomy and degree of functional impairment and rule out a coexistent esophageal tumor or structural lesion that will make endoscopy difficult.

4. Barium swallow may detect tumor in areas that are difficult for endoscopy, such as deep valleculae or pharyngoesophageal segment.

5. Do not start with videopharyngoesophagram in immunocompetent patients with acute sore throat. In patients with chronic sore throat, barium study is useful to rule out gastroesophageal reflux disease.

D. Differential Diagnostic Considerations

1. Bolus safety
   a. In the oral phase, thin liquids are manipulated better than thick liquids or barium paste.
   b. In the pharyngeal phase, a cohesive bolus such as barium paste is manipulated better than thick liquids, which are manipulated better than thin liquids.
   c. Thus, the safest bolus is a small bolus of cohesive, uniform texture. A large bolus of thin liquid or mixed texture is dangerous. THE MOST DANGEROUS BOLUS IS WATER!

2. Primary cricopharyngeal prominence

    a. Associated with abnormal pharyngeal contraction, infiltrating tumor, or postoperative patients.

3. Compensatory cricopharyngeal prominence
   a. Gastroesophageal reflux, functional obstruction such as achalasia, or mechanical obstruction (tumors, webs, strictures).

4. Lymphoid hyperplasia
   a. Aging, recent infection, allergy, prior tonsillectomy, adenoidectomy.
   b. Smooth ovoid 5–8-mm nodules symmetrically distributed over tongue base or palatine tonsil.

5. Lateral pharyngeal pouches
   a. Transient protrusions at level of thyrohyoid membrane.
   b. Common, normal variant in asymptomatic patients.
   c. Rarely associated with dysphagia due to stasis, late emptying, rare aspiration.
   d. If persistent, termed *lateral pharyngeal diverticula,* seen in patients with increased pharyngeal pressure (e.g., wind instrument players, glassblowers).

6. Zenker's diverticulum
   a. Through defect in cricopharyngeus muscle: Killian's dehiscence.
   b. Coughing after swallow, regurgitation.
   c. Some patients with normal upper esophageal sphincter pressure; others with spasm or elevated resting upper esophageal sphincter pressure.
   d. Sac is midline, behind cricopharyngeal bar and upper cervical esophagus.

7. Lateral cervical esophageal diverticula/pouches
   a. Protrusion through Killian-Jamieson space lateral to insertion of longitudinal tendon on cricoid cartilage.
   b. Unilateral or bilateral, transient pouch or persistent diverticulum.
   c. Sac is anterior and lateral to proximal cervical esophagus.

8. Webs
   a. Pharyngoesophageal segment or cervical esophagus.

    b. Anterior wall: patients usually asymptomatic; circumferential: may cause symptoms.

    c. Result of chronic gastroesophageal reflux?

  9. Pharyngeal cancer

    a. Squamous cell cancer 90%, related to smoking, alcohol.

    b. Lymphoma, 10%.

    c. Intraluminal mass: abnormal contour, extra barium coated lines, filling defect in barium pool, increased radiodensity of mass, mucosal irregularity, abnormal pharyngeal function.

References

Jones B, Donner MW (1991). Normal and Abnormal Swallowing: Imaging in Diagnosis and Therapy. New York: Springer-Verlag.

Rubesin SE (1995). Oral and pharyngeal dysphagia. Gastro Clin North Am 24: 331–352.

Rubesin SE, Jessurun J, Robertson D, Jones B, Bosma JF, Donner MW (1987). Lines of the pharynx. RadioGraphics 7:217–237.

Rubesin SE, Yousem DM (1995). Pharynx: normal anatomy and techniques. In Gore RM, Levine MS, Laufer I (eds): Textbook of Gastrointestinal Radiology. Philadelphia: WB Saunders, pp. 202–225.

Rubesin SE, Yousem DM (1995). Structural disorders [Pharynx]. In Gore RM, Levine MS, Laufer I (eds): Textbook of Gastrointestinal Radiology. Philadelphia: WB Saunders, pp. 244–276.

SUBSTERNAL OR SUBXIPHOID COMPLAINTS

A. Clinical Findings

  1. Esophageal disorders may have symptoms referred to neck, suprasternal notch, substernal area or subxiphoid region.

  2. Complaints: dysphagia (subjective awareness of difficulty swallowing), odynophagia (painful swallowing), heartburn, chest pain, vomiting.

B. Imaging Modalities

1. Upper gastrointestinal series: best approach for evaluation of structural and motor disorders.
2. Nuclear medicine studies: only of use in children.

C. Recommended Imaging Approach

1. If patient can stand, turn, and is mentally competent, start with double-contrast upper GI series before endoscopy.
2. Videopharyngoesophagram performed if laryngeal penetration, prominent cricopharyngeus, or Zenker's diverticulum seen.

D. Differential Diagnostic Considerations

1. Reflux esophagitis
   a. Barium study only 50% sensitive for detecting presence of gastroesophageal reflux. Detection of gastroesophageal reflux is not the purpose of the study, the purpose is to document complications of gastroesophageal reflux: esophagitis, stricture, Barrett's esophagus, adenocarcinoma.
   b. Associated with hiatal hernia; if not, suspect alcohol abuse, gastric disease, or scleroderma.
   c. Distal esophagus: granular mucosa, linear or punctate ulcers.
2. Feline esophagus
   a. Associated with gastroesophageal reflux.
   b. Transient contraction of muscularis mucosae.
   c. Thin transverse folds cross entire lumen.
3. Barrett's esophagus
   a. Normal double-contrast barium study: less than 1% have Barrett's esophagus.
   b. High risk (70%): reticular pattern, midesophageal stricture, or ulcer.
   c. Moderate risk (20%–40%): reflux esophagitis, distal esophageal stricture.
   d. Low risk (1%): gastroesophageal reflux, hiatal hernia.
4. Candida esophagitis

    a. Predisposing factors include immunosuppression, stasis due to scleroderma, or achalasia.

    b. Oropharyngeal thrush in 50%.

    c. Radiographic findings: sharply circumscribed plaques aligned longitudinally; shaggy esophagus, strictures, or ulcers very rare.

    d. Double-contrast esophagram detects about 95% of cases.

5. Herpes esophagitis

    a. Herpes simplex, type I.

    b. Immunosuppressed patients.

    c. Radiographic findings: discrete, small, apthoid-like ulcers separated by normal intervening mucosa.

    d. Barium studies specific in 50%, nonspecific esophagitis in 45%.

6. Drug-induced esophagitis

    a. Tetracyclines, quanidine, KCl.

    b. Usually self-limited, heals in 7–10 days.

    c. Radiographic findings: small, discrete ulcers in midesophagus at levels of normal extrinsic impression (aortic arch, left mainstream bronchus, left atrium).

7. Intramural pseudodiverticulosis

    a. 1–3-mm flask-shaped outpouchings (dilated submucosal glands and ducts).

    b. Upper or midesophageal stricture.

    c. Secondary candidal spores in 50% of patients.

    d. Few pseudodiverticula often associated with sequelae, gastroesophageal reflux disease (esophagitis, stricture) in lower esophagus.

8. Glycogenic acanthosis

    a. Asymptomatic elderly patients.

    b. Intracellular glycogen accumulation in squamous epithelial cells leads to 1–4-mm nodules or plaques up to 15 mm.

    c. Confused with candidal or reflux esophagitis.

9. Squamous cell carcinoma

    a. History of tobacco and alcohol abuse.

b. Associated head and neck squamous cell cancer in 10%–20%.

c. Radiographic findings
   - Infiltrating: irregular luminal narrowing
   - Polypoid: lobulated intraluminal mass
   - Ulcerative: meniscoid ulcer with nodular rim
   - Varicoid: thick, tortuous, fixed, folds
   - Superficial: coalescent nodules, plaques, small polyp

10. Adenocarcinoma
    a. Associated with Barrett's esophagus.
    b. Distal esophagus more frequent than midesophagus.
    c. Frequent invasion of gastric cardia, fundus.
    d. Radiographic findings: ulcerative, plaque-like, polypoid.

11. Spindle cell carcinoma
    a. Large polypoid or intraluminal mass without obstruction.

12. Inflammatory esophagogastric polyp
    a. Associated with changes of gastroesophageal reflux, reflux esophagitis.
    b. Smooth, ovoid polyp atop thick rugal fold at gastric cardia or protruding into distal esophagus from hiatal hernia.
    c. Need endoscopy if lobulated or irregular surface.

References

Gilchrist AM, Levine MS, Carr RF et al (1988). Barrett's esophagus: diagnosis by double contrast esophagography. AJR 150:97–102.

Levine MS (1988). Radiology of the Esophagus. Philadelphia: WB Saunders, pp. 1–373.

Levine MS, Loercher G, Katzka DA et al (1991). Giant, human immunodeficiency virus-related ulcers in the the esophagus. Radiology 180:323–326.

Levine MS, Macones AJ, Laufer I (1985). Candida esophagitis: accuracy of radiographic diagnosis. Radiology 154:581–587.

ABDOMINAL PAIN: GENERAL PRINCIPLES

1. Types of abdominal pain
   a. Visceral pain: pain arising from an abdominal viscus is poorly

localized because sensory afferents enter both sides of the spinal cord and innervation of viscera is multisegmental.
- C3–C5 (phrenic nerve): capsule of liver, central diaphragm, splenic capsule, pericardium
- T6–T9 (celiac axis, greater splanchnic nerve): periphery diaphragm, gallbladder, stomach, pancreas, small bowel
- T10–T11 (mesenteric plexus, lesser splanchnic nerve): colon, appendix, pelvic viscera
- Tll–L1 (lowest splanchnic nerve): sigmoid colon, rectum, renal pelvis, ureter, testes
- S2–S4 (hypogastric plexus): urinary bladder, rectum

   b. Parietal (somatic) pain: painful stimulus of parietal peritoneum. More intense, more precisely localized.

2. Common sites of perceived locations of pain by organ
   a. Esophagus: substernal or neck discomfort. Lower third of esophagus frequently subxiphoid.
   b. Stomach, mesenteric duodenum: midepigastric.
   c. Duodenal bulb: right upper quadrant pain, radiation to back.
   d. Jejunum, ileum: periumbilical, radiation to back. Terminal ileum: periumbilical, radiation to right lower quadrant.
   e. Colon: poorly localized to lower midabdomen.
   f. Gallbladder, common bile duct: right upper quadrant, midepigastric, referred to back.

3. The pain patterns of gallstone disease, gastric or duodenal ulcer, gastritis, esophagitis, and cancer of these organs frequently overlap. The imaging approach to these diseases will vary and will reflect the disorder that is most suspected.

References

Haubrich WS (1995). Abdominal pain. In Haubrich WS, Schaffner F, Berk JE (eds): Bockus Gastroenterology. Philadelphia: WB Saunders, pp. 11–29.

Klein KB (1995). Approach to the patient with abdominal pain. In Yamada T (ed). Textbook of Gastroenterology. Philadelphia: JB Lippincott, pp. 750–771.

DYSPEPSIA

A. Clinical Findings

Dyspepsia is defined as persistent or recurrent upper abdominal pain or discomfort and includes symptoms of nausea, upper abdominal bloating, early satiety, or postprandial fullness. Common causes of dyspepsia include gastroesophageal reflux disease (GERD), gastric and duodenal ulceration associated with *Helicobacter pylori* infection, peptic ulceration related to use of nonsteroidal antiinflammatory agents, gastric cancer, gallbladder and biliary tract disease, and pancreatic disease.

Workup and treatment of dyspepsia is changing due to (1) recognition of the strong association of *H. pylori* with many peptic disease states, (2) development of noninvasive tests to diagnose *H. pylori,* and (3) the need for a cost-effective approach to the diagnosis of peptic disease. Many patients should undergo empiric medical therapy before imaging. Two overriding principles suggest that barium is the modality of choice in many patients: (1) Endoscopy is only slightly more accurate than barium in diagnosis of lesions greater than 3 mm (95% vs. 90%), yet endoscopy is three to four times more extensive than barium studies and is less safe. (2) There is no correlation between symptoms, endoscopically diagnosed inflammation, and histology. As of late 1995, the consensus panel convened by the National Institutes of Health concluded that the value of antimicrobial therapy for *H. pylori*–infected patients with nonulcer dyspepsia is uncertain. Therefore, detection of minor mucosal abnormalities in dyspeptic patients is of uncertain and doubtful clinical significance.

This section discusses rational workup of patients who have not responded to empiric therapy or those patients who should be imaged first.

B. Imaging Modalities

Barium and Endoscopy—Principles of Diagnostic Accuracy: A "single-contrast upper gastrointestinal series" is clearly inferior to endoscopy in detection of gastric and duodenal ulcers and gastric cancers (about 75% vs. 95% accuracy). A double-contrast examination is superior to endoscopy in some respects, equal in others, and inferior in others.

1. GERD: Barium gives a broader view of GERD than endoscopy. Barium will demonstrate GE reflux in only 50%–70% of patients with GE reflux, but this is more than the number of patients with endoscopic esophagitis. If the question is "Does this patient reflux?", a pH probe study is the gold standard. Endoscopy is clearly superior in demonstrating mild reflux esophagitis and Barrett's esophagus. Barium is better in detecting motor disturbances related to GE reflux, mild strictures, Schatzki ring, cervical esophageal webs, and a prominent cricopharyngeus. If the barium swallow is normal, there is only a 1% chance of Barrett's esophagus. Therefore, a barium swallow is an excellent triage mechanism in workup of GERD, especially for those patients with dyspepsia rather than heartburn.

2. Gastric ulcer: Endoscopy is probably slightly superior in detection of gastric ulceration (95% vs. 90%). Endoscopy will be more accurate in postoperative patients and patients with large hiatal hernias. In the mobile patient, endoscopy and barium are roughly equivalent in diagnosis of gastric ulcer. One-half to two-thirds of patients have an unequivocally benign ulcer on barium studies. These patients can be followed radiographically to healing. Equivocally benign gastric ulcers are usually benign, but should be biopsied endoscopically. Suspicious or definitely malignant-appearing ulcers on barium studies should be evaluated endoscopically.

3. Duodenal ulcer: Endoscopy is slightly superior to upper GI series in detection of tiny duodenal ulcers (95% vs. 90%, respectively). If the duodenal bulb has been scarred by previous peptic disease, endoscopy is clearly superior in detection of duodenal ulcers.

4. Gastric cancer: Endoscopy and double-contrast upper GI series have approximately equal detection rates for early gastric cancer (96% vs. 95%, respectively). Barium is clearly superior to endoscopy in detection of scirrhous carcinoma (linitis plastica).

5. Patients with previous gastric or duodenal ulcers and recurrent symptoms: Endoscopy is superior in its ability to obtain histology and detect small ulcers in areas of scarring.

THE CLINICIAN MUST KNOW THE RADIOLOGISTS AND THEIR TECHNIQUES

If an upper GI series is to be performed to work up dyspepsia, an examination requires

- glucagon or anticholinergic agent to induce gastroduodenal hypotonia
- high-density barium for mucosal coating, effervescent agent for lumenal distension.

This exam is variously known as "double-contrast," "air-contrast," or "biphasic," as the exam also employs single-contrast techniques.

A double contrast upper GI series can only be easily obtained in

- patients who are mobile (can roll around in bed and stand up)
- patients who are able to understand the radiologist's instructions

IF A DOUBLE-CONTRAST UPPER GI IS NOT BEING PERFORMED FOR DIAGNOSIS OF DYSPEPSIA ON MOBILE, ALERT PATIENTS, EITHER FIND ANOTHER RADIOLOGIST OR DO ENDOSCOPY

Pancreatic Disease: See section on Pancreatitis and Pancreatic cancer.

Biliary Tract and Gallbladder Disease: See section on Right Upper Quadrant Pain

C. Recommended Imaging Approach

For dyspepsia after empiric medical therapy fails:

1. Endoscopy first
   - Immobile patients, patients who will not understand instructions
   - Previous benign duodenal or gastric ulcer and patient with recurrent symptoms refractory to medical treatment
   - Patients with dyspepsia and an acute upper GI bleed
   - Previous gastroduodenal surgery and dyspepsia if symptoms are not obstructive
   - Absence of radiologist capable of performing and interpreting double-contrast study
   - Young patient (<30 years) with refractory symptoms
2. Double-contrast upper GI first
   - Symptoms favor esophageal disease
   - Rule out cancer with associated weight loss, vomiting, or other signs of obstruction
   - Diabetic or other patients with suspected gastric motility disor-

der (nuclear medicine gastric emptying study with solids and liquids helpful)

- Patient with previous abdominal malignancy: pancreatic cancer, intraperitoneal metastasis
- Absence of monitoring and resuscitation facilities
- Older patient (>40 years with refractory symptoms)

References

Johnsen R, Bernersen B, Straume B et al (1991). Prevalences of endoscopic and histologic findings in subjects with and without dyspepsia. BMJ 302:749–752.

Levine MS, Creuteur V, Kressel HY et al (1987). Benign gastric ulcers: Diagnosis and follow-up with double contrast radiography. Radiology 164:9–13.

Low VHS, Levine MS, Rubesin SE, Laufer I (1994). Diagnosis of gastric carcinoma: Sensitivity of double contrast barium studies. AJR 162:329–334.

Stevenson GW (1994). Dyspepsia and epigastric pain. In Gore RM, Levine MS, Laufer I (eds): Textbook of Gastrointestinal Radiology. Philadelphia: WB Saunders, pp. 2494–2499.

ACUTE UPPER ABDOMINAL PAIN (CONFIRM PANCREATITIS, RULE OUT COMPLICATIONS)

A. Clinical Findings

Acute pancreatitis can be confused with acute cholecystitis, peptic disease, bowel obstruction or infarction, renal colic, appendicitis, or ruptured abdominal aortic aneurysm. Approximately 10%–20% of patients with acute pancreatitis do not have elevated serum amylase or lipase. Imaging is useful to confirm the diagnosis of pancreatitis, exclude other disorders that mimic pancreatitis, stage the disease with respect to prognosis, and image complications in patients who fail to respond to medical therapy. Patients with pancreatic necrosis involving more than 30% of the pancreatic parenchyma have significantly increased morbidity and mortality.

B. Imaging Modalities

By far, CT with technique dedicated toward imaging the pancreas is the most important modality in workup of acute pancreatitis.

1. Plain film
    a. Sentinel loop: a focally dilated loop of duodenum, left upper quadrant small bowel, or transverse colon ("colon cut-off").
    b. Abscess rarely detected by plain film.
2. Chest film
    a. One third abnormal. Elevated diaphragm(s). Pleural effusion(s). Basal atelectasis. Even pulmonary infiltrates. Patients may develop adult respiratory distress syndrome.
3. Upper gastrointestinal series
    a. Extrinsic mass effect and spiculation of contour where phlegmon secondarily involves stomach or duodenum. The duodenal C loop may be widened, the papilla enlarged, with an inverted 3 sign.
4. Endoscopic retrograde pancreatography
    a. Not usually performed in patients with acute pancreatitis, except in patients requiring sphincterotomy for choledocholithiasis.
5. Ultrasound
    a. Limited in at least 25%–33% of patients: bowel gas obscures visualization, limited visualization of spread of pancreatitis along fascial planes, will not recognize areas of necrosis, poor at visualizing complications such as abscess or pseudoaneurysm formation.
    b. Findings: diffusely enlarged, hypoechoic pancreas. Focal mass may represent fluid, phlegmon, or abscess.
6. Computed tomography
    a. Mild pancreatitis: Normal-appearing CT or gland that is slightly enlarged, with mild stranding of peripancreatic fat.
    b. Moderate: Enlarged pancreas with irregular contour, slightly heterogeneous parenchyma, small intrapancreatic fluid collections, peripancreatic inflammation and fluid, fascial plane thickening.
    c. Severe pancreatitis: Very enlarged, heterogeneous pancreas, necrotic areas do not enhance during arterial phase of contrast injection, large peripancreatic fluid collections or phlegmon involving anterior pararenal space, lesser sac, small bowel mesen-

tery, transverse mesocolon, posterior pararenal space, and less common sites; ascites.

d. Complications
- Abscess formation: May develop as infected fluid collection or in necrotic pancreatic parenchyma, occurs within a few days to weeks after onset, heterogeneous low attenuation collection 20–50 HU, poorly circumscribed or partly encapsulated, gas in 20%
- Pseudocyst: Localized collection of fluid confined by capsule of fibrous or granulation tissue; less than 4 cm in size frequently resolve spontaneously; larger pseudocyst may rupture, bleed, become infected, or erode an adjacent blood vessel
- Pseudoaneurysm: Inflammatory weakening of arterial wall, usually splenic or gastroduodenal artery; may lead to catastrophic hemorrhage
- Splenic vein thrombosis: Nonenhancing splenic vein with associated perigastric collaterals

C. Recommended Imaging Approach

1. CT: The modality of choice. Used to confirm equivocal clinical diagnosis, stage disease, or detect complications such as pancreatic necrosis, infected pseudocyst, hemorrhage, or pseudoaneurysm formation.
2. Ultrasound: Used in patients with mildly symptomatic or chemical pancreatitis and to image biliary tree.
3. Endoscopic retrograde cholangiopancreatography (ERCP): After pancreatitis has subsided, used to image biliary tree: common duct calculi, pancreas divisum, choledochocele, choledochal cyst, pancreas, biliary or ampullary cancers.
4. CT or ultrasound is also used to guide needle aspiration or percutaneous drainage of peripancreatic collections and abscesses.

References

Balthazar EJ, Robinson DL, Megibow AJ et al (1990). Acute pancreatitis: value of CT in establishing prognosis. Radiology 174:331–336.

Ranson JHC, Pasternak BS (1977). Statistical methods for qualifying the severity of clinical acute pancreatitis. J Surg Res 22:79–91.

ACUTE RIGHT LOWER QUADRANT PAIN (RULE OUT APPENDICITIS)

A. Clinical Findings

1. Periumbilical or epigastric abdominal pain that subsequently localizes to the right lower quadrant; anorexia, nausea, and vomiting
2. Right lower quadrant mass developing after 48 hours of onset of pain is highly suggestive of perforation
3. Perforation and mortality rates highest in infants and the elderly
4. Correct diagnosis made by experienced clinicians in only approximately 75% of cases

B. Imaging Modalities

1. Plain film
   a. Appendicolith: Only 10% of patients with acute appendicitis; round, ovoid, often laminated, usually 0.5–2.0 cm; often indicates either impending or present perforation
   b. Adynamic ileus: About 25% of patients have air/fluid levels in small bowel
   c. Thickening interhaustral folds of cecum and ascending colon
   d. Air-filled appendix: of no value
   e. Nonspecific obliteration psoas, obturator, properitoneal fat stripes
2. Computed tomography
   a. Definitive CT criteria for diagnosis of appendicitis
      - Abnormal appendix seen: Distended (>6 mm in diameter) tubular structure with circumferentially thickened and contrast enhancing wall; typically see periappendiceal inflammation except in the earliest/mildest cases
      - Calcified appendicolith seen in association with pericecal inflammation: Appendicolith seen by CT in 30% of cases (vs. 10% by plain film)

     b. Suggestive findings of appendicitis: Nonspecific inflammation seen without demonstration of abnormal appendix or appendicolith

     c. Associated findings: Periappendiceal, pelvic, mesenteric, or subhepatic abscess; reactive wall thickening of cecum and terminal ileum; secondary obstruction

3. Barium enema
     a. Filling of entire appendix excludes diagnosis of appendicitis
     b. Nonfilling or incomplete filling of appendix in association with mass effect on the cecum or distal ileum
     c. Nonfilling or incomplete filling of appendix alone is of no value and is seen in 10%–25% of normal patients

4. Ultrasonography
     a. Noncompressible aperistaltic tubular structure in right lower quadrant
     b. Appendiceal diameter greater than 6 mm
     c. Thickened appendiceal wall loses stratification of layers
     d. Appendicolith
     e. Pericecal fluid
     f. Prominent pericecal fat

C. Recommended Imaging Approach

1. Start with ultrasound in children, pregnant or ovulating women, or if gynecologic abnormality is more likely than appendicitis by history or physical examination. Ultrasound is limited in obese patients, patients in whom compression is painful, if gaseous distension limits visualization, if the appendix is in a retrocecal or other difficult location.

2. Start with CT in all other patients. CT is the modality of choice in adults if appendicitis is the most suspected diagnosis. CT requires oral contrast filling of terminal ileum and cecum to avoid false negatives. Use of intravenous contrast is preferable.

3. If an abnormal appendix or appendicolith is not identified, the etiology of a right lower quadrant inflammatory process cannot be ab-

solutely identified. A barium enema will then be of value to rule out Crohn's disease or other inflammatory disease of cecal or ileal origin.

References

Balthazar EJ, Megibow AJ, Siegel SE, Birnbaum BA (1991). High resolution CT in appendicitis. Prospective evaluation of 100 patients. Radiology 180:21–24.

Puylaert JBCM, Rutgers PH, Lalisang RI et al (1987). A prospective study of ultrasonography in the diagnosis of appendicitis. N Engl J Med 317:666–669.

ACUTE LEFT LOWER QUADRANT PAIN (RULE OUT DIVERTICULITIS)

A. Clinical Findings

1. Acute, persistent, left lower quadrant pain, often with extension to the back is typical description of pain in patients with diverticulitis. Pain may be suprapubic or localized to right lower quadrant.
2. Severe, gripping pain in the lower abdomen, more frequently on the left, often worse after meals, may be caused by diverticulosis with circular muscle thickening rather than diverticulitis.
3. A mass, tenderness, and guarding are seen in 50% of patients with diverticulitis. Fever is detected in only 30% of patients.
4. Diagnosis may be difficult in debilitated or elderly patients, patients with renal failure, or patients taking corticosteroids.

B. Imaging Modalities

1. Plain film
   a. Most plain films are normal in patients with diverticulitis.
   b. Plain films rule out ureteral calculi in most patients (85%–90%) with ureteral stones.
   c. Plain films demonstrate associated ileus or small bowel obstruction.
2. Barium enema

    a. Specific signs: extravasation contrast or air into walled-off abscess, fistula, or sinus tract. Free perforation into peritoneal space is rare.

    b. Inferred diagnosis
- Extrinsic mass effect of pericolic abscess on colon, with spiculation of luminal contour, tethered mucosal folds, sacculation of wall opposite inflammatory process.
- Distorted diverticula. Luminal narrowing.
- Mucosa is preserved.
- If complete retrograde obstruction to barium flow, distinguishing diverticulitis from cancer may be difficult (about 10% of patients).

3. Computed tomography

    a. Inflammatory changes in the pericolonic fat are the hallmark of diverticulitis (seen in almost all patients).

    b. Collections may be at the site or even a distance from the site of perforation.

    c. Induration and thickening or fluid tracking down sigmoid mesentery.

    d. Thickening of colonic wall greater than 4 mm.

    e. Complications seen by CT include pericolic abscess, intramural sinus tracts, colovaginal or colovesical fistulas, and secondary bowel obstruction.

C. Recommended Imaging Approach

Principles: Diverticulitis begins as focal inflammation at apex of diverticulum, which is located in the pericolonic fat. Microscopic or macroscopic perforation into pericolonic fat creates pericolic inflammatory process. The perforation is usually localized, contained by the sigmoid mesentery, pericolonic fat, and appendices epiploicae. Therefore, the diagnostic test of choice should examine the pericolic soft tissues.

1. Plain films are of little value.
2. CT is the procedure of choice in patients with acute pain. CT is less invasive than a contrast enema. It detects disease distant from the colon. It may distinguish a foreign body perforation.

3. The role of barium enema.
    a. Once diagnosis is established and patient is treated, after inflammatory process heals, a barium enema is helpful to differentiate perforated cancer from diverticulitis (10% of patients).
    b. Barium enema will distinguish conditions that may be confused with diverticulitis, such as Crohn's disease or ischemia.
    c. Barium enema is superior in demonstrating enteroenteric fistulae, intramural tracking, and blind sinus tracks. CT is superior in demonstrating presence of colovesical fistulae.
4. Endoscopy is used only if necessary after CT or contrast enema is performed in patients with acute left lower quadrant pain. Endoscopy will aid in diagnosis of small polyps hidden in areas of circular muscle thickening.

References

Balthazar EJ, Megibow, A, Schinella RA et al (1990). Limitations in the CT diagnosis of acute diverticulitis: Comparison of CT, contrast enema, and pathologic findings in 16 patients. AJR 154:281–285.

Cho CK, Morehouse HT, Alterman DD et al (1990). Sigmoid diverticulitis: Diagnostic role of CT: Comparison with barium enema studies. Radiology 176:11–115.

Hulnick DH, Megibow AJ, Balthazar EJ et al (1984). Computed tomography in the evaluation of diverticulitis. Radiology 152:481–495.

Wilson SR, Toi A (1990). The value of sonography in the diagnosis of acute diverticulitis of the colon. AJR 154:1199–1201.

ACUTE RIGHT UPPER QUADRANT PAIN (RULE OUT CHOLECYSTITIS)

A. Clinical Findings

1. Right upper quadrant pain and Murphy's sign.
2. Palpable gallbladder in one-third of patients.
3. Generally variable course, resolution (85%), emergent surgery (15%).

4. Approximately 25% with chronic and symptomatic cholecystitis develop acute symptoms.
5. Gallstones single most important factor; large stones > 2.5 cm in 72%, small stones in 28%.

B. Imaging Modalities

1. Plain films
   a. Limited value; nonspecific except with emphysematous cholecystitis (diabetics), gas in gallbladder.
2. Hepatobiliary scintigraphy
   a. Findings: nonvisualization of gallbladder (sensitivity, 90%–100%; specificity, 80%–95%).
   b. False positive: chronic cholecystitis, pancreatitis, ETOH, fasting, hyperalimentation, trauma, neoplasm, severe illness.
3. Sonography
   a. "Significant triad": positive Murphy's sign, thick wall with sonolucency, cholelithiasis.
   b. Complications: pericholicystic inflammation/abscess, gas in wall.
4. CT
   a. Generally not indicated in uncomplicated cholecystitis; useful to exclude other intraabdominal processes when diagnosis unclear.
5. Intravenous cholangiogram
   a. Not indicated (high mortality)!
6. ERCP
   a. Not primary method of diagnosis.

C. Recommended Imaging Approach

1. Sonography and scintigraphy most valuable exams; no clear general preference. Sonography can demonstrate any surrounding abscess in complicated cholecystitis. Scintigraphy is highly sensitive and not subject to limitations of sonography (bowel gas, large patient, overlying wounds).

2. Patients with history of chronic cholicystitis, acute exacerbation do not require imaging.

D. Differential Diagnostic Considerations

Comment: Approximately 16%–22% inappropriately initially diagnosed with cholecystitis.

1. Acalculous cholecystitis
   a. Very young, very old.
   b. 5%–15% acute cholecystitis.
   c. Mortality 2× calculous cholecystitis.
   d. Scintigraphy may be falsely negative in a sick patient.
2. Gangrenous cholecystitis
   a. Fulminant, mural necrosis.
   b. Sonography: wall irregular, debris.
   c. Scintigraphy: rim uptake 2° perihepatitis or hyperemia.
   d. Early surgical intervention.
3. Emphysematous cholecystitis
   a. Elderly, 20%–30% diabetic.
   b. Male/female 2:1, often acalculous.
   c. Perforation 5× simple acute cholecystitis.
   d. Sonography: echogenic wall, irregular shadowing, check plain film to exclude calcification.
4. Supperative cholecystitis
   a. Potential complication, secondary infected bile, empyema.
5. Mirizzi syndrome
   a. Stone impacted neck gallbladder or cystic duct surrounding inflammation, obstruction.
   b. Potentially adverse sequelae: erosion, fistula.
   c. Surgical complications, ligate CHD instead of cystic duct!
6. Bowel: appendicitis, ischemia, diverticulitis, Meckel's diverticulitis, ulcer, torsion epiploic appendices.
7. Liver: capsular distension, Fitz-Hugh–Curtis syndrome, perihepatitis, abscess.
8. Pancreas: pancreatitis.

9. Chest: pleuritis, pneumonia.
10. Renal: colic, nephritis.
11. Pelvic: pelvic inflammatory disease, ectopic, ovarian torsion.
12. Mesentery: lymphadenitis.

References

Baron RL, Stanley RJ, Lee JKT et al (1982). A prospective comparison of the evaluation of biliary obstructions using computed tomography and ultrasonography. Radiology 145:91–98.

Cooperberg P, Burhenne HJ (1980). Real-time ultrasonography: diagnostic technique of choice in calculous gallbladder disease. N Eng J Med 302:1277–1280.

Rheinhold C, Bret PM (1996). Current status of MR cholangiopancreatography. AJR 166:1285–1295.

Stewart ET, Vennes JA, Geenen JE (eds) (1977). Atlas of endoscopic retrograde cholangiopancreatography. Saint Louis: CV Mosby, pp. 1–354.

Zeeman RK, Burrell MI (1987). Gallbladder and Bile Duct Imaging. New York: Churchill Livingstone.

Zeeman RK, Lee C, Jaffe MH et al (1984). Hepatobiliary scintigraphy and sonography in early biliary obstruction. Radiology 153:793–798.

ADYNAMIC ILEUS AND OBSTRUCTION

A. Clinical Findings

1. *Ileus* is from the Greek word meaning to wrap or to roll. In practice, *ileus* means dilatation and may be due to functional dilatation or mechanical obstruction. Adynamic or paralytic ileus implies diminished motility.

2. Pseudoobstruction: idiopathic dilatation of the colon without anatomic cause of obstruction. Also known as Ogilvie's syndrome. Use terms adynamic ileus of colon.

3. Clinical findings depend on site. In general, adynamic ileus has only mild pain, moderate distension, and infrequent emesis. Gastric or proximal jejunal outlet obstruction has copious and frequent emesis, mild pain, and mild distension. Distal small bowel obstruc-

tion or colonic obstruction has moderate to severe pain and distension, but minimal emesis.

B. Imaging Modalities

1. Plain films
   a. Moderately effective to differentiate moderate/severe small
      bowel or colonic obstruction versus adynamic ileus. Somewhat
      effective at localizing the level of obstruction. Level of obstruc-
      tion frequently appears more proximal than indicated by plain
      film. Ineffective at determining underlying cause of obstruction
      or presence of strangulation.
   b. The value of plain films is in helping to determine whether a
      patient should be immediately operated on and for following up
      the amount of luminal distension if a patient is not operated on.
   c. Erect PA chest film for diagnosis of unsuspected intrathoracic
      disease; best view to detect free intraperitoneal gas.
   d. Erect abdominal film detects free intraperitoneal gas, examines
      lung bases, demonstrates air–fluid levels, and change in posi-
      tion of bowel loops.
   e. Decubitus views are alternative to erect views in patients unable
      to stand. Right side down decubitus position moves air into left
      colon. Left side down decubitus position moves air into rectum.
      Prone or prone cross-table lateral view also moves air into rec-
      tum.
2. Barium studies: Determine level and etiology of obstruction. Upper
   GI series best modality etiology for gastric outlet, duodenal or proximal jejunal obstruction. Barium enema best modality for colonic
   obstruction and may be of value for distal small bowel obstruction.
3. Computed tomography: Used for patients with distal small bowel
   obstruction, particularly if suspected etiology of obstruction is ex-
   tramucosal in origin, i.e., diverticulitis, intraperitoneal metastasis.

C. Recommended Imaging Approach

1. Rule out gastric outlet, duodenal, proximal jejunal obstruction: Bar-

ium study is the first modality, not endoscopy. If perforation suspected by plain film, use water-soluble contrast agent.

2. Suspected moderate- to high-grade distal small bowel obstruction: Start with CT. Barium enema with retrograde reflux into the small intestine to the site of obstruction is an excellent study, but barium will preclude a CT scan if this is immediately necessary. This retrograde small bowel study is usually performed after CT. DO NOT START WITH A SMALL BOWEL SERIES IF DISTAL OBSTRUCTION IS SUSPECTED BY PLAIN FILM. It will take many hours for oral barium to reach the site of high-grade small bowel obstruction, frequently overnight. Fluid in the obstructed bowel will degrade the study.

3. Suspected low-grade small bowel obstruction. For patients with crampy abdominal pain and relatively normal plain films, an enteroclysis is preferable over a small bowel series to shoe the site and etiology of lesions causing intermittent or minimal obstruction.

4. Rule out colonic obstruction. Barium enema is the modality of choice, not endoscopy. Since carcinoma of the colon is a much more common cause of obstruction than diverticulitis, barium usually suffices. If diverticulitis is suspected or perforation is suspected by plain film, start with CT. If an enema is to be performed and perforation is suspected by plain film, use water-soluble contrast.

D. Differential Diagnostic Considerations

1. Gastric outlet obstruction: Gastric dilatation and air–fluid levels may be absent due to vomiting.
2. Small bowel obstruction, plain film
   a. Disproportionate distension of small bowel with air–fluid levels.
   b. Fluid-filled bowel loops on plain films make obstruction seem more proximal than it is.
   c. Differential air–fluid levels (stepladder appearance) are of no value in distinguishing obstruction from adynamic ileus.
   d. A "string of pearls" sign strongly suggests obstruction.
   e. It takes 12–48 hours for gas and feces to be cleared from the colon distal to an obstructing lesion.

f. Look for sausage-shaped fluid densities—dilated fluid-filled loops.

g. Air-filled bowel below the superior ischiopubic ramus suggests a hernia.

3. Closed loop obstruction

a. Plain film occasionally shows a fixed, rigid, dilated loop.

b. Strangulation suggested by linear intramural gas, thick folds.

c. Clinical history, laboratory values, plain film may not suffice to rule out strangulation. If strangulation is suspected, get CT rather than angiogram or operate.

d. A closed loop is manifest on CT as a dilated C-shaped or U-shaped loop of small bowel surrounding a central portion of mesentery. The mesentery appears "whirled" due to rotated mesenteric vessels. Strangulation is suggested on CT by edema (increased attenuation) of mesenteric fat, fluid in mesenteric folds, thick and often contrast-enhancing bowel wall (target sign).

4. Colonic obstruction, plain film

a. Use decubitus and prone views to move air in colon distally, distinguish obstruction from adynamic ileus.

b. If the air refluxes retrogradely through ileocecal valve ("incompetent ileoceceal value"), plain film may mimic small bowel obstruction.

c. Cecal volvulus: Younger patients with cecum and ascending colon not fixed by a mesentery. Large dilated single loop, often in left upper quadrant, one air–fluid level.

d. Sigmoid volvulus: Older patients with redundant sigmoid. Inverted U-shaped loop arises from pelvis, three lines (walls) converge in pelvis, two air–fluid levels, absent rectal gas.

References

Herlinger H, Rubesin SE (1994). Obstruction. In Gore RM, Levine MS, Laufer I (eds): Textbook of Gastrointestinal Radiology. Philadelphia: WB Saunders, pp. 931–966.

Megibow AJ, Balthazar EJ, Cho KC et al (1991). Bowel obstruction: Evaluating with CT. Radiology 1890:313–318.

DIARRHEA

A. Clinical Findings

1. Acute diarrhea: Acute diarrhea, continuing less than 3 weeks in duration, is usually due to an infectious agent or drug effect. Radiology is usually of little value in the workup of acute diarrhea. Some patients with acute bloody diarrhea may have an unsuspected vascular disorder such as superior mesenteric artery or superior mesenteric vein thrombosis that may need ultrasonography, angiography, CT angiography, or MR angiography.

2. Chronic diarrhea: Patients with chronic diarrhea (longer than 3–6 weeks duration) may undergo radiologic examination. These patients have already undergone various tests including stool tests for ova and parasites, occult blood, fecal fat, and cultures.

B. Imaging Modalities

1. Barium enema: Endoscopy is superior to barium enema in evaluation for mild proctitis, collagenous colitis, and melanosis coli and should be performed before barium enema. Barium enema is superior to endoscopy, however, in demonstrating the distribution of disease and in visualizing the terminal ileum. Barium enema is mainly used to rule out

   a. A right sided colitis or terminal ileitis if only a flexible sigmoidoscopy has been performed or if colonoscopy failed to enter the terminal ileum, e.g., to rule out Crohn's disease

   b. Another cause of bloody diarrhea in patients with prior history of radiation proctitis

   c. Villous adenoma

2. Small bowel follow-through with per-oral pneumocolon: Obtains air-contrast views of terminal ileum in 85% of patients. Best test with barium enema to demonstrate morphology of terminal ileum. Single-contrast views of upper and middle small bowel.

3. Enteroclysis: Best test for imaging jejunum, overlapped pelvic ileal loops. Usually does not achieve double contrast in terminal ileum, however. Best test for thickening of small bowel folds or demonstration of small bowel tumors. Useful for demonstrating inflammatory or infiltrative disorders of small bowel causing diarrhea: Whipple's disease, mastocytosis, amyloidosis, radiation change, proximal extent and the skip lesions in Crohn's disease.

4. CT: Demonstration of the complications of Crohn's disease, especially abscess; enterovesical, enterocutaneous, enterovaginal fistulae. Useful for imaging large pancreatic islet cell tumors secreting glucagon, vasoactive intestinal polypeptide (VIP).

5. Endoscopic ultrasound: Procedure of choice to demonstrate gastrinoma.

C. Recommended Imaging Approach

1. Rule out Crohn's disease
   a. If sigmoidoscopy is the first study performed and is negative, perform double-contrast barium enema with reflux into the terminal ileum.
   b. If colonoscopy is the first study performed and fails to enter the terminal ileum or is equivocal about the terminal ileum, small bowel follow-through with per-oral pneumocolon is the first choice.
   c. If symptoms suggest irritable bowel syndrome and a morphologic disorder is to be ruled out, small bowel follow-through with per-oral pneumocolon and double-contrast barium enema probably suffice rather than starting with endoscopy.

2. Patient with known Crohn's disease
   a. It is always safer to start with CT. CT will document a complication of Crohn's disease in a surprisingly large number of patients, even those who have few symptoms. CT contrast is easier to evacuate than the denser barium used during barium enema or small bowel studies.
   b. If the patient has undergone bowel resection resulting in an ileocolic anastomosis, start with a double-contrast barium enema to

evaluate the neoterminal ileum. Do not start with a small bowel study. Overlap of small bowel loops may make evaluation of the neoterminal ileum difficult.

c. For demonstration of proximal extent of small bowel Crohn's disease, skip lesions, and fistulae, enteroclysis is the study of choice.

3. Patient with history of radiation therapy involving abdomen or pelvis: Start with enteroclysis.

4. Patient with suspected eosinophilic gastroenteritis: If patient has already undergone upper endoscopy or upper GI series, start with enteroclysis for best examination of small bowel folds.

5. Patient with suspected inflammatory or infiltrative disorder causing thick bowel folds (Whipple's disease, mastocytosis, etc.): Start with enteroclysis.

6. Patient with diarrhea suspected to be endocrine in origin, i.e., Zollinger-Ellison syndrome, VIPoma, glucagonoma, by serum tests.

    a. VIPoma, glucagonoma: Start with CT, as these are large pancreatic masses.

    b. Zollinger-Ellison syndrome: Start with endoscopic ultrasound. Follow with CT, MRI, angiography, even venous sampling for hormone, if necessary. Do not expect success finding primary tumor in large number of patients. Intraoperative ultrasound of pancreas or duodenal wall may be necessary.

7. Patient with history of prior vagotomy and partial gastrectomy: Enteroclysis may be difficult to perform—intubation may be very difficult if patient has an antecolic gastrojejunostomy on anterior wall of stomach. Small bowel follow-through may have to suffice.

8. Patient with short gut syndrome: Small bowel follow-through usually suffices.

9. Patient with diarrhea related to suspected fecal impaction: Start with plain film of abdomen. Evaluate drug list and S2–S4 reflex arc with anal manometry. See section on defecography.

D. Differential Diagnostic Considerations

1. Crohn's disease

    a. Nonstenotic phase: fine nodularity of small bowel mucosa,

prominent lymph follicles, aphthoid ulcers, cobblestoning, linear ulcers on mesenteric border small bowel, fibrofatty proliferation.
  b. Stenotic phase: string sign due to reversible edema, spasm, inflammation, or nonreversible fibrosis (true stricture), aneurysmal dilatation, fistula usually from distal ileum to cecum, sigmoid, other ileal loops; other fistulae to skin, vagina, bladder; abscesses, perianal tracking, and abscess

2. Zollinger-Ellison syndrome
  a. Often small, 3–5-mm tumors; secrete gastrin.
  b. Frequently multiple, extrapancreatic.
  c. More common in wall of duodenum than pancreas.
  d. Most (60%) malignant, with metastases at time of diagnosis.
  e. Endoscopic ultrasound best test for finding tumor in duodenum, pancreas.
  f. Angiography reveals dense, homogeneous, well-circumscribed blush in late arterial or capillary phase of selected arterial injection.

References

Engelholm L, DeToeuf MD, Herlinger H et al (1989). Crohn's disease of the small bowel. In Herlinger H, Maglinte DDT (eds): Clinical Radiology of the Small Intestine. Philadelphia: WB Saunders, pp. 295–334.

Fishman EK, Wolf EJ, Jones B et al (1987). CT evaluation of Crohn's disease: Effect on patient management. AJR 148:537–540.

Rubesin SE, Bronner M (1991). Radiologic-pathologic concepts in Crohn's disease. Adv Gastointest Radiol 1:27–55.

MALABSORPTION

A. Clinical Findings

1. Gastrointestinal: diarrhea, steatorrhea, flatulence, abdominal distension, weight loss
2. Vitamin, mineral deficiency: vitamin D or calcium—bone pain, paresthesia, tetany; folate or iron—pallor, glossitis, stomatitis, cheilosis; vitamin K—easy bruisability, petechiae, hematuria.

▲ TABLE 1. Anatomically Oriented Classification of Malabsorption

Organ	Diseases	Pathophysiology
Stomach	Zollinger-Ellison syndrome	Pancreatic enzyme inactivation by acid
	Postgastrectomy	Rapid transit of nutrients; dilution of pancreatic enzymes
	Pernicious anemia	Deficiency of intrinsic factor promoting vitamin B_{12} absorption
Pancreas	Chronic pancreatitis, cystic fibrosis, pancreatic carcinoma	Decreased pancreatic enzyme and bicarbonate release
Liver, biliary tree	Severe parenchymal liver disease	Decreased bile salt formation
	Cholestatic liver disease (primary biliary cirrhosis, drug-induced cholestasis), bile duct obstruction (bile duct carcinoma, pancreatic carcinoma, gallstones, sclerosing cholangitis)	Decreased bile salt delivery to the duodenum
Small intestine	Jejunal diverticulosis, scleroderma, small intestinal fistulae and strictures in Crohn's disease, intestinal pseudoobstruction, diabetes	Stasis with bacterial overgrowth, bile salt deconjugation
	Crohn's disease, small intestinal resection, cholecystocolonic fistula	Increased intestinal bile salt loss
	Lactase deficiency, Crohn's disease	Disaccharidase deficiency
	Celiac disease, tropical sprue, Whipple's disease, eosinophilic gastroenteritis, radiation enteritis, Crohn's disease, intestinal ischemia, ileal resection	Loss of normal epithelial cells
	Abetalipoproteinemia	Nonformation of chylomicrons
	Lymphangiectasia, lymphoma, tuberculosis, carcinoid	Lymphatic obstruction
	Diabetes mellitus, giardiasis, adrenal insufficiency, hyperthyroidism, hypogammaglobulinemia, amyloidosis, acquired immune deficiency syndrome	Multiple causes

Source: Rubesin SE, Rubin RA, Herlinger H (1992): Small bowel malabsorption: Clinical and radiological perspectives. Radiology 184:297.

3. An anatomically oriented classification of malabsorption is given in Table 1.

B. Imaging Modalities

1. Plethora of clinical tests include complete blood count; serum iron, folate, albumin; vitamins K, A, and B_{12}; qualitative or 24-hour quantitative fecal fat; C-14 xylose breath test
2. CT: If disease of pancreas, liver, mesenteric lymph nodes suspected
3. Ultrasound: If disease of biliary tree suspected
4. ERCP: If disorders of biliary tree, pancreas suspected
5. Enteroclysis (small bowel enema): Best barium study of small intestine. Far superior to small bowel follow-through to evaluate disease with abnormal bowel folds or mucosal nodularity. In patients with documented fat malabsorption and suspected small bowel abnormality, find a radiologist who can perform an enteroclysis rather than get a small bowel follow-through.

C. Recommended Imaging Approach

1. If small bowel disease is suspected, do enteroclysis and CT after small bowel biopsy. If proven fat malabsorption, do not do small bowel follow-through. DO ENTEROCLYSIS.

D. Differential Diagnostic Considerations

1. Jejunal diverticulosis: Diverticula primarily in jejunum, diminish in size and number as progress distally. Associated dysmotility. Complications: obstruction (stricture, volvulus, enterolith, diverticulitis), perforation (diverticulitis), hemorrhage. Get CT if suspect complication.
2. Systemic sclerosis: Small bowel changes in 60% with progressive systemic sclerosis. Dilated small bowel (primarily postbulbar duodenum, jejunum) with hypomotility. Hidebound (crowding of folds despite dilatation). Sacculations.
3. Gluten-sensitive enteropathy (celiac disease): If adult onset, frequently do not present with steatorrhea. Diagnosis: biopsy and response to gluten-free diet. Enteroclysis: decreased number of folds

per inch in jejunum (atrophy), mosaic pattern, and increased number folds per inch ileum (adaptation). If enlarged folds in jejunum or ileum, suspect complication: edema, ulcerative jejunoileitis, T-cell lymphoma. CT: hyposplenism, cavitary mesenteric lymph node syndrome. Also small bowel adenocarcinoma, squamous carcinoma esophagus, pharynx.

4. Giardiasis: Small bowel follow-through frequently normal. Some patients show hypermotility, thick duodenal/jejunal folds.

5. Whipple's disease: Multisystemic, insidious. Dementia, weight loss, pericarditis, endocarditis, arthralgias. Middle-aged white male. Enteroclysis: Large, nodular folds distal duodenum, proximal jejunum, finely nodular mucosa (enlarged villi). CT: Low attenuation lymph nodes.

6. Amyloidosis: Malabsorption (uncommon), deposition mucosa and submucosa: finely granular surface, 4–10 mm, large nodules. Muscle deposition: hypomotility, transient intussusception. Vascular deposition (infarction): erosions, 3–4 mm small nodules.

References

Herlinger H, Maglinte DDT (1986). Jejunal fold separation in adult celiac disease: Relevance of enteroclysis. Radiology 158:605–608.

Rubesin SE, Herlinger H, Saul SH et al (1989). Adult celiac disease and its complications. RadioGraphics 9:1045–1066.

Rubesin SE, Rubin RA, Herlinger H (1992). Small bowel malabsorption: Clinical and radiological perspectives. Radiology 184:297–305.

Tada S, Iida M, Matsui T et al (1991). Amyloidosis of the small intestine: Findings on double contrast radiographs. AJR 156:741–744.

ACUTE GASTROINTESTINAL HEMORRHAGE

A. Clinical Findings

1. Hematemesis: bright red blood or coffee ground vomitus; source in upper GI tract (above ligament of Treitz), negative nasogastric tube aspirate does not rule upper GI lesion as cause of bleed.

2. Melena: black, tarry, malodorous stool, usually degraded blood from upper GI source; source of blood may be small bowel or right colon.
3. Hematochezia: bright red blood per rectum. Source lower GI tract in 90%; in 10% source of blood is in upper GI tract, and there is rapid transit of blood.

B. Imaging Modalities

1. Endoscopy: Once patient with upper GI bleed is hemodynamically stabilized, endoscopy is the diagnostic study of choice and enables immediate therapeutic intervention. Do not use barium studies for acute GI bleeding in hemodynamically unstable patients. While excellent for diagnosis in chronic GI bleeding, double-contrast barium studies are degraded by blood, gastric contents, or feces. Patients are too ill to undergo a double-contrast examination. Barium will interfere with subsequent endoscopic or angiographic procedures. Barium studies will not diagnose mild varices and most Mallory-Weiss tears, and they cannot distinguish source of bleeding if multiple lesions are seen.

2. Radionuclide scans: For diagnosis of lower GI bleeding. Localize bleed to area of abdomen not specific location or etiology. Mainly used to determine if patients have ongoing bleeding at a rate sufficient to be detected during angiography.

   a. ^{99m}Tc sulfur colloid scan
   - Intravascular half-life is 2.5 minutes.
   - Early images (1–2 minutes) may reveal extravasation.
   - Detects bleeding at extravasation rates of 0.05–0.1 ml/min.
   - Study completed in 30 minutes.
   - Isotope must be seen to move to differentiate uptake from source in fixed tissue (accessory spleen, splenosis, uterine leiomyoma).
   - If examination is negative, angiography is deferred. If positive, there is a good probability angiography will visualize the bleeding site.

- Patient must be bleeding at time of study. Tracer uptake in spleen or liver may obscure bleeding site.
  b. ^{99m}Tc-labeled red blood cell scan
  - Continuous 5-minute scans for 30-minute period (total of six scans) and at 1 hour; delayed images if no bleeding identified.
  - Focus of tracer activity increases in intensity or changes location; or new area of tracer uptaked not seen on original images.
  - Red cell scan better than sulfur colloid in patients with intermittent bleeding. Red cell scan is less sensitive than sulfur colloid scan and is less able to determine site of origin if bleed noted on delayed images.
  - Unbound pertechnetate will be taken up in gastric mucosa, kidney, and bladder.
3. Angiography: Diagnostic modality if endoscopy has failed to diagnose source of upper GI bleed. May be used as primary modality for diagnosis lower GI bleed. Bleeding must be arterial, at rate of at least 0.5 ml/min, to detect extravasation.

C. Recommended Imaging Approach

1. Severe upper GI bleed
   a. Endoscopy first for severe acute upper GI bleed
   b. Angiography if upper endoscopy is inconclusive or if angiographic intervention is required.
2. Severe lower GI bleed
   a. Scintigraphic study before angiogram to determine if patient actively bleeding
   b. Colonoscopy or angiography for severe acute colonic bleeds.

D. Differential Diagnostic Considerations

1. Most frequent causes of acute upper GI bleed
   a. Gastric ulcer (21%), duodenal ulcer (24%), varices (10%); bleed may not spontaneously resolve.

   b. Erosive gastritis (23%), Mallory-Weiss tear (7%); bleed usually spontaneously resolves.
2. Most frequent causes of acute lower GI bleed: diverticulosis (40%) and angiodysplasia (20%), both easily treated by transcatheter embolization or vasopressin infusion.
3. Esophageal varices and transjugular intrahepatic portosystemic shunt (TIPS)
   a. First variceal bleed 30%–50% mortality and 66% mortality rate at 1 year
   b. 30%–50% rebleed rate after endoscopic sclerotherapy.
   c. Mortality rates not improved by surgical shunts.
   d. One year mortality rates in TIPS: Childs A, 0%; Childs B, 18%; Childs C, 40%. TIPS has statistically significant improvement in mortality over surgical shunts for Childs C, less definitive improvement for Childs A, B.
   e. TIPS: 30% increased hepatic encephalopathy.

References

Alavi A, Ring EJ (1981). Localization of gastrointestinal bleeding: Superiority of 99mTc sulfur colloid. AJR 137:741–748.

Coldwell DM, Ring EJ, Chet RR et al (1995). Multicenter investigation of the role of transjugular intrahepatic portosystemic shunt in management of portal hypertension. Radiology 196:335–340.

CHRONIC GASTROINTESTINAL BLOOD LOSS OR WEIGHT LOSS (RULE OUT OCCULT MALIGNANCY)

A. Clinical Findings
1. Occult GI bleeding
   a. There are numerous causes of occult GI bleeding that vary with age and locale of the patient.
   b. In undeveloped countries, the most common cause of occult GI blood loss is helminth infection.

     c. In developed countries, erosions or ulceration of the esophagus, stomach, or duodenum are the most common GI lesions causing occult GI bleeding.

     d. GI tumors are second to peptic diseases as causes of occult GI bleeding in adults, especially colonic carcinoma.

     e. Nonsteroidal antiinflammatory agents are the most frequent class of drugs that cause occult GI bleeding.

  2. Unintentional weight loss

     a. The most common causes of unintentional weight loss are cancer, psychologic disorders, or GI diseases. In the elderly, drug-induced effects and hyperthyroidism are two other common causes of weight loss.

B. Imaging Modalities

1. The approach to general workup of the GI tract varies depending on the skills, interest, and costs of both the local radiologist and endoscopist.

2. Double-contrast upper GI is equal to endoscopy in detection of upper GI cancer and ulcers. It is inferior to endoscopy in the detection of small varices, arteriovenous malformations, and Mallory-Weiss tears.

3. Double-contrast barium enema is equal to colonoscopy in detection of colonic cancer, approaches colonoscopy in detection of polyps larger than 1 cm (90% vs. 95%), and is inferior to colonoscopy in detection of small hemorrhoids, polyps less than 5 mm and arteriovenous malformations.

4. Enteroclysis (small bowel enema) is superior to small bowel follow-through in detection of thick fold diseases, tumors of the small intestine, and Meckel's diverticulum.

C. Recommended Imaging Approach

1. Rule out occult colonic malignancy

     a. If good double-contrast radiology is available and patient is candidate for double-contrast study (can communicate with radiologist and turn on fluoroscopic table), start with double-contrast barium enema. If moderate diverticulosis with circular muscle thickening is seen in sigmoid colon, add flexible sigmoidoscopy. If sigmoid colon is well seen and has only a few diverticula, flexible sigmoidoscopy is not needed.

  b. If patient is not a candidate for a double-contrast study or if the quality of the radiology is poor, start with colonoscopy. If colonoscopy is incomplete, perform double-contrast barium enema.

2. Rule out occult upper gastrointestinal malignancy

  a. If good double-contrast radiology is available and the patient is a candidate for a double-contrast examination, start with a double-contrast upper GI series.

  b. If patient has clinical history that suggests possibility of varices or Mallory-Weiss tear, start with endoscopy.

  c. If good double-contrast radiology is not available, or patient is not a candidate for a double-contrast study, start with endoscopy.

3. Rule out small bowel disease

  a. If small bowel must be examined for occult bleeding, start with enteroclysis.

  b. If malabsorption is suspected as a cause of unintentional weight loss, perform enteroclysis rather than small bowel series.

4. If an occult neoplasm is suspected in the pancreas, kidneys, or retroperitoneum, a CT scan should be performed, though this will have a relatively low yield. In the future, with improvement in cost and quality of MRI, MRI may replace CT for detection of subtle neoplasms of the pancreas and liver. However, a neoplasm that is large enough to cause weight loss will be detected on CT as well as on MRI.

D. Differential Diagnostic Considerations

Colorectal neoplasia and occult blood loss

1. Fecal blood testing is an insensitive and nonspecific marker for colonic carcinoma. Approximately 2%–10% of asymptomatic patients with heme positive stool will have colonic carcinoma.

2. Fecal blood is a very poor marker for adenomas of the colon. Only

5% of patients with colonic polyps are heme positive, a positivity rate no different that that for the general population.

3. Therefore, the majority of patients with heme-positive stool have non-neoplastic causes for fecal blood.

References

Levine MS, Kong V, Rubesin SE et al (1990). Scirrhous carcinoma of the stomach: Radiologic and endoscopic diagnosis. Radiology 175:151–154.

Moch A, Herlinger H, Kochman ML et al (1994). Enteroclysis in the evaluation of obscure gastrointestinal bleeding. AJR 163:1381–1384.

CONSTIPATION

A. Clinical Findings

1. Dietary intake causes stool frequency, weight, size, length, and consistency to vary tremendously.
2. Definition of constipation: Unsatisfactory defecation. Stools may be too hard, too small, too difficult to expel, or too infrequent.
3. Classification of constipation
   a. Neurogenic
      - Peripheral disorders: e.g., Hirschsprung's disease, Chagas' disease, autonomic neuropathy, spinal cord abnormality
      - Central: e.g., multiple sclerosis, cerebrovascular accident, Parkinson's disease, psychosocial disorders
   b. Drug-induced: Includes antacids (calcium or aluminum compounds), anticholinergics, anticoagulants, antidepressives, anti-Parkinsonian agents, opiates, psychotherapeutics
   c. Metabolic: Includes diabetes, uremia
   d. Endocrine: Includes hypothyroidism, pseudohypoparathyroidism, pheochromacytoma, glucagon-secreting tumors
   e. Structural lesions in colon: Include tumors, volvulus, hernia, diverticular disease and diverticulitis, strictures due to infection, ischemia, ulcerative colitis, scleroderma
   f. Structural lesions in rectum: Include rectal prolapse and inter-

nal intussusception, solitary rectal ulcer syndrome, anal canal disorders

B. Imaging Modalities

1. Colorectal transit (marker) studies: This is a study of physiology, not anatomy. In normal patients, 80% of markers are excreted within five days. Delayed transit in right colon is associated with colonic dysmotility; delay in left colon, "hindgut dysfunction"; delay in rectum, functional or mechanical outlet obstruction.
2. Colonic scintigraphy: Allows computerized quantification.
3. Defecography: Vaginal, small bowel, rectal and bladder opacification. Measure time to defecation, anal canal length, anorectal angle, level anorectal junction. This is an invasive study!

C. Recommended Imaging Approach

1. Rule out structural abnormality. Barium enema indicated before endoscopy in work-up of constipation.
2. Colonic marker studies are relatively inexpensive and noninvasive, but do not provide information about morphology.
3. Defecography and anal manometry are complimentary in workup of anorectal symptoms.

D. Differential Diagnostic Considerations

1. Defecography is still in its infancy as a modality. In normal persons, there is a high incidence of mucosal prolapse, intussusception, rectocele with barium entrapment, and broad ranges of anorectal angle measures and pelvic floor descent.
2. Mucosal prolapse syndromes include solitary rectal ulcer syndrome, colitis cystica profunda, inflammatory cloacagenic polyp. Barium enema is abnormal only in one-half to two-thirds of patients: thick valves of Houston, ulcers, mucosal nodularity, submucosal mass, especially involving anterior wall rectum.
3. Constipation from birth: Congenital abnormality, Hirschsprung's disease, meningocele. Constipation in children: Rule out sexual abuse. Constipation in adults: Rule out colonic cancer.

References

Ekberg O, Nylander G, Fork F-T (1985). Defecography. Radiology 155:45–48.

Mahieu P, Pringot J, Bodart P (1984). Defecography II. Contribution to the diagnosis of defecation disorders. Gastrointest Radiol 9:253–261.

JAUNDICE (RULE OUT BILIARY OBSTRUCTION)

A. Clinical Findings

1. The role of radiology in patients with suspected biliary obstruction (conjugated hyperbilirubinemia, isolated elevated alkaline phosphatase, etc.) is
   a. To determine whether obstruction is present
   b. To determine the location and etiology of the obstruction and, if the obstruction is treatable, by what approach: percutaneous, endoscopic, surgical, medical
2. Common causes of conjugated hyperbilirubinemia
   a. Hepatic parenchyma: Viral infection, alcohol, drug-induced, toxins, primary biliary cirrhosis
   b. Intrahepatic obstruction: Sclerosing cholangitis, hepatoma, metastases
   c. Hilar confluence and extrahepatic obstruction: Calculi; enlarged hilar lymph nodes due to metastases, lymphoma, etc.; choledochal cyst; inflammatory stricture due to prior stone passage, pancreatitis; bile duct, gallbladder, pancreatic, or periampullary malignancy
3. There may be coexistent hepatocellular and biliary disease, for example
   a. Increased incidence of gallstones in patients with cirrhosis
   b. 40% of patients with primary biliary cirrhosis have gallstones

B. Imaging Modalities

1. Ultrasound
   a. Fast, noninvasive, excellent visualization of major intrahepatic bile ducts and proximal common hepatic duct.

    b. Difficulty seeing distal common duct due to overlying gas in duodenum and hepatic flexure. Approximately 20%–40% of patients with common duct stones have normal-sized ducts; only two-thirds of common duct stones detected. Other disorders such as sclerosing cholangitis and cirrhosis prevent intrahepatic ducts from dilating in presence early obstruction.

2. Computed tomography
    a. As sensitive as ultrasound for ductal dilatation; identifies level of obstruction in 90%, etiology of obstruction in 70%. Superior to ultrasound in imaging distal common duct for calculi, pancreas for tumors, inflammatory processes.
    b. Slight risk of intravenous contrast; more expensive.
    c. Must modify technique, so radiologist must be alerted to clinical problem. Initially performed without oral or intravenous contrast. Oral contrast may cause artifact, obscure impacted calculus in ampulla, or fill periampullary diverticulum, mimicking a calculus. Thin (3–5 mm) collimation and close (3–5 mm) intervals. Follow with IV and oral contrast-enhanced scan.

3. Biliary scintigraphy (^{99m}Tc IDA scans)
    a. Of value in patients with early, functional obstruction, but no ductal dilatation.
    b. Rules out cystic duct obstruction or biliary leak.
    c. Does not image anatomy as well as other studies.

4. Percutaneous transhepatic cholangiography (PTC)
    a. Slightly more successful than ERCP at imaging biliary tree, 95% vs. 85%.
    b. Requires normal coagulation parameters (such as prothrombin time and platelet levels) so that hemorrhage will not occur. Cannot be performed in patients with large amounts of ascites.
    c. Preferred over ERCP for lesions involving confluence of right and left ducts or in patients with previous biliary-enteric surgery.
    d. Therapeutic options include biliary drainage, stone extraction, fragmentation of calculus by contact lithotripsy or laser, structure dilatation, stent placement.
    e. Complications include sepsis, biliary leak, pneumothorax, hematoma, arteriovenous fistula, abscess, peritonitis.

5. ERCP
   a. Preferred over PTC in patients with nondilated ducts, distal lesions, suspected pancreatic disease and when visualization of pancreatic duct will add to the diagnosis.
   b. Especially of value in diagnosis and simultaneous treatment of biliary calculus disease, drainage of untreatable distal malignancies, dilatation of benign strictures, sphincterotomy for papillary stenosis, stent placement.
   c. Failure to cannulate sphincter of Oddi approximately 10%–20%, especially in patients who have gastrojejunostomy.
   d. Complications include pancreatitis, pancreatic abscess, cholangitis.
6. MRI and MR cholangiography
   a. Currently slightly less sensitive in detection of etiology of obstruction than ERCP or CT; cannot detect calcification.
   b. More expensive than CT, but no risk of intravenous contrast.
   c. Does not demonstrate calcification in ductal calculi.

C. Recommended Imaging Approach

Tailor the order of tests to the clinical history, laboratory findings. The order of tests will depend on institutional preference, patient's body habitus, and the skills of the invasive gastroenterologist or radiologist.

1. Is biliary obstruction present? Equivocal liver enzyme and bilirubin levels.
   a. Ultrasound first. If dilated bile ducts are detected, CT or direct cholangiography.
   b. Early functional obstruction may precede ductal dilatation, especially in patients with choledocholithiasis. Therefore, if the initial ultrasound does not show a dilated biliary tree, either go directly to ERCP or perform cholescintigraphy or ultrasound using cholecystokinin or fatty meal.
2. Elderly patient with painless jaundice, rule out malignancy.
   a. CT first to show the extent of the pancreatic or hilar tumor, guide therapy. CT may miss a bile duct or periampullary cancer.
   b. If a lesion is suspected involving the hilum and both the right and left ductal systems need drainage, proceed to PTC. If a sus-

pected pancreatic, distal bile duct, or periampullary neoplasm is suspected, proceed to ERCP. If there is marked ascites or coagulopathy, proceed to ERCP.
3. Prior cholecystectomy, right upper quadrant pain, fever.
    a. Some physicians favor starting with ERCP to detect and treat distal common bile duct calculus disease.
    b. Other physicians start with a CT to rule out an abscess.
4. Biliary colic, fever. Rule out cholecystitis.
    a. Start with ultrasound or ^{99m}Tc IDA scan depending on institution's preference.

D. Differential Diagnostic Considerations

1. Normal intrahepatic ductal size on CT or ultrasound is 1–2 mm. Normal peripheral ducts are usually not visible on ultrasound, but central ducts may be visible.
2. Dilated intrahepatic ducts are parallel and usually anterior to portal venous tributaries and show acoustic enhancement posteriorly.
3. On ultrasound, a common hepatic duct larger than 6 mm is dilated; a common hepatic duct (CHD) 5–6 mm is equivocal.
4. On CT, a common bile duct larger than 8–9 mm is dilated; the duct wall is normally less than 1.5 mm in thickness. The ductal wall may normally show intravenous contrast enhancement.
5. Duct size and dilatation: Caveats
    a. Biliary obstruction without dilated ducts is seen in low-grade or intermittent obstruction, sclerosing cholangitis, or cirrhosis with coexistent cause for obstruction.
    b. Dilated ducts may be seen in absence of obstruction in patients with prior biliary surgery or prior, relieved obstruction.
    c. The extrahepatic tree dilates with age, approximately 1 mm per decade after age 50.

References

Baron RL, Stanley RJ, Lee JKT et al (1983). Computed tomograhic features of biliary obstruction. AJR 140:1173–1178.

Zeman RK, Lee C, Jaffe MH et al (1984). Hepatobiliary scintigraphy and sonography in early biliary obstruction. Radiology 153:793–798.

MASS LESIONS IN LIVER

A. Clinical Findings

1. Hepatic symptoms present in 50% of patients who die with hepatic metastases: hepatomegaly (31%), ascites (18%), jaundice (14.5%), varices (1%).

2. Liver function tests (LFTs) normal in 25%–50% of patients with metastases, underscoring need for imaging confirmation. LFT abnormalities often nonspecific; elevation of α-fetoprotein level strongly suggests hepatocellular carcinoma.

3. Metastases outnumber primary malignant hepatic tumors 18:1; most common nonlymphoma primaries include colon (42%), stomach (23%), pancreas (21%), breast (14%), and lung (13%). Carcinoma of pancreas, stomach, and lung most likely to present with silent primary and hepatic metastases.

4. Most common primary malignant hepatic tumors are hepatocellular carcinoma, intrahepatic cholangiocarcinoma.

5. Most common primary benign hepatic tumors are cavernous hemangioma (7%–20% prevalence in autopsy series), focal nodular hyperplasia (FNH), hepatocellular adenoma.

B. Imaging Modalities

1. General principles

   a. Multiple imaging techniques exist for detecting hepatic disease. The modality of choice will vary depending on the study indication, the available equipment, and the expertise of the radiology staff. CT is presently the best modality for detecting the simultaneous presence of hepatic and extrahepatic disease. Because studies have shown MRI to be equal or superior to CT for detecting both focal and diffuse hepatic disease, MR is being increasingly used as the study of choice when the liver is the primary site of evaluation. Ultrasound, CT, and MRI have replaced nuclear scintigraphy and angiography for the detection of focal hepatic masses. Although ultrasound has reasonably high diagnostic sensitivity (70%–90%) for detecting metastases, this modality is operator dependent, hepatic imaging may be compromised in regions of sonographic "blind spots," and study interpretation may be hindered in obese patients or patients with diffuse hepatic disease (e.g., fatty liver, cirrhosis). For these reasons, CT and MR have replaced ultrasound in many institutions as the preferred means of screening the liver for focal masses.

b. Multiple imaging techniques exist to characterize a known or suspected hepatic lesion. The imaging technique used is based on its ability to demonstrate characteristic imaging features that correspond to known pathophysiologic features of a benign or malignant neoplasm.

- Tumoral calcification: Plain films, CT, ultrasound.
- Solid vs. cystic vs. hemorrhage: Ultrasound, CT, MR.
- Tumor vascularity: Color Doppler ultrasound, contrast-enhanced CT or MR, angiography, nuclear scintigraphy flow, or blood pool studies (^{99m}Tc-labeled RBCs).
- Tumoral capsule: Contrast-enhanced CT, ultrasound, MR.
- Kupffer cell activity: ^{99m}Tc sulfur colloid scintigraphy, superparamagnetic iron oxide MR imaging.
- Hepatocyte function or biliary excretion: Mn-DPDP–enhanced MR, ^{99m}Tc IDA derivative scintigraphy.
- Hepatic vessel patency: Color Doppler ultrasound, contrast-enhanced CT or MR, CT angiography, MR angiography, conventional angiography.

2. Plain film examination
   a. Limited value; diffuse disease or large focal mass may present with hepatomegaly.
   b. Less sensitive than CT for detecting calcification.
3. Nuclear scintigraphy

    a. No longer used for routine detection of hepatic metastases that appear as photopenic defects with ^{99m}Tc sulfur colloid scintigraphy.

    b. ^{99m}Tc-labeled RBC study: most specific means of diagnosing hemangiomas. Limited for hemangiomas ≤ 2 cm (unless triple-headed SPECT available) and for small hemangiomas adjacent to inferior vena cava and intrahepatic branches of portal/hepatic veins.

    c. Sulfur colloid scintigraphy used to demonstrate reticuloendothelial cell function in FNH: normal tracer uptake in 50%; increased uptake in 10%. Hepatocellular adenomas may also possess Kupffer cells and show uptake in 20%.

    d. [99m]Tc IDA derivative scintigraphy: See IDA uptake and excretion in FNH; IDA uptake only in hepatocellular adenomas that lack biliary ductules and do not excrete agent.

    e. Gallium citrate scintigraphy: Increased uptake seen in up to 90% cases of hepatocellular carcinoma; occasionally used to confirm hepatic lymphoma.

3. Angiography

    a. Provides preoperative vascular "road map" for hepatic surgeons.

    b. Often used as last resort to help characterize neoplasms when noninvasive techniques are nondiagnostic or percutaneous biopsy indeterminate.

4. Ultrasound

    a. Least expensive cross-sectional modality. Used to screen liver in institutions where CT and MR are unavailable or where particular expertise in sonographic imaging exists.

    b. Diagnostic sensitivity of intraoperative ultrasound approaches 96%; provides important data that may affect surgical decision making in patients thought to be candidates for segmental hepatic resection of metastases or hepatocellular carcinoma.

    c. Sonographic features of most focal hepatic lesions are nonspecific, limiting ultrasound role in lesion characterization. Metastases may demonstrate hyperechoic, hypoechoic, cystic, target, and calcified patterns. Ultrasound used to help characterize hypoattenuating CT masses as simple cysts, distinguish simple from complex cystic masses, and determine lesion vascularity (color Doppler).

5. CT

  a. Currently competing with MR as preferred means to study patients with suspected hepatic disease. Test of choice to survey both hepatic and extrahepatic disease.

  b. Detection sensitivity: CT arterial portography (CTAP) > helical (spiral) contrast-enhanced CT > conventional contrast-enhanced dynamic incremental CT (DICT) > noncontrast CT (NCCT) > enhanced CT with intravenous drip infusion technique.

  c. CTAP detects 20%–25% more lesions than conventional CT; invasive requiring superior mesenteric artery or splenic artery injection; most sensitive imaging modality to detect number and location of hepatic tumor foci; reserved for patients considered for segmental hepatic resection, hepatic artery chemotherapy infusion, or chemoembolization.

  d. Noncontrast CT is used to detect calcification and hypervascular malignancies (hepatocellular carcinoma and metastases from breast, carcinoid, islet cell, pheochromocytoma, renal cell, thyroid, and choriocarcinoma).

  e. Biphasic helical CT (hepatic arterial and portal venous phase imaging): best CT technique to detect hypervascular malignancies and to characterize hepatic lesions; often used with NCCT.

6. MRI

  a. Sensitivity of lesion detection $\geq$ CT; capable of detecting and characterizing many hepatic lesions in single study; most commonly used as "problem solving" technique to help characterize lesions found by CT and ultrasound.

  b. Best technique to detect focal masses within cirrhotic livers: MR sensitivity > conventional CT sensitivity (68%) for detecting hepatocellular carcinoma, regenerating nodules, and malignant degeneration of regenerating nodules.

  c. Study of choice to identify or confirm fatty liver or to detect metastases in fatty liver.

  d. Study of choice in patients unable to undergo contrast-enhanced

CT; can determine vessel patency without use of intravenous contrast; can administer intravenous gadolinium-DTPA as needed in patients with renal insufficiency.

e. Direct multiplanar imaging capabilities superior to conventional CT.

f. Limited ability to detect calcification; very sensitive to presence of hemorrhage and iron.

C. Recommended Imaging Approach

1. Rule out focal hepatic mass

   a. Patient without a known primary or patient with known "hypovascular" primary lesion (e.g., colon, stomach, lung, pancreas): Start with contrast-enhanced helical CT.

   b. Patient with a known or suspected "hypervascular" primary (breast, carcinoid, islet cell, pheochromocytoma, renal cell, thyroid, choriocarcinoma): Start with CT (unenhanced CT followed by biphasic helical CT) to diagnose both hepatic and extrahepatic disease; may start with MR if liver is the only organ of interest.

   c. Patient with known cirrhosis: Start with MR.

   d. Any patient unable to receive iodinated intravenous contrast: Start with MR.

2. Characterize hepatic lesion

   a. Suspected hemangioma: Start with ^{99m}Tc-labeled RBC SPECT; use MR if lesions <2 cm or if nuclear scintigraphy unavailable or expertise is lacking. Near totally thrombosed lesions may require angiography.

   b. Suspected hepatocellular carcinoma: Start with MR in cirrhotic livers; use biphasic helical CT if MR unavailable.

   c. Suspected focal nodular hyperplasia: Start with sulfur colloid scintigraphy (with SPECT if available) or MR with and without gadolinium DTPA; use biphasic helical CT if foregoing unavailable.

   d. Suspected hepatocellular adenoma: May start with either CT or

MR to identify hemorrhage; imaging features often otherwise nonspecific.

D. Differential Diagnostic Considerations

1. Calcification
   a. Metastases: Mucinous carcinomas of colon, stomach, pancreas; pancreatic islet cell; breast; leiomyosarcoma; and papillary serous ovarian cystadenocarcinoma.
   b. Calcified central scars: Hemangioma, fibrolamellar hepatocellular carcinoma.
   c. Hepatic amyloidosis, rare.
2. Hemangioma
   a. CT: Peripheral, globular enhancement isodense with aorta on single-pass contrast-enhanced CT (67% sensitive, 100% specific to differentiate from metastasis); 55% show classic pattern of centripetal "fill-in" with delayed isodensity.
   b. MR: "Light bulb" sign on heavily T2-weighted images; peripheral globular enhancement with gadolinium DTPA; overall accuracy ≈ 90%.
   c. Labeled-RBC SPECT imaging: "Perfusion-blood pool mismatch"; specificity and positive predictive value approach 100%; reduced sensitivity for lesions <2 cm, particularly if adjacent to major intrahepatic vessels.
   d. Ultrasound: Hyperechoic (70%, homogeneous (58%–73%), well marginated (90%) with or without posterior acoustic enhancement.
   e. Angiography: Persistent contrast puddling within lesion beyond venous phase.
3. Focal nodular hyperplasia
   a. CT: Markedly hypervascular in hepatic arterial and early portal venous phase; homogeneous except for central scar that does not calcify. Differential includes fibrolamellar hepatocellular carcinoma.
   b. MR: Signal intensity nearly isointense with liver, high-intensity

central scar on T2-weighted images, which enhances with gadolinium DTPA due to blood vessels.

c. Scintigraphy: Sulfur colloid uptake (normal or increased) in 60%.

d. Ultrasound: Variable nonspecific appearance.

e. Angiography: Hypervascular lesion with "spoke-wheel" pattern in 70%.

4. Hepatocellular adenoma

a. Best clue: Hemorrhagic mass in female taking oral contraceptives.

b. Imaging features typically reveal hypervascular mass (nonspecific); specificity rises if internal hemorrhage or fat seen on either CT or MR. Sulfur colloid uptake noted in up to 20%.

5. Hepatocellular carcinoma

a. CT: Hyperdense enhancement in non-necrotic regions; enhancing rim when present; with or without central scar; arterioportal shunting; coexistent cirrhosis (60%) or hemochromatosis in non-Asian population.

b. MR: Variable appearance depending on degree of necrosis, fibrosis, fatty change present; vascular invasion, peripheral rim, and hemorrhage well detected; can differentiate small hepatocellular carcinoma from regenerative nodules.

c. Scintigraphy: Although majority gallium avid, scintigraphy has been replaced by CT/MR/percutaneous biopsy.

d. Ultrasound: Variable nonspecific appearance; color Doppler useful to exclude tumor thrombus in portal and hepatic veins and to assess lesion vascularity.

e. Angiography: Hypervascular tumors with neovascularity, arteriovenous shunting, and portal and hepatic venous involvement.

References

Choi BI, Takayasu K, Han MC (1993). Small hepatocellular carcinomas and associated nodular lesions of the liver: Pathology, pathogenesis, and imaging findings. AJR 160:1177–1187.

Heiken JP, Weyman PJ, Lee JKT et al (1989). Detection of focal hepatic masses:

Prospective evaluation with CT, delayed CT, CT during arterial portography and MR imaging. Radiology 171:47–51.

Miller WJ, Baron RJ, Dodd III GD, Federle MP (1994). Malignancies in patients with cirrhosis: CT sensitivity and specificity in 200 consecutive transplant patients. Radiology 193:645–650.

Nelson RC, Chezmar JL (1990). Diagnostic approach to hepatic hemangiomas. Radiology 176:11–13.

Ros PR (1993). Benign liver tumors. In Gore RM, Levine MS, Laufer I (eds): Textbook of Gastrointestinal Radiology. Philadelphia: WB Saunders, pp. 1861–1896.

CHAPTER 3

Genitourinary Disease

Richard H. Cohan, MD
Nirish R. Lal, MD
James H. Ellis, MD
University of Michigan Medical Center

Imaging Handbook for House Officers, Edited by Paul M. Silverman and Douglas J. Quint.
ISBN 0-471-13767-7 © 1997 Wiley-Liss, Inc.

CONTRAST MATERIAL

All iodinated radiographic contrast material is similar. This includes contrast agents used for excretory urography, computed tomography, retrograde urethrography, cystography, retrograde pyelography, sinus or fistulae injections, and water-soluble iodinated contrast agents used for hysterosalpingography and gastrointestinal tract studies.

Currently, two major groups of contrast material are used: conventional ionic media (high osmolality contrast media [HOCM], which have been marketed for many years), and low osmolality contrast media, including nonionic agents (LOCM), which have been widely available for 10–15 years. The latter produce fewer adverse reactions; however, they are much more expensive than the former. It is for this reason that most institutions administer LOCM selectively to patients identified to be at increased risk (see below) for having an adverse reaction to contrast media.

Manifestations of Contrast Reactions

1. Nonidiosyncratic (dose-dependent reactions due to physiologic effects of contrast media)
   a. Mild: Warmth, metallic taste in mouth, nausea, vomiting.
   b. Moderate: Vasovagal reaction (mild hypotension and bradycardia), severe vomiting, angina.
   c. Severe: Contrast-induced renal failure, pulmonary edema, cardiac arrhythmias, myocardial infarction, hypertensive crises, seizures.
2. Idiosyncratic (nondose-dependent reactions that are allergic-like in nature): These almost always occur within 20 minutes of contrast medium injection
   a. Mild: Hives (urticaria).
   b. Moderate: Severe hives, mild bronchospasm, transient hypotension.
   c. Severe: Marked bronchospasm, laryngeal/airway edema, prolonged hypotension, respiratory or cardiac arrest.
3. Other: Delayed reactions may occur 30 minutes or more after administration of contrast media. Symptoms include rigors, fevers, abdominal

pain, rash, and hypotension. The etiology of these reactions is un-known.

Incidence of Adverse Reactions to Contrast Media

Reactions	HOCM	LOCM
All	4%–13%	1%–3%
Moderate–severe	0.2%–1%	0.04%–0.1%
Very severe	0.04%–0.4%	0.004%–0.02%
Fatal	1:15,000–1:170,000	1:170,000

Patients at Increased Risk of Having an Adverse Reaction to Contrast Media

1. Previous idiosyncratic ("allergic-like") reactions to any iodinated contrast agent. Dramatically increases the chance of having a similar or other severe acute reaction to the same or another iodinated contrast agent in comparison with the general population, provided that the agent reaches the vascular system (3–11× relative risk of acute reaction).
2. Asthmatics (1.2–8× relative risk of acute reaction). When reactions occur, they are also more likely to be severe.
3. Food or medication allergies (1.5–3× relative risk of acute reaction).
4. Azotemia (particularly if azotemia is due to diabetic nephropathy) (risk of developing contrast induced renal failure).
5. Other patients at risk for developing contrast induced renal failure include
   a. Patients who are dehydrated
   b. Elderly
   c. Patients who have multiple contrast-enhanced studies within a short period of time
   d. Patients receiving other nephrotoxic drugs
   e. Patients in severe congestive heart failure
6. Severely debilitated patients (includes patients with American Heart

Association Class IV congestive heart failure), cardiac arrhythmias, sickle cell anemia, pheochromocytoma, myasthenia gravis.

Medications Associated With an Increase Risk of Adverse Reaction to Contrast Medium

1. Metformin (Glucophage): Should contrast-induced renal failure occur in patients on this oral antihyperglycemic agent, patients may rarely develop lactic acidosis that can be fatal. (The drug package insert recommends that metformin use be discontinued at least 48 hours prior to contrast medium injection. Metformin should not be reinstituted until renal function is documented to be normal 48 hours or more after contrast medium injection.)
2. Interleukin-2: There are an increased number of delayed reactions in patients receiving this drug (or who have received this drug previously) as part of antitumor chemotherapy. Reactions are most likely if the interleukin-2 was administered within 2 weeks of contrast media injection. We recommend that all patients on interleukin-2 be closely monitored after contrast material administration. Alternative studies should be considered in any patient who has previously had a delayed reaction.
3. Nephrotoxic medications: Aminoglycoside antibiotics and nonsteroidal antiinflammatory agents. Use of these substances may increase the likelihood of the patient developing contrast-induced renal failure.
4. β-adrenergic blockers: Patients may have an increased incidence of adverse reactions.

Premedication

Should be considered for patients who have had previous allergic-like reactions to contrast material. Must be given, whenever feasible, to all patients whose prior reactions included a respiratory component.

1. Corticosteroids should be included as part of all pretreatment protocols. Studies have shown that a single dose of corticosteroids 1–2 hours prior to a contrast-enhanced study does not reduce the frequency of subsequent reactions. Suggested regimens: Methylprednisolone 32 mg PO 12 and 2 hours prior to study or prednisone 50 mg PO 13, 7, and 1 hour prior to study.
2. H1 antihistamines (usually used in conjunction with corticosteroids):

Diphenhydramine 50 mg PO/IM/IV 1 hour prior to study. *Note:* Can produce drowsiness. When given intravenously may produce or exacerbate hypotension.

3. H2 antihistamines (may be used in addition to H1 antihistamines in patients who have had previous severe adverse reactions): Cimetidine 300 mg PO or IV 1 hour prior to study or Ranitidine 50 mg PO or IV 1 hour prior to study.

4. Other agents: Ephedrine 25 mg PO 1 hour prior to study (reduces reaction rate; however, can produce angina or hypertension so not widely used).

5. Efficacy of corticosteroid pretreatment according to previously published studies:
   a. When used in all patients, reduces incidence of all reactions from 10% to 6%.
   b. When used in all patients, reduces incidence of severe reactions from 2% to 1%.
   c. When used in previous reactors, reduces incidence of repeat reactions from about 35% to <10%.

6. LOCM is preferred as a contrast material for patients who have had a previous allergic-type reaction to contrast material.

Interviewing the Patient Prior to Administration of Intravascular Contrast Media

1. Determine whether patient has had contrast material previously (any prior reaction and if so, what). Premedication should be instituted if the patient had a previous allergic-like reaction.

2. Determine whether there are any other risk factors for an adverse reaction (asthma, allergies, other medical conditions).

3. Assess medical history: Does the patient have diabetes mellitus, renal disease, cardiac disease, hypertension? If patient is at risk for renal disease or has known renal disease, obtain a serum creatinine level.

4. Obtain a list of currently taken medications (to determine whether the patient is receiving metformin, interleukin-2, other nephrotoxic agents, or cardiac medication). Metformin must be discontinued. If patient is at risk for contrast-induced renal failure, nephrotoxic medications should be stopped.

5. If the patient is a woman of childbearing age, ask her if she could be pregnant (since radiation to the fetus is not desirable). If patient is not sure, obtain a β-HCG blood test.

Management of Patients Having an Allergic-Like Reaction to Contrast Material

1. Assessment of the acutely reacting patient
   a. Interview the patient.
   b. Obtain vital signs.
   c. Oxygen (if reaction has a respiratory or cardiovascular component): Administer high doses (10–12 L/min by partial nonrebreathing mask).
   d. Suction (if patient is vomiting).
   e. Secure intravenous access.
2. Institute appropriate specific treatment
   a. Urticaria: No treatment needed if mild. Diphenhydramine (50 mg PO/IM/IV) can be used to reduce pruritis. *Note:* Diphenhydramine can cause drowsiness and exacerbate or produce hypotension.
   b. Bronchospasm: Albuterol inhaler (2–3 puffs). If symptoms do not improve, add epinephrine (1:1000): 0.1–0.3 ml SC (if patient is normotensive) repeated q10–15 min prn.
   c. Laryngeal edema: Epinephrine (1:1000) 0.1–0.3 ml SC (if patient is normotensive), repeated q10–15 min prn.
   d. Hypotension (with tachycardia); Elevate legs as high as is practical, isotonic intravenous fluids (Ringer's lactate or 0.9% [normal] saline) infused at a rapid rate (may need 1 L within 20 minutes). If patient also has a respiratory reaction, add epinephrine (1:10,000) 1–3 ml IV over 5–15 minutes. May be repeated q5–15 min prn. If hypotension is isolated and there is no response to leg elevation and isotonic fluids, add vasopressors.
   e. Hypotension (with bradycardia): Elevate legs as high as is practical. Isotonic intravenous fluids (Ringer's lactate or 0.9% [normal] saline) infused at a rapid rate (may need 1 L within 20 minutes). If patient remains symptomatic, add atropine (0.5–1 mg IV) to reverse bradycardia.

f. Delayed reactions: Symptomatic treatment (antipyrexic medications for fevers, meperidine for rigors, fluid for hypotension).

References

Bush WH, Swanson DP (1991). Acute reaction to intravascular contrast media: Types, risk factors, recognition, and specific treatment. AJR 157:1153–1161.

Cohan RH, Leder RA, Ellis JH (1996). Treatment of adverse reactions to radiographic contrast media in adults. Radiol Clin North Am 34:1055–1076.

PAINLESS HEMATURIA

A. Clinical Comment

Painless hematuria can be either gross or microscopic. Typically encountered in middle-aged and elderly men and women.

B. Imaging Modalities

1. Plain Radiographs

Advantages

- Low cost.

Disadvantages

- Rarely identifies cause of hematuria.

2. Excretory Urography

Advantages

- Can identify large renal masses.
- Can identify filling defects (usually either tumors, blood clots, or calculi in the renal collecting systems).
- Demonstrates obstruction easily.
- Relatively inexpensive.
- Screens both the renal parenchyma and the collecting systems.

Disadvantages

- Requires intravenous contrast material.

- Utilizes ionizing radiation.
- Limited evaluation of the kidneys (small [<3 cm] renal masses are frequently missed).
- Limited evaluation of the bladder. Since the vast majority of cases of hematuria result from bladder or prostate disease, excretory urography demonstrates the cause of hematuria in only a small minority of patients.

3. Sonography

Advantages

- Does not require ionizing radiation.
- Identifies renal masses with greater sensitivity than urography.
- Identifies most larger (>5 mm) renal calculi.
- Can demonstrate small prostatic cancers when performed using a transrectal approach.

Disadvantages

- Isoechoic solid renal masses (many of which are cancers) may be difficult or impossible to detect.
- Cannot reliably distinguish between renal angiomyolipomas and renal adenocarcinomas (the former are nearly always echogenic, and the latter are occasionally echogenic, particularly when small).
- Assessment of renal collecting system is extremely limited. Ureters are frequently not visualized. Small filling defects in renal calices, infundibulae, and renal pelvis are easily missed.
- Evaluation of bladder is limited.
- Transrectal ultrasound of the prostate misses many cancers and also makes false-positive diagnoses.

4. CT

Advantages

- Excellent visualization of renal parenchyma. When performed using thin-image collimation (5 mm or less) after intravenous contrast material administration it is the most sensitive imaging modality for renal mass detection.

- Stages renal cancers with 90% accuracy.
- Usually able to distinguish between angiomyolipomas and renal cancers.

Disadvantages

- Requires intravenous contrast material (for optimal study).
- Requires ionizing radiation.
- Can miss small abnormalities in the renal collecting systems.
- Evaluation of the prostate and bladder is limited. Cannot distinguish prostate cancer from benign prostatic hyperplasia. Many bladder abnormalities produce focal or diffuse bladder thickening and cannot be differentiated from one another.

5. MRI

Advantages

- Does not use ionizing radiation.
- Does not use iodinated radiographic contrast material (so it can be performed as an alternative in patients in whom radiographic contrast material is contraindicated due to prior contrast reaction or elevated serum creatinine level).
- When performed with gadolinium, rivals CT in its ability to detect renal masses and stage renal adenocarcinoma.
- Transrectal MR coils are reasonably accurate in detecting and locally staging prostatic neoplasms.
- MR urography can assess the collecting systems for filling defects and obstruction with detail approaching that of excretory urography.

Disadvantages

- Expensive.
- Offers no additional benefit to CT in most instances.
- Transrectal coil is usually used only as part of a dedicated exam of the prostate.
- MR urography is not routinely performed
- New technique. More experience necessary to evaluate efficacy.
- Standard MR is not sensitive for evaluation of the renal collecting systems.

6. Retrograde Pyelography

Advantages
- Offers an exquisite view of the renal collecting systems.
- Likely represents the most sensitive imaging modality for visualization of the collecting systems.
- Although this procedure uses iodinated contrast media, it can be performed with relative safety in patients who have had prior adverse reactions to intravascular contrast material, since little or no contrast material is absorbed through intact uroepithelial cells.

Disadvantages
- Cannot evaluate the kidneys.
- Invasive procedure. The ureteral stent is inserted by a urologist during cystoscopy.

7. Arteriography/Venography

Advantages
- Arteriovenous fistulae can be easily demonstrated during arteriography.
- Pressure tracings can be obtained in the left renal vein during venography, permitting a diagnosis of renal vein hypertension to be made or excluded in patients in whom no other source of bleeding has been identified.

Disadvantages
- Does not image the intraabdominal organs. Arteriography is only recommended once other imaging studies have been performed.

C. Recommended Imaging Approach

If a patient has painless gross or microscopic hematuria and no evidence of infection/cystitis and/or if the patient's hematuria persists after a course of antibiotics, the patient should be referred to a urologist. Since the cause of the hematuria is usually in the lower urinary tract, cystoscopy is diagnostic in most patients. However, many urologists prefer to have an excretory urogram performed prior to cystoscopy despite the low yield of this study. This is because if the urogram demonstrates any findings suspicious of upper tract filling defects (i.e., possible uroepithelial tumors), a retrograde pyelogram can be performed at the time of the cystoscopy. If the excretory urogram is delayed until after cystoscopy, it is conceivable that a second cystoscopic procedure may be needed.

If the excretory urogram and cystoscopy fail to identify the source of hematuria, then CT can be used to assess the kidneys for renal masses. MRI (with gadolinium) should be reserved for patients who cannot receive intravenous contrast material for a CT. An unenhanced CT is not an acceptable study in a patient who is being evaluated for a renal mass. Sonography does not play a role in the standard evaluation of patients with painless hematuria. In instances where symptomatic hematuria remains unexplained after urography, cystoscopy, and cross-sectional imaging studies are completed, renal arteriography and venography can then be performed, with pressure tracings obtained from the renal vein, if bleeding is demonstrated to be coming from the left ureteral orifice. In some patients, the source of hematuria is never identified. These patients are usually closely followed; however, the exhaustive work up described has essentially excluded the most worrisome causes of hematuria.

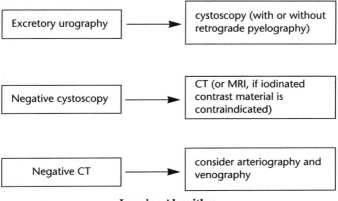

Imaging Algorithm

D. Differential Diagnostic Considerations

1. Lower urinary tract disease

   a. Benign prostatic hyperplasia: Most common etiology in older males.

   b. Prostatitis: May also cause perineal or pelvic pain.

   c. Cystitis: Most common etiology in women and young men. Is usually uncomplicated, although a number of variants exist.

   d. Transitional cell carcinoma of the bladder: Irritative neoplasm, encountered more often in smokers, coffee drinkers, individuals with industrial toxin exposure.

2. Upper urinary tract disease

   a. Renal adenocarcinoma: Most common solid renal neoplasm. Patients usually do not present with hematuria until neoplasm is large.

   b. Transitional cell carcinoma of the ureters, renal pelves, calices, or renal infundibula.

   c. Renal angiomyolipoma: Benign tumors that are more common in patients with tuberous sclerosis (in which case they are multiple and bilateral) and in middle-aged females.

   d. Occult stone disease: Usually stones are proximal and do not produce any obstruction.

   e. Arteriovenous fistula: Seen most commonly after renal biopsy or other penetrating trauma.

   f. Arteriovenous malformation: Extremely rare.

   g. Renal vein hypertension: Nearly always found in the longer left renal vein, perhaps resulting from compression by the crossing superior mesenteric artery. This is usually a diagnosis of last resort.

References

Nishimura Y, Fushiki M, Yoshida M, et al (1986). Left renal vein hypertension in patients with left renal bleeding of unknown origin. Radiology 160:663–667.

Warshauer DM, McCarthy SM, Street L (1988). Detection of renal masses: Sensitivities and specificities of excretory urography/linear tomography, US, and CT. Radiology 169:363–365.

ACUTE FLANK PAIN

A. Clinical Comment

Acute flank pain is often severe. Patients may have nausea and vomiting. Onset is usually sudden. Symptoms may wax and wane.

B. Imaging Modalities

1. Plain Radiographs

Advantages
- Easy to obtain.
- Low cost.
- Most renal or ureteral calculi can be identified.

Disadvantages
- 10%–20% of genitourinary calculi are radiolucent.
- May be difficult to determine if pelvic basin calcification is genitourinary tract calculus or a phlebolith.
- Does not assess functional significance of a stone (i.e., obstruction).

2. Intravenous Urography

Advantages
- Provides functional and anatomic information that assesses presence or absence of obstruction.
- Identifies etiology of calcification (i.e., inside or outside urinary tract) in most instances.

Disadvantages
- Requires use of contrast media to which some patients can severely react. Contrast media is not recommended in unprepared patients who have had prior allergic-like reactions.
- Uses ionizing radiation. To be avoided when possible in pregnant patients.
- May take several hours to identify level of obstruction since excretion is delayed on the obstructed side.

3. Ultrasound

Advantages

- Easily identifies dilatation of collecting system.
- Resistive index (ratio of peak systolic pressure minus end-diastolic pressure divided by peak systolic pressure) elevates in obstructed kidneys (above 0.7).
- Well-hydrated patients have reduced or absent ureteral jets on the obstructed side. Ureteral jets can be identified with color-flow Doppler imaging.

Disadvantages

- Resistive index does not immediately rise in patients with obstruction (may take up to 4–6 hours).
- Dilatation of collecting system is not always present.

4. CT

Advantages

- Virtually all genitourinary calculi are visible (including stones that are lucent on plain film).
- Identifies collection system dilatation.
- Does not require use of intravenous contrast material for this indication.
- Instantaneous diagnosis.

Disadvantages

- Expensive.
- Requires many images.
- Difficult to distinguish pelvic phleboliths from small stone, especially when there is minimal ureteral dilatation.

5. MR Urography

Advantages

- No ionizing radiation.
- Rapid diagnosis.
- Radiographic contrast media is not needed.

Disadvantages
- Expensive.
- Experimental. Sensitivity and specificity not assessed.
- May require hydration and diuretic for adequate visualization.
- Stone itself cannot be seen (calcification does not produce signal).

C. Recommended Imaging Approach

An abdominal radiograph followed by an excretory urogram is the traditional (and still very effective) way in which to evaluate patients with acute flank pain. Given the risks of adverse reactions to urography, in general we recommend that, whenever possible, urography not be performed as an emergency in the middle of the night (at a time when staff support

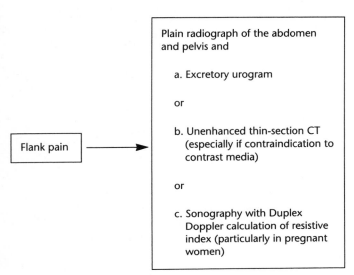

Imaging Algorithm

might be reduced). In most instances, the patient can be hydrated and studied the following morning. An abdominal plain radiograph followed by either a sonogram (during which Duplex Doppler is performed so that resistive indices can be calculated) or a limited noncontrast CT is also an appropriate examination and can be performed as an alternative. Although it is not effective in imaging the entirety of the ureters, sonography is preferred in pregnant women, since attempts should be made to avoid radiation exposure to the fetus. Unenhanced CT should be performed as the procedure of choice in nonpregnant patients in whom there is a contraindication to use of intravascular contrast material, such as those who have had previous reactions or who are severely azotemic. After an initial dose of antibiotics, nephrostomy should be performed emergently in any patient with infected urine and/or sepsis in whom imaging studies (urography, sonography, or CT) suggest that one of the collecting systems is obstructed.

D. Differential Diagnostic Considerations

1. Urolithiasis
   a. 85% of patients with genitourinary calculi will have microscopic hematuria.
   b. 80%–90% of genitourinary calculi are radiopaque and visible on abdominal radiographs.
   c. Obstructing calculi can be located anywhere in the ureter but are most commonly at the ureterovesical junction, followed by the ureteropelvic junction or pelvic inlet.
2. Acute pyelonephritis
   a. Patients usually have evidence of sepsis (fever, chills, leukocytosis) and exquisite flank tenderness.
   b. Urine is usually infected (containing white blood cells and bacteria). Predisposing factors include diabetes mellitus, prior instrumentation, obstructive uropathy, bacterial endocarditis.
3. Pyonephrosis (obstructed/infected collecting system).
   a. Can be due to stone/stricture.
   b. Patients usually have evidence of infection (pyuria, bacturia, leukocytosis, and fever).

    c. Primary indication for emergency percutaneous nephrostomy or ureteral stenting.

4. Non-genitourinary related causes
    a. Musculoskeletal.
    b. Gastrointestinal.

References

Haddad MC, Sharif HS, Shahed MS et al (1992). Renal colic: diagnosis and outcome. Radiology 184:83–88.

Platt JF, Ellis JH, Rubin JM (1995). Role of renal Doppler imaging in the evaluation of acute renal obstruction. AJR 164:379–380.

Smith RC, Rosenfield AT, Choe KA et al (1993). Acute flank pain: Comparison of non-contrast enhanced CT and intravenous urography. Radiology 194:789–794.

ELEVATED PROSTATE-SPECIFIC ANTIGEN

A. Clinical Comment

Prostate-specific antigen (PSA) levels are now frequently obtained as a screen for prostate cancer in men over the age of 50 years. In general, PSA serum levels under 4 ng/ml are considered normal. PSA levels between 4 and 10 are worrisome for prostate cancer, but can be seen in patients with benign prostatic hyperplasia (BPH), particularly if prostate volumes are large. In contrast, once the PSA level exceeds 10 ng/ml, the likelihood of a cancer is extremely high. It should also be remembered that some prostate cancers do not secrete PSA. Therefore, some patients with cancers will not have elevated PSA levels.

Sonography and MR are the only imaging studies that can detect small prostate cancers. All other modalities are reserved for patients after a diagnosis of cancer is established. While the other studies may be helpful (if metastatic disease is detected), they are frequently negative. In these instances, patients may go on to have surgery, at which time metastatic disease may be detected that could not be seen with any of the imaging modalities.

B. Imaging Modalities

1. Plain Radiography

Advantages

- Can identify bone metastases (the vast majority of which are at least partially sclerotic).
- Inexpensive and easy to obtain.

Disadvantages

- Often not helpful. Many patients with prostate cancer do not have bone metastases. For this reason, plain radiographs are best obtained as a follow up to a positive bone scan to evaluate bones that demonstrate increased uptake of radiotracer (to differentiate between malignant and benign causes of increased uptake).
- Does not image prostate gland or abdominal or pelvic cavity contents.
- Uses ionizing radiation.

2. Sonography

Advantages

- Identifies 70% of prostate cancers, most of which are hypo-echoic lesions in the peripheral zone.
- Can direct biopsy of a suspicious lesion detected during sonography.
- Can direct systematic biopsies of a prostate gland in which no lesions are detected during sonography.
- Can obtain an accurate prostate gland volume, permitting determination of PSA density (PSA divided by the volume of prostate gland). An elevated PSA density (>0.15) suggests that PSA elevation is likely due to a cancer.

Disadvantages

- Misses a significant minority of prostate cancers.

3. MRI

Advantages

- When performed with a transrectal coil can detect and accurately locally stage many prostate cancers.
- Can also detect enlarged pelvic lymph nodes.
- Can detect bone metastases in the spine (provided that the spine is imaged).

Disadvantages

- Expensive. Not feasible as a first imaging test in patients with elevated PSA levels.
- Fails to detect some prostate cancers.
- Makes some errors in local staging, when there is no gross extracapsular spread of tumor.
- Fails to detect lymph node involvement in some tumors. Prostate cancer tends to spread to lymph nodes without grossly enlarging them, at least at first, preventing detection of lymph node metastases in these cases.
- Assesses only the bones included in the imaging protocol. Does not provide a survey of all osseous structures.

4. Radionuclide (Bone) Scan

Advantages

- Sensitive for detecting bone metastases.
- Provides a survey of the entire skeleton.

Disadvantages

- Not specific. Any bone in which there is increased turnover will show increased radiotracer uptake.
- Not recommended routinely. Many patients with prostate cancers, especially if the PSA is under 10 ng/ml, do not have bone metastases.

5. CT

Advantages

- Can be used for identifying distant metastatic disease (i.e., involvement of retroperitoneal lymph nodes, liver, and adrenal masses).
- Occasionally visualizes sclerotic bone metastases.

Disadvantages

- Of little or no utility in evaluating the prostate gland itself. Cannot distinguish between BPH and prostate cancer.
- Extremely inaccurate in locally staging prostate cancer.
- Insensitive for detection of lymph node metastases. *Note:* Many urologists now reserve computed tomography for patients in whom there is clinical suspicion of metastatic disease or with very elevated PSA levels (>30 ng/ml), since these patients are more likely to have identifiable metastases. CT is only helpful if it demonstrates metastatic disease.
- Utilizes ionizing radiation and iodinated radiographic contrast media.

C. Recommended Imaging Approach

A digital rectal examination of the prostate gland should be performed in any patient in whom a PSA level is obtained. If the digital rectal examination demonstrates a focal nodule in the prostate gland, then a transrectal biopsy of the prostate gland can be performed (in the absence of any imaging). If digital rectal exam does not demonstrate a nodule, then sonography should be obtained. If sonography identifies a focal hypoechoic lesion, gland asymmetry, or a contour bulge, the abnormal area should be biopsied under ultrasound guidance. If sonography does not detect a focal abnormality, PSA density can be determined. If the PSA density is less than 0.15 ng/ml/cc the urologist may elect merely to follow the patient. Alternatively, if the PSA density is elevated or if there is clinical concern for a prostate cancer, systematic biopsies of the peripheral portion of the prostate gland can be performed under ultrasound guidance. Currently, at least three biopsies are obtained from the right and left sides of the prostate gland (base, mid gland, and apex).

Additional imaging should be deferred to those patients in whom a diagnosis of prostate cancer is established. MRI can be performed for local staging of tumors. As already stated, bone scans and CT scans are reserved for patients in whom the PSA levels are most elevated (>10 ng/ml and >30 ng/ml respectively, for example). Plain radiographs should only be obtained as a follow-up to a positive bone scan.

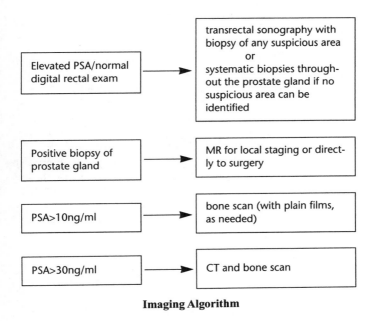

Imaging Algorithm

D. Differential Diagnostic Considerations

1. Prostatic carcinoma: Extremely common neoplasm in men.
2. BPH: Affects the majority of men over the age of 50 years.

ACUTE TESTICULAR PAIN

A. Clinical Comment

Acute testicular pain may occur either in the absence or as a result of trauma. Identification of the cause is crucial, since some etiologies require emergent surgery. Unfortunately, clinical distinction among the common causes can be exceedingly difficult. Imaging plays a crucial role in evaluating many of these patients.

B. Imaging Modalities

1. Sonography

Advantages

- Gray-scale sonography may distinguish between torsion and orchitis. Early on, torsed testes become hypoechoic. Inflamed testes also become hypoechoic; however, the epididymal heads are also usually involved and tend to become hyperechoic. Ruptured testes usually have a heterogeneous echotexture.
- Color-flow Doppler sonography can often distinguish between torsion and epididymoorchitis. In the former instance there is dramatically reduced or absent blood flow in the affected testis. In the latter instance blood flow is usually increased.
- Focal testicular abscesses, an occasional complication of orchitis, can be detected.

Disadvantages

- Distinction between torsion and infection can occasionally be difficult. When torsion is partial, flow is not completely eliminated. Occasionally, torsion only involves the appendix testis.
- Faulty settings can lead to false-positive diagnoses of torsion. Studies should be performed and interpreted by an experienced sonographer. Blood flow in the abnormal testis should always be compared with the contralateral normal testis.

2. Nuclear Medicine (Tagged Red Blood Cell) Scanning

Advantages

- Acute complete torsion has a characteristic appearance in which there is lack of radiotracer uptake in the affected side of the scrotum. In comparison, blood flow is increased in the affected side of the scrotum in patients with epididymoorchitis.

Disadvantages

- Areas of diminished tracer uptake can also be produced by hydroceles, hematomas, or tumors.
- When torsed testes are not diagnosed acutely, reactive hyperemia may develop around the hypoperfused testis, leading to increased radiotracer activity on the nuclear medicine scan.
- Increased radiotracer in the symptomatic hemiscrotum is a nonspecific finding. A variety of other abnormalities can produce increased radiotracer uptake, including varicoceles and tumors.

C. Recommended Imaging Approach

Combined use of sonography and nuclear medicine tagged red blood cell scans permits differentiation between testicular torsion and epididymoorchitis in the vast majority of patients. Either test can be performed initially. If there is any question about the results of the test or if the patient's clinical condition raises questions about the imaging findings, the other test should be obtained.

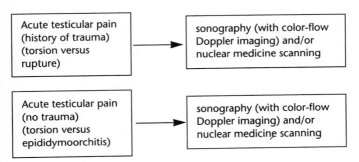

Imaging Algorithm

D. Differential Diagnostic Considerations

1. Epididymoorchitis: Most common inflammatory process in the scrotum. Usually produced by bacteria (*Escherichia coli* and *Pseudomonas*). Patients may have a discharge from the urethra. On physical examination the scrotum is extremely tender and edematous. Most patients respond to treatment with antibiotics.

2. Testicular torsion: Results from anomalous attachment of the epididymis to the scrotal wall. Usually seen in young men. May develop spontaneously or as a result of trauma. May be partial or complete. Surgical repair is required within 24 hours of complete torsion in order to save the testis. Repair usually includes orchiopexy of the contralateral nontorsed testes, since the anomaly is generally bilateral. Clinical distinction of torsion from epididymoorchitis is not possible in up to one-half of patients.

3. Testicular rupture: Rare injury that more often occurs as a result of sports injuries rather than after other blunt trauma. Emergent surgical repair is indicated within 72 hours.

Reference

Dunnick NR, McCallum RW, Sandler CM (1991). Textbook of Uroradiology. Baltimore: Williams & Wilkins.

SCROTAL MASS

A. Clinical Comment

Distinction between intratesticular and extratesticular masses is very important, since the majority of the former are malignant, while most of the latter are benign.

B. Imaging Modalities

1. Sonography

Ultrasound evaluation is recommended as major imaging modality for evaluation of the scrotum and its contents.

Advantages
- Lack of ionizing radiation and contrast material.
- Usually easily distinguishes between intra- and extratesticular lesions.
- Duplex Doppler or color-flow Doppler imaging can demonstrate flow in varicoceles, allowing for a specific diagnosis to be made. *Note:* Flow in varicoceles is often not seen unless the patient is placed in an upright position and/or asked to perform a Valsalva maneuver.
- Spermatoceles can occasionally be specifically suggested, as they have no flow and often contain internal echoes.

Disadvantages
- Many intratesticular lesions look similar using gray-scale and Doppler imaging (e.g., focal orchitis and neoplasm are both commonly hypoechoic).
- When tumors are isoechoic with normal testis or infiltrative (altering the echotexture of the entire testis), identification is difficult.
- Extratesticular lesions can look similar.

2. MRI

Advantages
- Easily depicts testicular and epididymal anatomy.
- Does not utilize ionizing radiation.

Disadvantages
- Expensive.
- Offers little advantage over sonography in most patients.

C. Recommended Imaging Approach

Patients with scrotal masses should be referred to the urology service. Occasionally, a mass can be identified as intratesticular on physical examination, in which case no imaging evaluation is needed prior to surgery. Instead, imaging (usually with CT) may be performed to determine whether a patient with a testicular malignancy has metastatic disease in the abdomen and/or pelvis. In the remaining patients, sonography is usually the preferred imaging study.

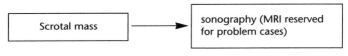

Imaging Algorithm

D. Differential Diagnostic Considerations

1. Intratesticular

   a. Testicular carcinoma: Most common in 20–45-year-old men. Over 90% are of germ cell origin. Seminomas are the most common germ cell tumors (40%–50%), with embryonal cell carcinoma (15%–35%), teratomatous tumors (10%), and choriocarcinomas (<5%) being less frequently encountered. Gonadal stromal tumors (Leydig or Sertoli cell tumors) are uncommon. Unlike germ cell tumors, most stromal tumors are benign.

   b. Metastases: More common than germ cell tumors in older men. Can spread from any primary neoplasm, but most commonly from urogenital tract tumors.

   c. Lymphoma: May be primary or secondary. Rare in young men, but may account for up to 25% of testicular malignancies in males over 50 years old.

   d. Testicular cysts: Very rare. Usually under 1 cm in maximal diameter. Result from trauma or inflammation or may be idiopathic.

   e. Orchitis: May be focal or diffuse, acute or chronic.

   f. Testicular abscess: Results from epididymoorchitis. Frequently in diabetics.

   g. Testicular adrenal rests: Rarely encountered in patients with elevated ACTH levels.

2. Extratesticular
   a. Varicocele: Represents dilated veins draining the testis (usually in the pampiniform plexus). May be idiopathic or due to incompetent valves in the left testicular vein. Present in about 40% of infertile males. New onset varicocele can result from sudden renal vein thrombosis (often due to renal adenocarcinoma).
   b. Epididymal cyst: Reported in up to 25% of males. Represents retention cyst resulting from dilated epididymal tubules. Rarely exceeds 2 cm in diameter.
   c. Spermatocele: Represents retention cyst, usually in the epididymal head. Contains thick fluid with sperm.
   d. Hydrocele: Can be diagnosed by transillumination. A small hydrocele can be present normally.

Reference

Dunnick NR, McCallum RW, Sandler CM (1991). Textbook of Uroradiology. Baltimore: Williams & Wilkins.

HYPERTENSION

A. Clinical Comment

While there are a large number of causes of hypertension, most patients have essential hypertension and require medical treatment. While many of the other etiologies can also be controlled with medication, renovascular hypertension can be cured with angioplasty, renal parenchymal disease cured by tumorectomy or nephrectomy, and adrenal adenomas and carcinomas potentially cured by adrenalectomy. Therefore, it is important to identify curable causes of hypertension, when possible.

B. Imaging Modalities

1. Excretory Urography

Advantages

- Can identify large renal masses.

- Can detect abnormal renal anatomy (contour, collecting system) or function.

Disadvantages

- Does not assess abdominal and renal vasculature.
- Does not optimally assess adrenal glands (may detect large tumors).
- Can easily miss small renal masses.
- Requires use of iodinated contrast material and ionizing radiation.

2. Sonography

Advantages

- Inexpensive.
- No need for radiographic contrast material.
- No ionizing radiation.
- Can be performed to determine size of kidneys and presence of collecting system dilatation.
- Identifies many renal and some adrenal masses.
- Easily visualizes perinephric fluid collections.
- Color-flow and duplex Doppler ultrasound has shown promise in identifying patients with renal artery stenosis.

Disadvantages

- Limited evaluation of the adrenal glands in some patients. Can miss small adrenal masses.
- Can miss small isoechoic renal masses.
- Use of Doppler ultrasound for detection of renal artery stenosis remains investigational.

3. CT

Advantages

- One of the most sensitive modalities for detecting renal or adrenal masses.
- Adrenal CT does not require intravenous contrast material administration. CT can also identify extraadrenal pheochromocy-

tomas (which tend to be quite large even when the patient first presents).
- Often able to distinguish between benign and malignant adrenal masses (since the former are often of or below water attenuation).
- Can identify renal subcapsular fluid collections or masses.
- When performed in the helical mode using very thin-image collimation can evaluate the abdominal vasculature, including the renal arteries for stenosis. This special examination must be planned at the time the patient is scanned.

Disadvantages
- Cannot distinguish among most types of solid renal masses.
- Some benign adrenal masses cannot be differentiated from malignant adrenal masses (since both may be of soft tissue attenuation).
- Aldosteronomas can be so small (<5 mm) that they can be missed even on thin section CT examinations. In addition, nodules in patients with macronodular hyperplasia may be confused for adenomas. In these patients, adrenalectomy is not curative.
- Unless a specific helical vascular protocol is used, CT cannot evaluate the renal arteries for stenosis. Even when helical techniques are employed, stenoses may be underestimated or overestimated due to limitations of the reconstruction algorithms. Stenoses in branch vessels may be missed.
- When CT is performed for assessment of the renal parenchyma or vessels, use of intravenous contrast material is mandatory.

4. MRI

Advantages
- Permits good visualization of adrenal glands, kidneys, and retroperitoneum.
- Can distinguish between many benign and malignant adrenal masses.
- Can evaluate the abdominal vasculature.
- Does not require use of ionizing radiation or iodinated radiographic contrast media.

Disadvantages
- Expensive.
- Offers little imaging advantage over CT (other than the lack of need for iodinated contrast media).
- As with CT, renal artery stenoses can be overestimated, underestimated, or missed.

5. Renal Arteriography

Advantages
- Still accepted as the gold standard for evaluation of the renal arteries and their branches.
- Percutaneous transluminal angioplasty can be performed to treat a renal artery stenosis immediately after a diagnostic arteriogram.

Disadvantages
- Invasive procedure with small, but definite, morbidity.
- Requires use of iodinated contrast material and ionizing radiation.
- Plays little or no role in evaluation of the adrenal glands or renal parenchyma.

6. Venous Sampling

Advantages
- Adrenal vein sampling (for aldosterone levels) permits definitive identification of the hypersecreting adrenal gland in patients in whom cross-sectional imaging does not identify an adrenal aldosteronoma.
- Renal vein renin levels can be obtained from both kidneys in order to determine whether a visualized renal artery stenosis is responsible for hypertension.

Disadvantages
- Sampling of the right adrenal vein is extremely difficult (the right adrenal vein originates directly from the inferior vena cava and is difficult to cannulate, especially in inexperienced hands).
- Renal vein renin levels do not necessarily correlate with the like-

lihood of a successful angioplasty. Some patients with nonlateralizing renins will still be cured by angioplasty. For this reason, renin levels are no longer commonly measured.

7. Nuclear Medicine Scanning

Advantages
- Radionuclide renography with captopril can detect renal artery stenoses in many patients.
- Radioactive iodine-labeled metaiodobenzylguanidine (MIBG) is effective in detecting pheochromocytomas.
- Does not require injection of iodinated contrast material.

Disadvantages
- Radionuclide renography does not provide an anatomic picture of the renal vasculature.
- MIBG is not widely available.

C. Recommended Imaging Approach

Many patients with hypertension are treated medically. If hypertension is refractory to medical treatment, if it develops in a young (<25–30-year-old) patient, if hypertension develops or increases rapidly, if a renal bruit is heard on auscultation, or if the patient has persistent hypokalemia, labile blood pressure, or other signs and symptoms suggestive of a secondary cause, additional workup is usually performed. If renovascular hypertension is suspected, arteriography remains the study of choice. MRI can be obtained in patients in whom there is a contraindication to iodinated contrast material. We do not recommend sonography as part of the routine workup of these patients.

If there is clinical concern for an adrenal or renal parenchymal etiology, abdominal CT should be obtained. Thin-section images can be obtained through the adrenal glands and/or kidneys. Intravenous contrast material administration is not required for imaging of the adrenal glands and, in fact, is not recommended in patients in whom a pheochromocytoma is a possible diagnosis (since intravenous contrast material can trigger norepinephrine release and a hypertensive crisis in occasional patients who are not pretreated with α-adrenergic blocking medication). Aldosteronomas are quite small and, as already stated, may not be detected even on thin-section CT studies; however, the remaining adrenal masses that produce hypertension are usually quite large at the time of presentation and are easily identified. Intravenous contrast material administration is recommended for imaging of the kidneys. Adrenal venous sampling can be performed in patients with biochemical evidence of aldosteronomas (decreased serum potassium and renin or increased urinary aldosterone levels) if the CT examination is unrevealing.

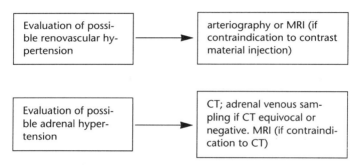

Imaging Algorithm

D. Differential Diagnostic Considerations

1. Essential hypertension: Most common etiology, accounting for >90% of cases.

2. Renal artery stenosis: Accounts for less than 5% of hypertension. Stenosis results in secretion of renin by the kidney (due to ischemia), which in turn eventually promotes the conversion of angiotensin I to angiotensin II, leading to aldosterone secretion.

   a. Atherosclerotic disease: Accounts for two-thirds of cases. Usually in older men. Stenoses are commonly near the renal artery ostia.

   b. Fibromuscular dysplasia: Most commonly occurs in young to middle-aged women. Most common type (medial fibroplasia) produces a typical beaded pattern on arteriography.

   c. Neurofibromatosis: Characteristic café-au-lait spots on skin. Hypertension results from renal artery dysplasia as well as a 5% incidence of pheochromocytoma.

3. Other vascular causes of hypertension

   a. Takayasu's aortitis: Usually seen in young females. Affects major branches of the aorta.

   b. Renal artery aneurysm: Associated with but possibly not responsible for hypertension in some patients.

   c. After renal transplantation: Etiology is often unclear.

4. Adrenal gland hyperfunction

   a. Aldosteronoma (usually due to adrenal adenoma): Excess levels of aldosterone result in abnormal retention of sodium and excretion of potassium and hydrogen ions, producing metabolic alkalosis and hypokalemia. Aldosteronomas are quite small and may be difficult to detect on imaging studies (CT and MRI). Patients have decreased plasma renin and increased urinary aldosterone levels.

   b. Adrenal hyperplasia (usually due to Cushing's disease): Affected patients usually have other cushingoid manifestations, including hirsutism, truncal obesity, abdominal striae, buffalo hump, acne, hyperglycemia (20%), and osteoporosis. Diagnosis is made with dexamethasone suppression test.

   c. Pheochromocytoma: Adrenal medullary tumors produce either episodic (40%) or sustained (60%) blood pressure elevation in the vast majority of patients. Classic associated symptoms include headache, sweating, and palpitations. While most of these neuroendocrine tumors originate in the adrenal glands, about 10% arise elsewhere along the sympathetic chain. Produces elevated urinary and serum catecholamine levels. Elevated urinary catecholamines, metanephrine, or vanillylmandelic acid levels are more sensitive and specific than elevated serum catecholamines.

   d. Adrenal carcinoma (when causing hypertension usually secretes glucocorticoids).

5. Renal parenchymal disorders

   a. Renal adenocarcinoma/Wilm's tumor: May produce hypertension by compressing the renal artery. Some tumors secrete renin. Arteriovenous shunting may also produce hypertension.

b. Juxtaglomerular tumors: Rare benign renin-secreting solid renal tumor seen in young patients.

c. Unilateral ureteral obstruction: Rarely activates the renin–angiotensin system.

d. Chronic pyelonephritis/reflux nephropathy: Rarely activates the renin–angiotensin system.

e. Renal cysts: Isolated cysts rarely produce hypertension by compressing the main renal artery or a branch vessel. However, adult polycystic kidney disease is typically associated with hypertension.

f. Ask-Upmark kidney: Hypoplasia of a segment of the kidney. Existence of this entity is somewhat controversial, as it may merely represent an area of scarring due to reflux nephropathy.

6. Chronic subcapsular hematoma (Page kidney): Due to compression of parenchyma by a chronic fibrotic reaction.

7. Other
   a. Neurologic causes

ACUTE RENAL FAILURE

A. Clinical Comment

Acute renal failure (ARF) is a rapid decline in glomerular filtration rate over hours to weeks. Specific etiologies are innumerable. By grouping etiologies into three main categories and using the information from history, physical exam, and laboratory data, a likely etiology can often be determined. When this fails to disclose a likely etiology of the ARF, radiologic evaluation, which has a very limited role in this disorder, may be of utility.

B. Imaging Modalities

1. Plain Films

Advantages.
- Low cost.

- May detect large vesical or renal calculi.
- May detect renal osteodystrophy—would suggest chronic renal failure.

Disadvantages
- Almost never will detect etiology of ARF.

2. Sonography

Advantages
- Inexpensive.
- No ionizing radiation or contrast.
- Can detect upper tract obstruction.
- Small kidneys suggest chronic renal failure.
- Detects distended bladder if cannot pass Foley catheter.
- Can detect renal vein thrombosis.
- Doppler studies may assist in distinguishing among type of medical renal disease.

Disadvantages
- Upper tract obstruction is rare cause of ARF, particularly without reason to suspect it, so will rarely reveal etiology.

3. Excretory Urography

Advantages
- Can demonstrate obstruction.

Disadvantages
- Intravenous contrast may worsen renal function.
- Unlikely to get good study with standard dose of contrast.
- Unlikely to reveal etiology of ARF.

4. CT

Advantages
- May reveal renal vein thrombosis or renal artery occlusion.
- Will see evidence and possibly etiology of postrenal azotemia.
- Small kidneys would suggest a chronic process.

Disadvantages

- Will not reveal etiology in vast majority of cases, unless postrenal azotemia.
- Ionizing radiation.
- While intravenous contrast is required for optimal study, its use is relatively contraindicated due to patient's azotemia.
- Expensive.

5. MRI

Advantages

- No ionizing radiation or iodinated contrast material.
- MR urography may demonstrate evidence and possibly etiology of postrenal azotemia.
- May see renal vein thrombosis or renal artery occlusion.

Disadvantages

- Will not reveal etiology in vast majority of cases. MR urography not routinely performed. Most radiologists have no experience with this latter technique.

6. Angiography

Advantages

- Can demonstrate renal vein thrombosis or renal artery occlusion.

Disadvantages

- Invasive and expensive.
- Uses ionizing radiation and iodinated contrast material.
- Will not reveal etiology in vast majority of cases.

7. Retrograde Pyelography/Urethrography

Advantages

- Can identify etiology in postrenal azotemia.

Disadvantages

- Will not reveal etiology in vast majority of cases.
- Invasive and expensive.
- Rarely offers additional information. If sonography shows no di-

latation, retrograde pyelography is unlikely to be positive. If sonography shows dilatation, retrograde pyelography is unlikely to be more informative.

C. Recommended Imaging Approach

The probable etiology of ARF can often be elicited through medication history, (e.g., current use of gentamycin) past medical history (e.g., systemic lupus erythematosis), signs and symptoms (e.g., fever or orthostatic hypotension), laboratory data (e.g., elevated BUN or creatinine level), and microscopic urinalysis (e.g., presence of red blood cell casts). Catheterization of the bladder can assess distal postrenal azotemia.

If etiology of ARF is still not apparent, there are a few uncommon eti-

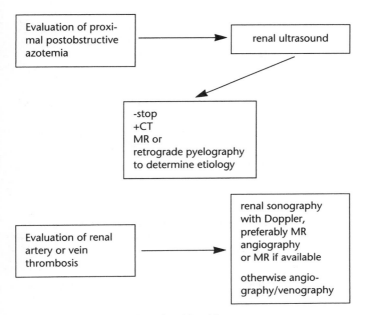

Imaging Algorithm

ologies of ARF for which radiologic evaluation may be of benefit, although the diagnostic yield is low without some reason to suspect these etiologies. One is proximal postrenal azotemia. Ultrasound is a good first test to look for pelvocaliectasis because ultrasound is inexpensive, avoids contrast and ionizing radiation, and is sensitive to this finding. It is important to remember that this is an uncommon cause of ARF, as the process must be bilateral in a patient with two functioning kidneys. If pelvocaliectasis is seen, further delineation of its cause with CT, retrograde pyelography, or MR urography should be considered.

The second etiology of ARF for which radiologic evaluation is helpful is renal vein thrombosis or renal arterial occlusion: Angiography/venography is the gold standard to diagnose these abnormalities, but sonography with gray-scale and duplex or color-flow Doppler or MR venography can detect renal vein thrombosis. In many patients MR angiography may detect renal artery stenoses or occlusions. MR is preferred over CT since the former can be performed without administering iodinated contrast material.

D. Differential Diagnostic Considerations

1. Prerenal azotemia—most common
   a. Categories
      - Volume depletion: Dehydration, hemorrhage, diuretics, third spacing fluid.
      - Decreased cardiac output: Left ventricular dysfunction, valvular disease, pericardial tamponade.
      - Vasodilatation: Sepsis.
   b. Clues
      - Restoration of renal perfusion leads to prompt resolution of ARF.
      - Fractional excretion of sodium <1%, urine sodium <20 mg/L, BUN/creatinine ratio >20/1, orthostatic hypotension.
2. Intrarenal azotemia—common
   a. Categories
      - Acute tubular necrosis: Ischemia, drugs (aminoglycosides, amphotericin), rhabdomyolysis, contrast agents, crystals.
        Most common form of acute renal failure.

"Muddy brown" casts on microscopic urinalysis in approximately 75% cases.

- Acute interstitial nephritis: Nonsteroidal antiinflammatory agents, β-lactam antibiotics, sulfonamides, infection.

    Fever, rash, peripheral eosinophilia.

    On microscopic urinalysis, white blood cells (WBC), WBC casts, eosinophils on Hansel stain.

- Acute glomerulonephritis

    On microscopic urinalysis, red blood cells (RBC) and RBC casts.

- Vascular: Renal vein thrombosis, severe renal artery stenoses, or renal artery occlusion.

3. Postrenal azotemia—uncommon
    a. Distal: Urethral stricture, neurogenic bladder, prostatic hyperplasia, blood clot, or calculus at bladder neck.
        - Catheterize bladder: Very high urine volume.
    b. Proximal: Renal calculi, blood clots, sloughed papillae, retroperitoneal fibrosis.
        - Must involve both ureters if have two functioning kidneys.

References

Dunnick NR, McCallum RW, Sandler CM (1991). Textbook of Uroradiology. Baltimore: Williams & Wilkins.

Platt JF, Ellis JH, Rubin JM (1991). Examination of native kidneys with duplex Doppler ultrasound. Semin US CT MR 12:308–318.

Stuck KS, White GM, Granke DS et al (1987). Urinary obstruction in azotemic patients: Detection by sonography. AJR 149:1191–1193.

ACUTE RENAL FAILURE AFTER TRANSPLANTATION

A. Clinical Comment

ARF after renal transplantation is generally heralded by an increased serum creatinine level and diminished urinary output. Although determining the etiology can be difficult clinically, as the signs and symptoms are generally not specific, it is important to determine the underlying process so that appropriate treatment can be started expeditiously. Radiologic evaluation plays a major role in this workup.

B. Imaging Modalities

1. Plain Radiography

Advantages
- Low cost.
- May see a calculus.

Disadvantages
- Extremely unlikely to reveal cause.

2. Sonography

Advantages
- Inexpensive.
- Sensitive for obstruction.
- Can see fluid collections adjacent to transplantation that may be compressing ureter or renal transplant vessels.
- Use of duplex or color-flow Doppler can assess renal artery for stenosis or thrombosis or renal vein for thrombosis.
- Identifies edema, hypoechoic renal pyramids, and/or loss of distinction between renal sinus and renal parenchyma in the transplanted kidneys of occasional patients who are rejecting their transplants.
- Used to guide renal transplant biopsy, transplant nephrostomy, or percutaneous aspiration and/or drainage of peritransplant fluid collections.

Disadvantages
- Unable to distinguish among the various causes of renal parenchymal dysfunction (rejection, acute tubular necrosis, cyclosporine toxicity).
- Cannot distinguish among various peritransplant fluid collections.

3. Nuclear Medicine (^{99m}Tc MAG3) Imaging

Advantages

- Can identify absence of perfusion in patients with hyperacute rejection, renal artery thrombosis, and renal vein thrombosis.
- Detects normal perfusion and diminished function in patients with acute tubular necrosis, cyclosporine toxicity, and obstruction.
- Decreased perfusion and function is characteristic of rejection.

Disadvantages

- Cannot distinguish among hyperacute rejection, renal artery thrombosis, and renal vein thrombosis.
- Cannot distinguish among acute tubular necrosis, cyclosporine toxicity, and obstruction.
- Is neither highly sensitive nor specific for detecting transplant rejection.

4. CT

Advantages

- Can detect transplant collecting system dilatation.
- Can detect peritransplant fluid collections.
- Can be used to guide transplant biopsy, percutaneous nephrostomy, or percutaneous drainage of peritransplant fluid collections.

Disadvantages

- Expensive.
- Utilizes ionizing radiation.
- Cannot evaluate patency of renal artery or vein (since intravenous material would not be administered in the setting of azotemia).
- Offers essentially no advantage over sonography, and, in fact, is more limited than sonography.

5. Angiography

Advantages

- Gold standard study for detection of renal artery stenosis or thrombosis and renal vein thrombosis.
- Therapeutic angioplasty may be performed in patients in whom renal artery stenoses are detected.

Disadvantages
- Invasive.
- Injected radiographic contrast material may contribute to deteriorating renal function.
- Cannot distinguish among renal parenchymal causes of acute dysfunction.
- Cannot evaluate peritransplant region for fluid collections.
- Involves use of ionizing radiation.

6. MRI

Advantages
- Does not require use of iodinated contrast material or ionizing radiation.
- Can assess transplant for obstruction (especially if MR urography is performed).
- Can evaluated renal transplant vessels for stenoses or thromboses.
- Can evaluate peritransplant region for fluid collections.

Disadvantages
- Expensive.
- Cannot distinguish among renal parenchymal causes of acute transplant dysfunction. Offers essentially no advantage over sonography.

C. Recommended Imaging Approach

An ultrasound examination is a good initial study to assess renal transplant patients with elevated serum creatinine levels and/or diminished urine output. It can identify collecting system dilation, suggesting obstruction, or peritransplant fluid collections. Both types of abnormalities can be promptly treated. Obstruction can be treated with percutaneous nephrostomy. Occasionally, the obstructed segment of ureter (usually at the ureterovesical anastomosis) can be successfully dilated percutaneously. Peritransplant fluid collections can be percutaneously aspirated. Peritransplant lymphoceles can often be successfully treated by percutaneous drainage (although the drainage catheters may have to be left in place for long periods of time). While peritransplant urinomas can also be success-fully drained, if they have resulted from breakdown at the ureterovesical anastomosis (usually due to ischemic necrosis), surgery will likely be re-quired.

Duplex and color-flow Doppler ultrasound can also assess renal trans-plant arterial and venous blood flow. Since the renal vessels are quite su-perficial (in the iliac fossa) they are usually much more easily and accu-rately imaged than are native renal vessels. Angiography and percutaneous angioplasty can then be performed in patients in whom renal artery stenoses are identified.

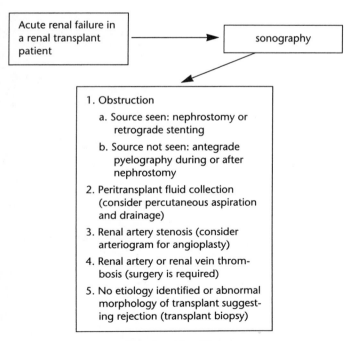

Imaging Algorithm

If the ultrasound evaluation is unrewarding, the patient most likely will need a renal transplant biopsy to differentiate among the other causes of ARF.

Some use nuclear scintigraphy as the initial test in evaluating patients with malfunctioning renal transplants. Although there are characteristic scintigraphic findings for many of the causes of transplant failure, none are entirely specific. Often, a combination of imaging studies and biopsy are required to determine the etiology of ARF in the transplant patient.

D. Differential Diagnostic Considerations

1. Rejection of transplanted kidney
   a. Hyperacute rejection: Antibody-mediated process that is uncommon with current screening of donor and recipient compatibility. Irreversible process that is usually evident at the time of the initial surgery and is treated with nephrectomy.
   b. Accelerated acute rejection: Antibody-mediated process occurring in first several days after transplantation surgery. The transplanted kidney may be salvageable with aggressive immunosuppression.
   c. Acute rejection: Cell-mediated process occurring within the first 3 months of surgery. The kidney can often be salvaged with immunosuppression.
   d. Signs and symptoms of rejection: Fever, oliguria, graft tenderness, graft swelling.
2. Acute tubular necrosis
   a. Related to period of ischemia prior to revascularization of the transplanted kidney. Therefore, common with cadaver transplants and rare with living donor transplants.
   b. Manifests within the first 48 hours after transplantation and usually resolves within 1 to 3 weeks.
3. Cyclosporine toxicity: Acute form is dose related (serum levels of cyclosporine are usually elevated). Manifestations are reversible if dose of cyclosporine is decreased.
4. Renal artery thrombosis: Caused by intimal flap at anastomotic

site, kinked renal artery, hyperacute rejection, extrinsic compression of renal artery (by hematoma, for example).
5. Renal artery stenosis: Related to problem at the anastomotic site.
6. Renal vein thrombosis
   a. May be related to problem at anastomosis or to external compression (by hematoma, urinoma, or lymphocele).
   b. Serious problem in transplanted kidneys (because there is no collateral circulation).
7. Ureteral obstruction: Possibly related to problem at ureterovesical anastomosis, postoperative edema, blood clot, sloughed papillae, calculi, external compression (by hematoma, urinoma, or lymphocele).

URINARY TRACT INFECTION

A. Clinical Comment

Most patients who present with urinary tract infections have an acute cystitis that responds to a brief course of antibiotics. Recurrent episodes of cystitis in girls or women or even one episode of cystitis in boys may lead to additional evaluation, since predisposing conditions may be present, including vesicoureteral reflux, urolithiasis, congenital urinary tract abnormalities, neurogenic bladder, or ureteral obstruction.

B. Imaging Modalities

1. Abdominal Radiograph

Advantages
- Easy to obtain and inexpensive.
- Identifies 80%–90% of all urinary tract calculi.
- Can detect air in the bladder wall or around the kidneys.

Disadvantages
- Uses ionizing radiation.
- Cannot evaluate kidneys or ureters.

2. Voiding Cystourethrography

Advantages
- Assesses bladder capacity.
- Detects and grades severity of vesicoureteral reflux.
- Can identify some urethral diverticula.
- Assesses degree of bladder emptying.

Disadvantages
- Cannot specifically diagnose cystitis.
- Fails to detect some urethral diverticula.
- Does not evaluate kidneys and ureters (unless reflux is present).
- Uses ionizing radiation.
- Should not be performed during acute phase of infection, since active infection can be spread in a retrograde fashion into the upper genitourinary tract.

3. Radionuclide Cystography

Advantages
- Assesses bladder capacity.
- Excellent sensitivity for detecting vesicoureteral reflux.
- Assesses degree of bladder emptying.

Disadvantages
- Does not provide an anatomic image of the bladder.
- Should not be performed during acute phase of infection.

4. Excretory Urography

Advantages
- Identifies 80%–90% of urinary tract calculi.
- Identifies dilation and obstruction of renal collecting systems.
- Can determine degree of renal parenchymal loss.
- Visualizes congenital or acquired abnormalities predisposing the patient to infection, including pelvic kidney, horseshoe kidney, medullary sponge kidney, calyceal diverticula, primary or congenital megaureter.

Disadvantages
- Cannot determine whether vesicoureteral reflux is present.
- Does not assess perirenal region (for extension of inflammatory processes).
- Limited evaluation of bladder and urethra.
- Utilizes iodinated contrast material and ionizing radiation.

5. Sonography

Advantages
- Images bladder (including bladder wall thickness).
- Can evaluate perineum. Can identify urethral diverticula.
- Visualizes kidneys and proximal renal collecting systems. Can determine whether there is any renal parenchymal loss or collecting system dilation.
- Detects renal or perirenal fluid collections.
- Can sometimes distinguish pyonephrosis from sterile dilated renal collecting system due to the presence of echoes in infected urine.
- By use of resistive indices can determine whether collecting system dilatation is due to obstruction.
- Identifies most renal calculi.
- Can visualize many congenital abnormalities, including an ectopically located or horseshoe kidney.
- Can identify air in bladder wall or in renal collecting system.

Disadvantages
- May miss small renal or any ureteral calculi.
- Cannot differentiate urethral diverticula from dilated periurethral glands that do not communicate openly with the urethra.
- Cannot determine whether vesicoureteral reflux is present.

6. CT

Advantages
- Identifies many congenital renal anomalies.
- Permits assessment of the entire abdominal cavity, including the

kidneys and retroperitoneum, allowing for assessment of the extent of a renal and/or perirenal inflammatory process.

- May be used to direct percutaneous aspiration or drainage of infected renal or perirenal fluid collections.
- All genitourinary calculi are of high attenuation on CT and are therefore detectable if appropriate technique is used.

Disadvantages

- Offers limited evaluation of the ureters, bladder, and urethra.
- Cannot determine whether vesicoureteral reflux is present.

C. Recommended Imaging Approach

In general, if imaging work up of a patient with recurrent urinary tract infections is required, a plain abdominal radiograph can be obtained in order to identify any renal, ureteral, or bladder calculi or any abnormal gas collections (especially in patients with diabetes mellitus). Voiding cystourethrography is performed as the initial examination in children and is also helpful in women. Radionuclide cystography can be performed as an alternative study. If no reflux is identified during voiding cystourethrogra-

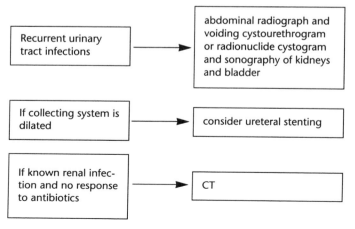

Imaging Algorithm

phy, additional imaging with either excretory urography or sonography or both is performed. If the renal collecting system is dilated, pyonephrosis must be suspected (particularly if the urine in the dilated collecting system has internal echoes), and ureteral stenting (either in a retrograde fashion via cystoscopy or in an antegrade fashion via nephrostomy) should be considered. CT should be reserved for patients in whom relatively extensive renal and perirenal infection is suspected in order to depict the complete extent of the inflammatory process and to direct subsequent therapy, which may include percutaneous procedures.

Imaging is not routinely required for evaluation of patients with pyuria and flank pain, since a diagnosis of acute pyelonephritis is made clinically. Imaging with sonography and/or CT should only be obtained in a patient with acute pyelonephritis if there has been no response to an appropriate course of antibiotics.

D. Differential Diagnostic Considerations

1. Acute bacterial cystitis: Most common cause of urinary tract infection. Usually responds to antibiotic treatment.
2. Emphysematous cystitis: Most commonly caused by *E. coli*. Often seen in diabetics. Usually responds to aggressive antibiotic treatment.
3. Urethral diverticula: Can serve as a nidus for recurring infections in women. Can also produce dysuria.
4. Acute pyelonephritis: Usually results from retrograde spread of infection from the bladder. A clinical diagnosis. Patients most often have severe flank pain.
5. Renal abscess: Can develop as a complication of acute pyelonephritis. Should be suspected if a patient with pyelonephritis fails to respond to antibiotics.
6. Pyonephrosis: Results from infection of an obstructed collecting system. Treatment consists of emergent percutaneous nephrostomy or ureteral stenting.
7. Xanthogranulomatous pyelonephritis: Most often occurs in a renal collecting system obstructed by a large calculus. Symptoms are usually of long duration, in up to half of patients lasting for more than 6 months.

8. Emphysematous pyelonephritis: Often occurs in diabetics. Has a very high mortality when gas is produced in the renal parenchyma and/or retroperitoneum.

9. Genitourinary tract tuberculosis: Results from hematogenous spread of disease from the lungs in most instances. Spreads antegrade from kidneys to ureters and then bladder. Can be suspected in patients with pyuria if routine cultures do not identify an offending organism.

10. Genitourinary tract fungal infections: Usually occur as opportunistic infections in patients with chronically indwelling catheters (into the bladder or proximal renal collecting systems) or patients who are immunocompromised. *Candida albicans* is the most frequent offending organism.

11. Malacoplakia: Results from an abnormal granulomatous response to infection (due to a lysosomal enzyme defect). Most common in the bladder.

12. Prostatis/seminal vesiculitis: Usually made as a clinical diagnosis.

Reference

Dunnick NR, McCallum RW, Sandler CM (1991). Textbook of Uroradiology. Baltimore: Williams & Wilkins.

DECREASED URINARY STREAM/DIFFICULTY VOIDING

A. Clinical Comment

This problem is much more common in males. Evaluation of patients with decreased urinary stream or difficulty voiding usually involves assessment of bladder and urethral function.

B. Imaging Modalities

1. Retrograde Urethrography

Advantages

- Easily and rapidly performed.
- Determines whether an anterior urethral stricture is present.

- Identifies stricture location, severity, and length.
- Can identify complications of strictures or coexisting abnormalities.

  Fistulae.

  Diverticula: Can represent abscess that has excavated into urethra.

  Urethral calculi: Most urethral stones have migrated from upper tract.

  Carcinoma: Usually suggested only by worsening of known stricture.

Disadvantages

- Limited evaluation of posterior (prostatic and membranous) urethra. Intact urogenital diaphragm usually prevents much retrograde visualization of this portion of the urethra.
- Utilizes ionizing radiation.
- Uncomfortable procedure for patient.

2. Voiding Cystourethrography

Advantages

- Permits assessment of bladder (including identification of bladder capacity, which may be significantly increased).
- Also evaluates both anterior and posterior urethra.
- Can visualize some markedly enlarged prostate glands.

Disadvantages

- Usually not required in assessment of patients with urethral strictures, since the vast majority of strictures not related to pelvic trauma occur in the anterior urethra.
- Requires insertion of Foley catheter into bladder (may not be possible in patients with tight urethral strictures).
- Not indicated in patients with suspected prostatic enlargement. Many patients with normal cystograms can have significant outlet obstruction due to BPH.
- Utilizes ionizing radiation.

3. Excretory Urography

Advantages

- Can visualize some markedly enlarged prostate glands.
- Large post-void residuals may indicate inability to empty the bladder completely.
- Occasionally identifies coincidental upper urinary tract disease.

Disadvantages

- Inaccurate assessment of prostate gland. Many patients with normal urograms can have significant bladder outlet obstruction due to BPH.
- Large post-void residuals are a nonspecific finding. May indicate an unwillingness rather than an inability to void.
- Does not evaluate any portion of the urethra.
- Utilizes intravenous injections of iodinated contrast media and ionizing radiation.

4. Sonography

Advantages

- Has been used to image urethra and perineum using a transperineal or endourethral approach.
- Transrectal sonography can accurately determine prostate volume and can also assess the prostate gland for neoplasms.
- Can assess bladder (capacity, bladder wall thickness, bladder lumen, and post-void residual).

Disadvantages

- Evaluation of urethra and perineum remains largely investigational and is not performed at many medical centers.
- Transrectal determination of prostatic volume offers little advantage over digital rectal exam for assessing prostate gland size (unless extremely accurate calculations are required to evaluate patient response to medical therapy).

4. MRI

Advantages

- When performed using a transrectal coil, identifies many prostate cancers.

- Most accurate imaging modality for local staging of prostate cancer.

Disadvantages
- Despite initial enthusiasm, accuracy in detecting and staging prostate cancers has been disappointing. Not routinely used for this purpose by many urologists.
- Offers no advantage to sonography in patients with BPH.
- No utility for evaluation of the urethra.

C. Recommended Imaging Approach

Patients presenting with decreased urinary stream or difficulty voiding fall into two main groups. The most common etiology (usually seen in males over the age of 50) is BPH. Enlarged prostates are easily detected by digital rectal examination. In general, no imaging is required in patients with BPH, unless careful follow-up of prostate size is required for proto-

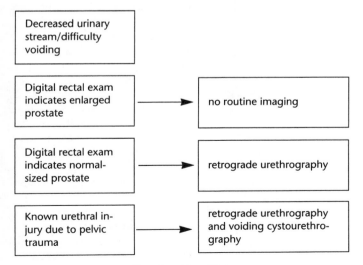

Imaging Algorithm

cols involving medical treatment (in which case sonography can be used to measure volume).

Urethral strictures are often suggested by patient history (i.e., of sexually transmitted disease, instrumentation, trauma, etc.). In addition, urethral strictures are much more common causes of decreased urinary stream than BPH in younger males (<40). Imaging evaluation of suspected urethral strictures is best performed with retrograde urethrography. Voiding cystourethrography is reserved for patients with posterior urethral injuries, usually in conjunction with retrograde urethrograms (in order to determine the length of an occlusion in patients after urethral injuries).

Difficulty voiding in women is usually due to bladder dysfunction and is usually evaluated by urologists with urodynamic studies. Voiding cystourethrography may occasionally be obtained as an adjunctive study.

D. Differential Diagnostic Considerations

1. Benign prostatic hyperplasia (BPH): Affects 80% of all men. Approximately 10% require treatment, most commonly with transurethral resection.

2. Prostate carcinoma: Difficulty urinating is a late manifestation of this disease, since the vast majority of prostate cancers affect the outer portion (peripheral zone) of the prostate, a region removed from the urethra. When present in patients with prostate cancer, it is usually secondary to superimposed BPH.

3. Urethral stricture: In the United States, approximately 50% are traumatic and 50% are inflammatory. The vast majority of urethral strictures not due to pelvic trauma are in the anterior (cavernous or bulbar) urethra. Specific etiologies are as follows:

    a. Inflammatory
       - Gonorrheal: Often involves a long segment of bulbocavernous urethra.
       - Nonspecific urethritis: Presumed diagnosis when etiology of an inflammatory stricture cannot be determined.
       - Tuberculosis: Usually develops as a descending infection from the upper urinary tract. Typically also produces multiple fistulae ("watering can" perineum).

- Schistosomiasis: Usually develops secondary to fistulae. Strictures most commonly occur in the bulbar urethra.
- Condyloma acuminata: Viral infection that may require multiple treatments. If suspected, no retrograde procedures should be performed: Infection can spread proximally as a result of retrograde urethrography or even Foley catheterization.

b. Traumatic
- Blunt pelvic trauma: Usually associated with pelvic fractures. Affects prostatic and sometimes membranous urethra (see Lower Genitourinary Tract Trauma).
- Instrumentation: May result from traumatic Foley catheterization (in which case the urethra is often injured at the penoscrotal junction. Other Foley-related urethral strictures are believed to be due either to pressure necrosis by the catheter or to a reaction to material in the catheter itself. May also result from injuries during cystoscopy, most often caused by the resectoscope used for transurethral resections. Resectoscope injuries are most common at the bulbomembranous junction.
- Surgery: Can occur after abdominal–perineal resection.
- Straddle injury: See Lower Genitourinary Tract Trauma.

c. Neoplastic: Account for <5% of urethral strictures.
- Malignancies: 80% are squamous cell carcinomas. Many patients have a history of urethral stricture. Can be suspected in a patient with a urethral stricture if symptoms suddenly worsen.
- Benign: Rare. Include transitional cell papilloma, fibrous polyp.

d. Congenital: Rare.

4. Medications: Include some antipsychotics.
5. Neurogenic bladder: See Urinary Incontinence.

Reference

Dunnick NR, McCallum RW, Sandler CM (1991). Textbook of Uroradiology. Baltimore: Williams & Wilkins.

URINARY INCONTINENCE

A. Clinical Comment

Patients with urinary incontinence may complain of inability to control urine flow at all times (complete loss of function), of persistent dribbling, or merely of leakage of urine during stress. There are two urinary sphincters, the internal sphincter at the bladder base and the external sphincter at the urogenital diaphragm. Involuntary muscles are located at both sphincters; however, voluntary muscles are present only in the external sphincter. Disruption of both of these sphincters inevitably leads to incontinence; however, continence is maintained if only one of these sphincters is destroyed.

B. Imaging Modalities

1. Voiding Cystourethrography

Advantages

- Confirms the presence of incontinence.
- Identifies phase during which incontinence occurs (e.g., during filling, straining, coughing).
- Can be used to classify type of incontinence.
- Assesses size, contour, capacity, and contractility of bladder.
- Can identify some urethral diverticula.

Disadvantages

- Cannot identify, classify, and quantitate abnormalities in bladder function.
- Utilizes ionizing radiation.

2. Sonography

Advantages

- Assesses size, contour, capacity, and contractility of bladder.
- Can determine bladder wall thickness.
- Can evaluate kidneys for proximal collecting system dilation or parenchymal loss.

- Can identify all urethral diverticula (when transducer is placed directly on the perineum).

Disadvantages
- Cannot directly visualize urine loss. Does not identify phase during which incontinence occurs.
- Cannot identify, classify, and quantitate abnormalities in bladder function.
- Does not distinguish between dilated periurethral glands and urethral diverticula.

C. Recommended Imaging Approach

Evaluation of the incontinent patient should begin with a careful medical history. The patient should be questioned about any neurologic conditions and prior trauma. A complete list should be obtained of medications the patient is taking. Female patients should be questioned about any potential relationship between symptoms and childbearing. The patient should also be questioned about the type of incontinence that is present. Subsequent workup then usually includes urodynamic studies (usually performed by urologists) and/or voiding cystourethrography. No other imaging is performed. Treatment of incontinence depends on the etiology. Medications causing incontinence can be discontinued. Cystoceles can be surgically repaired. In some patients intermittent straight catheterizations of the bladder are helpful. In others, a chronically indwelling catheter or a condom catheter may be used. Occasionally, artificial urethral sphincters can be inserted.

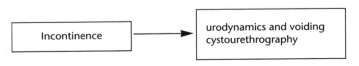

Imaging Algorithm

D. Differential Diagnostic Considerations

1. In females
   a. Pelvic relaxation: Typically occurs after childbearing. Associated with a cystocele. Usual symptoms are of stress incontinence only.
   b. Urethral diverticulum: Often with symptoms of dysuria and frequency. May have history of recurrent urinary tract infections.
   c. Urethritis/cystitis: Also often associated with dysuria and frequency.
2. In females and males
   a. Medications: Including diuretics and antipsychotics
   b. Neurogenic bladder: May be post-traumatic or due to neurologic diseases such as multiple sclerosis. Basic types of neurogenic bladders are summarized below (many neurogenic bladders are complex in terms of mechanism).
      - Classic upper motor neuron injury: Intact urinary reflex. Results in overflow incontinence.
      - Classic lower motor neuron injury: Interrupted urinary reflex arc. Bladder becomes atonic.
      - Sensory loss: Inability to determine when bladder is full.
      - Detrusor-sphincter dyssynergia: Lack of coordination between contraction of bladder muscle and relaxation of urethral sphincters.
3. In males
   a. Following prostatectomy: Prostatectomy removes internal sphincter. Incontinence develops when the nerve supply to the external sphincter is damaged or in patients who have previously had injuries to their external sphincters (due to blunt pelvic trauma).
   b. Following repair of urethral stricture: 30% incidence.

Reference

Dunnick, NR, McCallum RW, Sandler CM (1991). Textbook of Uroradiology. Baltimore: Williams & Wilkins.

RENAL TRAUMA

A. Clinical Comment

Trauma may be blunt or penetrating. Minor injuries from blunt traumas, such as renal contusions, are most common, accounting for 85% of renal injuries. Moderately severe injuries, encountered in 10% of patients, include renal lacerations, which are tears in the renal parenchyma extending through the renal capsule, fractures that are lacerations extending completely through the kidney, and segmental injuries to renal vessels. Major injuries are unusual, occurring in 5% of patients. These include multiple renal lacerations, renal pedicle injuries (avulsion or intimal tears leading to renal artery thrombosis), and ureteral avulsions (usually occurring at the ureteropelvic junction). Only major injuries usually require surgery. It is generally accepted that revascularization of a devitalized kidney (due to pedicle injury) must be performed within 6–12 hours if any residual renal function is to be preserved. Injuries from penetrating trauma, occurring after stab or gunshot wounds or after iatrogenic injury, can be similar to those seen after blunt trauma; however, patients may also develop pseudoaneurysms and arteriovenous fistulae.

B. Imaging Modalities

1. Plain Radiograph of the Abdomen

Advantages
- Rapidly obtained study that permits assessment of lumbar spine and pelvic bones.

Disadvantages
- Does not permit evaluation of the genitourinary tract.

2. Excretory Urography

Advantages
- Easily demonstrates findings in patients with major injuries. Absence of perfusion/visualization of a kidney suggests renal pedicle injury, while extravasation of contrast material from the collecting system indicates significant collecting system disruption.

- Rapidly obtained. Can even be done using portable equipment in the emergency room.

Disadvantages

- Nonvisualization of a functioning kidney is a nonspecific sign. Nontraumatic causes such as obstruction, ectopically located kidney, agenesis, renal artery stenosis, renal vein thrombosis, and multicystic dysplastic kidney are more often responsible. For this reason, a cross-sectional imaging study is required after a urogram fails to demonstrate a functioning kidney in order to confirm its presence and lack of perfusion.
- Portable studies are often of limited quality.

3. Sonography

Advantages

- Alterations in blood flow may be detected in patients with pseudoaneurysms or arteriovenous fistulae after penetrating trauma. The pseudoaneurysms and fistulae themselves are often detected.

Disadvantages

- Offers limited evaluation of the kidneys and renal collecting system. Essentially has no role in evaluating patients with suspected blunt renal trauma.

4. CT

Advantages

- Single most helpful examination. Clearly delineates kidneys. Parenchymal and pedicle injuries are easily identified. Allows for assessment of other abdominal organs.

Disadvantages

- Extravasation from the renal collecting system can be missed if patients are scanned dynamically only prior to excretion of contrast material into the renal collecting system. Delayed scans must be obtained during renal excretion in any patient in whom there is a renal injury or in whom perinephric or subcapsular fluid is noted.

- Injuries resulting from penetrating trauma are not always easily identified. For example, pseudoaneurysms may be small and are easily missed.
- Requires iodinated contrast material and ionizing radiation.

5. Arteriography

Advantages
- Permits identification of the site of a disrupted (avulsed or thrombosed) renal pedicle.
- Can easily identify arteriovenous fistulae or pseudoaneurysms developing as a result of penetrating trauma.
- Detected pseudoaneurysms and arteriovenous fistulae may be treated (embolized) at the time the diagnostic study is performed.

Disadvantages
- Does not allow for optimal evaluation of renal parenchyma or of other abdominal organs.

C. Recommended Imaging Approach

Recent studies have indicated that imaging of any kind need not be performed in a hemodynamically stable patient who has only microscopic hematuria after blunt abdominal trauma. While some of these patients have renal or parenchymal collecting system injuries, it is extremely unlikely that any will require surgery. Instead, imaging of patients with blunt trauma should be performed if there is gross hematuria or if patients with microscopic hematuria are hemodynamically unstable. Imaging may be required for any patient (regardless of the type of hematuria that is present) after penetrating trauma, depending on wound location.

When imaging is performed, CT scanning provides the most comprehensive evaluation of the abdomen and pelvis and is preferred, particularly if there is concern for other organ injury. Excretory urography should be reserved for patients in whom there is suspicion of isolated renal or renal collecting system trauma. Occasionally, limited, portable excretory urograms are obtained in unstable patients immediately before they are brought to the operating room. In these instances, the urograms serve to identify or exclude major renal injuries. Arteriography is most appropriate for evaluating selected patients after penetrating renal trauma either in conjunction with or instead of a CT examination or perhaps for selected cases of renal pedicle injury. Sonography is probably best reserved for patients who experience iatrogenic renal trauma (such as renal biopsy).

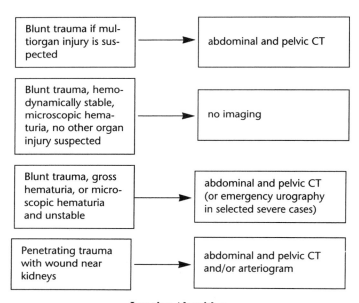

Blunt trauma if multiorgan injury is suspected	→ abdominal and pelvic CT
Blunt trauma, hemodynamically stable, microscopic hematuria, no other organ injury suspected	→ no imaging
Blunt trauma, gross hematuria, or microscopic hematuria and unstable	→ abdominal and pelvic CT (or emergency urography in selected severe cases)
Penetrating trauma with wound near kidneys	→ abdominal and pelvic CT and/or arteriogram

Imaging Algorithm

D. Differential Diagnostic Considerations

1. Blunt trauma
    a. Subcapsular hematoma
    b. Perinephric hematoma
    c. Renal contusion
    d. Renal laceration
    e. Renal fracture

    f. Partial disruption of the renal collecting system

    g. Complete ureteral avulsion

2. Penetrating trauma

    a. Traumatic Foley catheterization

    b. Subcapsular hematoma

    c. Perinephric hematoma

    d. Renal contusion

    e. Renal laceration

    f. Pseudoaneurysm

    g. Arteriovenous fistula

Reference

Mee SL, McAninch JW, Robinson AL et al (1989). Radiographic assessment of renal trauma: A 10-year prospective study of patient selection. J Urol 141:1095–1098.

LOWER GENITOURINARY TRACT TRAUMA

A. Clinical Comment

Lower genitourinary tract trauma must be suspected when there is blunt trauma to the pelvis, usually after a motor vehicle accident. It can also result from penetrating (stab or gunshot) wounds or be iatrogenic (due to a traumatic Foley catheterization).

B. Imaging Modalities

1. Retrograde Urethrography

Advantages

- Easily and rapidly performed.
- Allows for recognition of urethral injuries after blunt or penetrating trauma.
- Identifies urethral injuries in patients with cavernosal tears (penile fractures).
- Must precede Foley catheter insertion in patients with suspected

urethral injury whenever possible (since Grade I injuries can be converted to Grade II or III injuries).

Disadvantages
- Often cannot be performed because patients may arrive in the emergency room with Foley catheters already in place. Pericatheter urethrograms are occasionally helpful for visualization of the anterior urethra. Many pericatheter urethrograms are not successful, however.
- Allows for assessment of only the urethra.

2. Cystography

Advantages
- Easily and rapidly performed.
- Allows for detection of most (over 85% of) bladder injuries.

Disadvantages
- Small tears in the bladder wall, as can sometimes be seen in patients with gunshot wounds, are occasionally not identified.
- Does not assess the integrity of other abdominal and pelvic organs.

3. Excretory Urography

Advantages
- Identifies catastrophic injuries of the upper urinary tract (renal pedicle injuries) that may require emergency surgery.

Disadvantages
- Many bladder injuries are missed, because contrast material in the bladder is not directly instilled under pressure. For this reason, urography should not be performed instead of cystography in any patient in whom a bladder injury is suspected.
- Permits assessment of only the urinary tract. Does not visualize other abdominal organs for injury
- Utilizes ionizing radiation and iodinated radiographic contrast material.

4. CT

Advantages

- Permits a survey of all abdominal and pelvic organs.
- Can identify extraperitoneal or intraperitoneal fluid in the pelvis.
- Bladder extravasation is easy to recognize once the bladder has been filled with contrast material.

Disadvantages

- Sensitivity for bladder tears is unknown. Bladder injuries conceivably could be missed, because contrast material in the bladder is not directly instilled under pressure. Conventional cystography or CT cystography (whereby dilute contrast material is instilled through a Foley catheter, which is then clamped immediately prior to the CT) should be performed if bladder injury is suspected and the CT is negative.
- Utilizes iodinated radiographic contrast material and ionizing radiation.

5. Cavernosography

Advantages

- Can detect the site of a cavernosal tear in a patient with a suspected penile fracture, making subsequent surgical repair easier.
- Easy to perform.

Disadvantages

- Some cavernosal tears are not detected (possibly because they are partial). There are, therefore, some falsely negative studies.

6. Sonography

For suspected testicular rupture. See Acute Testicular Pain.

C. Recommended Imaging Approach

Imaging of patients without any inserted urethral catheters in whom lower genitourinary tract trauma is suspected should begin with retrograde urethrography. If a Grade I urethral injury is present, a catheter should be inserted under the direction of a urologist (since the treatment of such injuries is urethral stenting). Blind catheter insertion in such patients can significantly worsen a Grade I injury (transforming it into a Grade II or III injury). Patients with Grade II or III urethral injuries require suprapubic bladder catheters. These patients are most commonly treated by delayed surgical repair. If no urethral injury is present, a Foley catheter can be inserted normally. If multiorgan injury is suspected, plain films and an abdominal and pelvic CT are usually obtained. If bladder injury is suspected, the urinary catheter should be clamped at the time of the CT and, if possible, dilute contrast material instilled through the catheter into the bladder in order to perform a CT cystogram. Otherwise, a conventional cystogram should be performed at some time after the CT is completed if the CT is negative. Both sonography and MRI essentially have no role in the evaluation of patients with possible injuries to the lower genitourinary tract, except for possible testicular rupture.

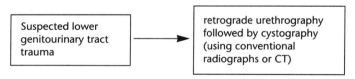

Imaging Algorithm

D. Differential Diagnostic Considerations

1. Urethral injury: Patients may present with blood/clot at the urethral meatus. Results from stretching or disruption of the urethra near the urogenital diaphragm (after blunt trauma) or in the bulbar urethra (after straddle injury). Posterior urethral injuries are graded as follows:

   Grade I: Stretch injury (no extravasation of contrast material during retrograde urethrography).

   Grade II: Urethral disruption with intact urogenital diaphragm. Contrast material extravasates into extraperitoneal tissues in pelvis.

Grade III: Urethral and urogenital diaphragm disruption. Contrast material extravasates into pelvic and perineal tissues. Most common injury.

2. Bladder injury: Hematuria is almost always present. Other signs of bladder injury are not specific. Bladder injuries are graded as follows:

Grade I: Contusion (incomplete tear of bladder wall).

Grade II: Intraperitoneal rupture. Occurs at dome of bladder. Most common when a patient with a full bladder is in a motor vehicle accident.

Grade III: Interstitial bladder injury (incomplete perforation of serosal surface of bladder wall).

Grade IV: Extraperitoneal rupture. Usually associated with pelvic fractures.

Grade V: Combined bladder injury.

3. Penile fracture (rupture of the corpus cavernosum): Rare injury, generally occurs during sexual activity.

4. Testicular rupture: Rare injury most frequently resulting from athletic injury.

References

Kane NM, Francis IR, Ellis JH (1989). The value of CT in the detection of bladder and posterior urethral injuries. AJR 153:1243–1246.

Sandler CM, Harris JH, Carriere JN et al (1981). Posterior urethral injuries after pelvic fracture. AJR 137:1233–1237.

RETROPERITONEAL HEMORRHAGE

A. Clinical Comment

Patients with sudden retroperitoneal hematomas present with abdominal or back pain. They may have symptoms of hypotension (light headedness and tachycardia). Hematocrit levels may be decreased. In some instances a combination of patient history and the location of the hemorrhage may suggest its etiology. For example, anterior pararenal space bleeding may be due to pancreatitis, and perinephric hematomas can be due to ruptured abdominal aortic aneurysms, renal masses, or trauma. Subcapsular renal hematomas can be due to renal masses, trauma, or anticoagulation.

B. Imaging Modalities

1. Abdominal Radiography

Advantages

- Sometimes suggests the presence of a retroperitoneal mass (due to deviation of kidneys or obliteration of a portion of one psoas shadow).
- Can identify bone injuries in trauma patients.

Disadvantages

- Cannot identify the hemorrhage. Almost never diagnostic.
- Plain radiograph signs of retroperitoneal masses are very insensitive.
- Uses ionizing radiation.

2. Sonography

Advantages

- Imaging study of choice for evaluation of the groin after femoral arterial puncture. Can detect arteriovenous fistulae and pseudoaneurysms within groin hematomas. Can be used to treat pseudoaneurysms via ultrasound-controlled compression.
- Can often determine whether a large retroperitoneal mass is present.
- Can occasionally detect the etiology of the hematoma (aortic aneurysm or renal mass).

Disadvantages

- Hematoma has a variable sonographic appearance (hypoechoic or hyperechoic).
- Differentiation of hematoma from other retroperitoneal masses (tumor, abscess) may be impossible.

- Sonographic imaging of the retroperitoneum is limited. Visualization of the retroperitoneum may not be possible in some patients, particularly those who are obese.
- Not as sensitive for leaking aneurysm as CT.

3. CT

Note: use of intravenous contrast material is often preferred, but is not mandatory.

Advantages
- Offers rapid and thorough evaluation of the retroperitoneum. Considered by many to be the imaging study of choice.
- Easily determines presence, location, size, and extent of the hematoma.
- May identify etiology of hematoma (aneurysm, renal mass, peripancreatic inflammation, retroperitoneal tumor).

Disadvantages
- Fails to detect retroperitoneal hemorrhage in some symptomatic patients with large aortic aneurysms who have hematomas identified during subsequent surgery, probably because these patients have not yet actively ruptured their aneurysms at the time of the imaging study. For this reason, a symptomatic patient with a large aortic aneurysm should still be closely monitored and, probably, at least semi-electively repaired, even if the CT fails to identify any evidence of a rupture.
- Utilizes ionizing radiation.

4. MRI

Advantages
- Provides complete visualization of the retroperitoneum.
- As with CT, determines presence, location, size, and extent of the hematoma.
- May identify etiology of hematoma.
- Does not use ionizing radiation.

Disadvantages
- Offers little imaging advantage over CT, but is more expensive.

- Acutely ill patients are often not easily monitored in the MR suite.

5. Angiography

Advantages

- Can identify and treat (by embolization) an abnormal/bleeding artery or pseudoaneurysm due to either pancreatitis or trauma.
- Can identify and treat (by embolization) a bleeding artery in patients with hemorrhagic angiomyolipomas.
- Can identify abdominal aortic aneurysms and determine their location with respect to the renal arteries. This information may be helpful to the vascular surgeon.

Disadvantages

- Cannot directly visualize the retroperitoneum. Best performed after CT, if the CT indicates an abnormality that may be treatable by embolization.
- Rarely detects active leakage of blood into retroperitoneal space.
- Invasive procedure. Utilizes ionizing radiation and iodinated contrast material.

C. Recommended Imaging Approach

Imaging is performed in hemodynamically stable patients in whom the clinical diagnosis of ruptured abdominal aortic aneurysm is considered but uncertain. The imaging study of choice in these patients is CT. If the CT demonstrates an aneurysm and a rupture, the patient should be sent immediately to the operating room. If the CT demonstrates a large aneurysm (>5 cm maximal diameter) but no rupture, the patient should be closely monitored and aortic aneurysm repair performed on a semi-elective basis, since free rupture may subsequently occur at any time. If the CT fails to detect an aneurysm or a rupture, another etiology of the patient's pain should be considered.

CT is also the imaging study of choice in patients in whom other causes of retroperitoneal hemorrhage are considered. Arteriography can be obtained after CT if the CT suggests an etiology amenable to embolization (bleeding angiomyolipoma or pseudoaneurysm, for example).

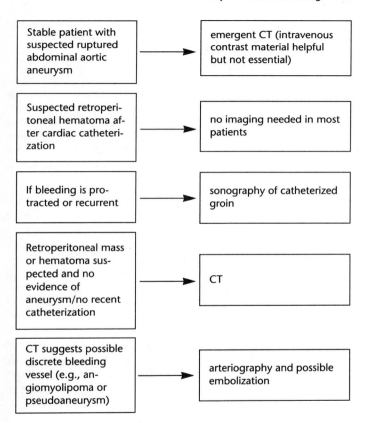

Imaging Algorithm

CT is rarely helpful in patients in whom retroperitoneal hemorrhage is suspected after cardiac catheterization and need not be performed in this setting on a routine basis. While CT can determine whether a decrease in the patient's hematocrit is due to a retroperitoneal hematoma, its effect on subsequent treatment is minimal. Usually, therapy does not change even if a hematoma is present. Instead, groin sonography (with duplex and color-flow Doppler imaging) should be performed in these patients. This is the procedure of choice for detecting arteriovenous fistulae and pseudoaneurysms. In fact, prolonged sonographic compression of pseudoaneurysms can produce complete thrombosis of these structures and effectively treat patients in whom these complications develop.

D. Differential Diagnostic Considerations

1. Iatrogenic: Retroperitoneal hematomas can develop after groin punctures are made for arteriography/cardiac catheterizations. Hematoma dissects up from the pelvis in the extraperitoneal space and can spread into any of the retroperitoneal compartments.

2. Rupture of abdominal aortic aneurysm: Usually does not occur until the aneurysm reaches a diameter of at least 5 cm. Patients who survive to be admitted to the emergency room usually complain of severe back pain. Many patients are hypotensive. Emergent surgical repair is required.

3. Hemorrhage of renal mass: Most common cause of idiopathic perinephric hemorrhage. Common presentation of patients with large angiomyolipomas; however, renal adenocarcinomas can also bleed.

4. Coagulopathy: Due to either intrinsic blood dyscrasia or anticoagulant medication.

5. Trauma: Occasionally mild trauma can produce significant hemorrhage.

6. Pancreatitis: Hemorrhage likely results from erosion of the inflammatory process into peripancreatic vessels. Occasionally, pancreatitis can produce pseudoaneurysms of the superior mesenteric or splenic artery.

7. Hemorrhagic retroperitoneal neoplasm: Rarely, primary or metastatic retroperitoneal tumors may spontaneously bleed. Hemorrhage

may also result when patients with these neoplasms are anticoagulated.

References

Siegel CL, Cohan RH (1994). CT of abdominal aortic aneurysms. AJR 163:17–29.

Siegel CL, Cohan RH, Korobkin M, Alpern MB, Courneya DL, Leder RA (1994). Abdominal aortic aneurysm morphology: CT features in patients with ruptured and nonruptured aneurysms. AJR 163:1123–1129.

► CHAPTER 4

Obstetrics and Gynecology

Barbara Hertzberg, MD
Duke University Medical Center

Imaging Handbook for House Officers, Edited by Paul M. Silverman and Douglas J. Quint.
ISBN 0-471-13767-7 © 1997 Wiley-Liss, Inc.

FIRST TRIMESTER PAIN
(SUSPECTED ECTOPIC PREGNANCY)

A. Clinical Findings

1. Positive β-HCG.
2. Classic clinical triad of amenorrhea, pain, and palpable adnexal mass is frequently not present.
3. Occasionally: Tachycardia, hypotension, subjective symptoms of pregnancy (breast tenderness, nausea).
4. All women with a positive β-HCG should be considered at risk for ectopic pregnancy, but the following indicate especially high risk:
   a. History of pelvic inflammatory disease.
   b. Intrauterine contraceptive device.
   c. Prior ectopic pregnancy.
   d. Prior tubal reconstructive surgery.
   e. In vitro fertilization.
   f. Prior tubal ligation.

B. Imaging Modalities

1. Sonography
   a. Ultrasound is generally the only imaging procedure necessary for patient with suspected ectopic pregnancy.
   b. Transabdominal sonography, endovaginal sonography, or both can be performed depending on individual physician preference, laboratory protocol, and initial ultrasound findings.
2. MRI
   a. May be helpful if abdominal pregnancy is suspected by sonography: Potentially can better differentiate compressed empty uterus separate from advanced abdominal pregnancy.
3. Plain films, CT, radionuclide studies—not indicated.

C. Recommended Imaging Approach

1. A β-HCG level should be obtained prior to ordering ultrasound for ectopic pregnancy. The β-HCG is necessary to interpret the ultra-

sound examination. A negative serum β-HCG effectively excludes the diagnosis of ectopic pregnancy.

2. A minority of patients with ectopic pregnancy are critically ill and hemodynamically unstable owing to massive intraabdominal hemorrhage. They require rapid fluid resuscitation and immediate laparotomy, and there may be no time for ultrasound.

3. If transabdominal ultrasound is done, it is performed with a full urinary bladder. Flanks are scanned for free intraperitoneal blood. If a live intra- or extrauterine gestation is seen, examination is considered complete.

4. If a live pregnancy is not seen by transabdominal sonography, endovaginal ultrasound should be performed. Alternately, endovaginal ultrasound can be done as the initial test.

D. Differential Diagnostic Considerations

1. One of the main goals of ultrasound is to determine if there is an intrauterine pregnancy:
   a. If intrauterine pregnancy is seen, coexistent ectopic pregnancy is extremely unlikely (1/4,000 to 1/30,000).
   b. Likelihood of coexistent intrauterine and ectopic pregnancy higher in patients undergoing ovulation induction or in vitro fertilization.

2. Fluid collection in uterine cavity is not sufficient to document intrauterine pregnancy because hormonal stimulation of ectopic pregnancy can result in fluid in the uterus ("pseudogestational sac").

3. Intrauterine cardiac activity and yolk sac or gestational sac separate from uterine cavity ("double decidual sac sign" or "intradecidual sign") are necessary for confident diagnosis of intrauterine pregnancy by ultrasound.

4. Only ultrasound finding that is 100% diagnostic of ectopic pregnancy is extrauterine embryo with cardiac activity.

5. Echogenic ring in adnexa ("adnexal ring sign") or large amount of echogenic blood in conjunction with complex adnexal mass are highly suggestive of ectopic pregnancy.

6. Negative pelvic ultrasound (empty uterus, no adnexal masses, no free fluid) does not exclude ectopic pregnancy. Up to 20% of patients with ectopic pregnancy have completely "normal"-appearing pelvic ultrasound.

7. Correlation of ultrasound findings with serial quantitative serum β-HCG levels is helpful when sonography is not definitive.

References

Frates MC, Laing FC (1995). Sonographic evaluation of ectopic pregnancy: An update. AJR 165:251–259.

Hertzberg BS (1994). Ultrasound evaluation for ectopic pregnancy. Radiologist 1:11–18.

Parvey HR, Maklad N (1993). Pitfalls in the transvaginal sonographic diagnosis of ectopic pregnancy. J Ultrasound Med 3:138–144.

FIRST TRIMESTER BLEEDING (THREATENED ABORTION)

A. Clinical Findings

1. Approximately one-fourth of pregnant patients have vaginal bleeding early in pregnancy.

2. Mild cramping or pain. Loss of symptoms of pregnancy (nausea, breast tenderness, etc.). Many patients asymptomatic.

3. In some patients with gestational trophoblastic disease: Passage of vesicles per vagina, hyperemesis, toxemia, or uterus large for gestational dates.

B. Imaging Modalities

1. Ultrasound: Imaging procedure of choice in patient with first trimester bleeding.

2. CT, MRI, plain films, radionuclide studies: Not indicated.

C. Recommended Imaging Approach

1. β-HCG should be obtained prior to ordering sonography to evaluate for first trimester bleeding. A thorough physical examination should be performed to search for abdominal tenderness, adnexal masses, uterine enlargement, dilatation of the cervical os, and cervical lesions.

2. Ultrasound examination can be done with either transabdominal (usually requires a full urinary bladder) or endovaginal approach. If a live pregnancy is not seen by transabdominal sonography, endovaginal ultrasound will usually be necessary.

3. If ultrasound findings are not definitive, a follow-up study may be necessary in 3–7 days. Quantitative serum β-HCG level should be obtained and correlated with ultrasound findings.

D. Differential Diagnostic Considerations

1. Causes of first trimester bleeding include blighted ovum, threatened or incomplete abortion, ectopic pregnancy, incorrect menstrual dating, gestational trophoblastic disease, and lesions of the cervix.

2. Approximately one-half of pregnancies with first trimester bleeding eventually abort. Sonographic demonstration of intrauterine embryonic cardiac activity greatly improves prognosis for a viable pregnancy.

3. Sonographic demonstration of an intrauterine yolk sac or an intrauterine gestational sac separate from the uterine cavity indicates there is an intrauterine pregnancy, but, in the absence of fetal cardiac activity, follow-up is necessary to evaluate for viability.

4. Ultrasound demonstration of an embryo measuring greater than 5 mm without cardiac activity is considered diagnostic of embryonic death. If an embryo without cardiac activity measures less than 5 mm, a follow-up study should be done in 3–4 days.

5. Ultrasound findings that adversely affect prognosis include an intrauterine hematoma (particularly if it is large or located immediately under the placenta), an abnormally large yolk sac, or an abnormally slow embryonic heart rate.

6. Typical ultrasound appearance of a molar pregnancy is soft tissue mass containing numerous small cystic spaces enlarging the uterine cavity. Some patients also have bilateral multicystic ovarian enlargement due to theca lutein cysts.

References

Lindsay DJ, Lyons EA, Levi CS, Zheng XH (1992). Endovaginal appearance of the yolk sac in early pregnancy: Normal growth and usefulness as a predictor of abnormal pregnancy outcome. Radiology 183:115–118.

Nyberg DA, Laing FC, Filly RA (1986). Threatened abortion: Sonographic distinction of normal and abnormal gestation sacs. Radiology 158:397–400.

Nyberg DA, Mack LA, Laing FC et al (1987). Distinguishing normal from abnormal gestational sac growth in early pregnancy. J Ultrasound Med 6:23–26.

UNKNOWN GESTATIONAL AGE

A. Clinical Findings

1. Usual reasons for uncertainty in clinical estimation of gestational age:
   a. Inability to recall last menstrual period.
   b. Irregular menstrual cycles.
   c. First trimester bleeding.
   d. Recent pregnancy.
   e. Breastfeeding.
   f. Uterine size inconsistent with last menstrual period.
   g. Oral contraceptives.

B. Imaging Modalities

1. Ultrasound: Imaging method of choice to estimate gestational age. Indicated when historical dates are in question, obstetric intervention or elective delivery is considered likely, or there is a discrepancy between fundal height and dates.
2. Plain films, CT, MRI, radionuclide studies: Not indicated.

C. Recommended Imaging Approach

1. Sonographic estimation of gestational age can be done by transabdominal or endovaginal sonography during first trimester. During second and third trimesters, transabdominal sonography is generally used.

2. First trimester:

   a. Mean sac diameter: Average internal diameter of the sac. Only used before embryo is seen. Provides an early estimate of gestational age but much less accurate than measuring embryo itself.

   b. Crown–rump length: Highly reliable predictor of gestational age (accuracy ±3–5 days in mid first trimester, more variation later in the first trimester) because there is little biologic variability in fetal size early in gestation.

3. Second and third trimesters: Combinations of specific fetal measurements are used. Usually the gestational age indicated by biparietal diameter (BPD), corrected BPD, or head circumference (HC) is averaged with gestational age corresponding to femur length (FL).

D. Differential Diagnostic Considerations

1. Ultrasound estimates of gestational age are reported in terms of menstrual age. Menstrual age is equivalent to conceptual age plus 2 weeks.

2. Sonographic estimation of gestational age is based on fetal size. Biologic variability in fetal size increases as gestation advances, so sonographic estimates of gestational age become progressively less accurate late in pregnancy. Third trimester ultrasound estimates of gestational age should be viewed with caution.

3. Abnormal portions of fetal anatomy (such as the head in a fetus with hydrocephalus or the femur in a fetus with a skeletal dysplasia) should not be used in estimating gestational age.

4. Once an estimated gestational age has been assigned by ultrasound early in pregnancy, it should be used as the standard for gestational age in subsequent studies. Thus, the gestational age at a follow-up study would be equivalent to the gestational age at the time of the

initial study plus the number of weeks elapsed. Gestational age should be not reassigned based on the ultrasound measurements obtained each time the fetus returns for follow-up.

References

Hadlock FP (1990). Sonographic estimation of fetal age and weight. Radiol Clin North Am 28(1):39–50.

Hadlock FP, Harrist RB, Martinez-Poyer J (1991). How accurate is second trimester fetal dating? J Ultrasound Med 10:557–561.

Hadlock FP, Shah YP, Kanan DJ, Lindsey JV (1992). Fetal crown–rump length: Reevaluation of relation to menstrual age (5–18 weeks) with high-resolution real-time US. Radiology 182:501–505.

SIZE LARGER THAN DATES (SUSPECTED MULTIPLE GESTATION)

A. Clinical Findings

1. Fundal height measurement larger than expected for estimated gestational age.
2. Clinical findings in patients with multiple gestations: More than one fetal heart audible, sensation of greater than expected fetal activity, hyperemesis, history of fertility pills.

B. Imaging Modalities

1. Ultrasound: Imaging method of choice to evaluate etiology of larger than expected uterine size during pregnancy.
2. Plain films, CT, MRI, radionuclide studies: Not indicated.

C. Recommended Imaging Approach

1. During first trimester, transabdominal or endovaginal ultrasound can be performed. During second and third trimesters, transabdominal ultrasound is usually done, although endovaginal ultrasound can be used as a complementary technique when necessary.

2. The ultrasound examination should include careful assessment of fetal number, amniotic fluid volume, and uterine wall and adnexa, looking for masses.

3. If multiple gestations are identified, the pregnancy should be examined for the presence of a separating membrane, fetal gender, and number of placental sites in order to assess amnionicity and chorionicity.

D. Differential Diagnostic Considerations

1. Main differential considerations are inaccurate dates, multifetal gestation, large for gestational age (LGA) fetus, polyhydramnios, pelvic mass such as uterine fibroid or ovarian neoplasm, and gestational trophoblastic disease. Ultrasound can usually distinguish between these possibilities, although in some cases a combination of factors is present.

2. Most common etiology of mild polyhydramnios is idiopathic. Maternal causes of polyhydramnios include gestational diabetes (also causes LGA fetuses) and isoimmunization syndromes. Wide variety of fetal anomalies can cause polyhydramnios; the most common include CNS malformations, high gastrointestinal tract obstructions, and cardiovascular anomalies. There is a very high incidence of fetal anomalies (up to 75%) in pregnancies with severe polyhydramnios.

3. Multiple gestations should only be diagnosed when there is more than one fetus with cardiac activity. A number of entities can give false impression of multiple gestational sacs during first trimester, including uterine contraction distorting sac, bicornuate uterus, subchorionic hematoma, and incomplete fusion between amnion and chorion.

4. Diagnosis of LGA fetus is based on measurement of fetal abdominal circumference and estimation of fetal weight. The measured abdominal circumference and estimated fetal weight are then compared with the values expected for the fetus' assigned gestational age; if above the 90th percentile, the fetus is considered LGA.

5. Ultrasound identification of LGA fetus can be pivotal finding in determining that a fetus should be delivered by cesarean section rather than vaginally.

6. When uterus is large for dates due to gestational trophoblastic disease, ultrasound typically reveals soft tissue mass with multiple cystic spaces enlarging the uterine cavity. A fetus is usually not seen, although a live fetus can coexist with molar tissue in a partial mole or when there is a complete mole with coexistent fetus (a form of twin pregnancy).

References

Boyd ME, Usher RH, McLean FH (1983). Fetal macrosomia: Prediction, risks, proposed management. Obstet Gynecol 61:715–722.

Davis JL, Ray-Mazumder S, Hobel CJ et al (1990). Uterine leiomyomas in pregnancy: A prospective study. Obstet Gynecol 75:41–44.

Doubilet PM, Benson CB (1990). Fetal growth disturbances. Semin Roentgenol 25(4):309–316.

SIZE LESS THAN DATES (SUSPECTED INTRAUTERINE GROWTH RETARDATION)

A. Clinical Findings

1. Fundal height measurement less than expected for estimated gestational age.

2. Hypertension, smoking, placental abruption, sensation of decreased fetal movement in some patients with intrauterine growth retardation.

B. Imaging Modalities

1. Ultrasound is imaging method of choice to evaluate etiology of smaller than expected uterine size during pregnancy.

2. If intrauterine growth retardation is suspected after initial ultrasound evaluation, tests of fetal well-being, including biophysical

profile, nonstress and contraction stress test, serial ultrasounds for growth and amniotic fluid volume, and Doppler interrogation of blood flow are performed.

3. Plain films, CT, MRI, and radionuclide studies are not indicated.

C. Recommended Imaging Approach

1. Ultrasound imaging of the pregnancy with size less than dates should include careful assessment of amniotic fluid volume and fetal size.

2. Fetal bladder and kidneys should be carefully documented, particularly in the setting of oligohydramnios.

D. Differential Diagnostic Considerations

1. Major diagnostic considerations include inaccurate dates, intrauterine growth retardation (IUGR), oligohydramnios, and fetal descent into pelvis as term approaches.

2. Unlike polyhydramnios, oligohydramnios is always abnormal. Etiologies include fetal demise, renal anomalies, premature rupture of membranes, IUGR, abdominal pregnancy, and postmaturity syndrome.

3. IUGR is associated with a dramatic increase in perinatal morbidity and mortality. This is because the adverse intrauterine conditions causing growth restriction can lead to fetal hypoxia and demise.

4. Conventional definition of IUGR is fetal weight less than the 10th percentile for gestational age. This encompasses a heterogeneous group of fetuses who are small for gestational age for a variety of different reasons. Only some of these fetuses are small due to adverse intrauterine conditions. Other etiologies include low (but normal) inherited potential for growth and intrinsic limitations on growth such as chromosomal abnormalities or in utero infection.

5. When fetus is suspected of IUGR based on ultrasound measurements, serial tests are performed to evaluate fetal well-being. Goal is to determine optimum time for delivery, that is, when risks of remaining in utero due to adverse intrauterine conditions outweigh risks of prematurity.

References

Hadlock FP, Harrist RB, Martinez-Poyer J (1991). In utero analysis of fetal growth: A sonographic weight standard. Radiology 181:129–133.

Hertzberg BS (1995). US evaluation of fetal growth. Radiologist 2:95–102.

Smith CV (1990). Amniotic fluid assessment. Obstet Gynecol Clin North Am 17:187–200.

PAINLESS THIRD TRIMESTER VAGINAL BLEEDING (SUSPECTED PLACENTA PREVIA)

A. Clinical Findings

1. Painless third trimester vaginal bleeding.
2. Abnormal fetal lie.
3. Digital exam of cervix: Should not be done unless ultrasound has excluded placenta previa.

B. Imaging Modalities

1. Ultrasound is imaging procedure of choice for third trimester vaginal bleeding. Sonography accurately depicts placental location and frequently demonstrates intrauterine hematomas arising from placental abruption.
2. MRI can be complementary to ultrasound, but is usually not necessary.
3. Plain films, CT, and radionuclide studies are not indicated.

C. Recommended Imaging Approach

1. Transabdominal ultrasound is performed first to evaluate location of placenta relative to cervix. Goal is to image both lower edge of placenta and cervix.
2. If transabdominal ultrasound fails to identify both lower edge of placenta and cervix, transperineal or endovaginal ultrasound is performed. If endovaginal sonography is done, it should be performed cautiously to avoid inducing vaginal bleeding if patient has placenta previa.

3. If ultrasound suggests placenta previa but maternal urinary bladder is distended with urine, imaging should be repeated after bladder has been emptied.

D. Differential Diagnostic Considerations

1. Differential diagnosis of painless third trimester bleeding includes placenta previa, placental abruption, labor, cervical erosion, polyps, trauma, and coagulation disorders. In many cases, etiology of third trimester bleeding is never determined.

2. Potential sources of ultrasound false-positive results for placenta previa include distortion of lower uterus by contractions or full urinary bladder, echogenic subchorionic hematoma overlying cervix, and lower uterine fibroid. These false-positive results can usually be excluded by careful ultrasound examination.

3. Sonographic visualization of lower edge of placenta is not sufficient to rule out placenta previa. The cervix must also be visualized to rule out a succenturiate (accessory) lobe overlying the cervix.

4. Placenta previa is graded based on amount of cervix covered with overlying placental tissue. Grading varies from institution to institution. A typical grading system is
   a. Complete previa: Internal os completely covered by placenta.
   b. Partial previa: Internal os partially covered by placenta.
   c. Marginal previa: Placental tissue extending onto a portion of cervix but not involving internal os.

5. Follow-up sonography is indicated in patients with suspected placenta previa. Marginal and partial previas sometimes improve with advancing pregnancy.

References

Artis AA III, Bowie JD, Rosenberg ER, Rauch RF (1985). The fallacy of placental migration: Effects of sonographic techniques. AJR 144:79–81.

Hertzberg BS, Bowie JD, Carroll BA, Kliewer MA, Weber TM (1992). Diagnosis of placenta previa during the third trimester: Role of transperineal sonography. AJR 159:83–87.

Leerentveld RA, Gilberts ECAM, Arnold MJCWJ, Wladimiroff JW (1990). Accuracy and safety of transvaginal sonographic placental localization. Obstet Gynecol 76:759–762.

THIRD TRIMESTER VAGINAL BLEEDING AND PAIN (SUSPECTED PLACENTAL ABRUPTION)

A. Clinical Findings

1. Vaginal bleeding.
2. Pelvic pain.
3. With severe abruptions: Pelvic tenderness, back pain, uterine rigidity, and fetal demise. These findings are present in only a minority of placental abruption. Majority of abruptions are milder and associated only with vaginal bleeding.
4. Predisposing factors: Hypertension, trauma, multiparity, previous abruption, maternal cocaine use.
5. Complications: Hypovolemic shock, acute renal failure, disseminated intravascular coagulation (DIC), postpartum hemorrhage, Couvelaire uterus (extravasation of blood into uterine musculature).

B. Imaging Modalities

1. Ultrasound: Used to detect intrauterine hematomas, evaluate amount of placental elevation by hematoma, and rule out placenta previa.
2. Plain films, CT, MRI, radionuclide studies: Not indicated.

C. Recommended Imaging Approach

1. Transabdominal ultrasound to evaluate uterine contents for hematoma and rule out placenta previa.
2. If lower edge of placenta or cervix not seen, transperineal or endovaginal ultrasound to rule out placenta previa.

D. Differential Diagnostic Considerations

1. Ultrasound evaluation for placental abruption focuses on detecting *intrauterine* hematomas. Negative sonography does not rule out

placental abruption; bleeding may not be detected if it is predominantly external or similar in echogenicity to placenta.

2. The two most commonly detected locations for hematomas: retroplacental and subchorionic.

3. Retroplacental hematomas need to be distinguished from retroplacental uterine contractions (transient), retroplacental fibroids, and the normal subplacental hypoechoic venous complex (conforms to contour of the uterus and does not have mass effect on placenta).

4. Placental thickening should be viewed with suspicion because acute retroplacental hematoma can be similar in echogenicity to placenta. When in doubt, a follow-up sonogram will show evolution in ultrasound appearance of hematoma if this was explanation for apparent placental thickening.

5. Subchorionic hematoma that extends over cervix can give false impression of placenta previa.

6. Chronic subchorionic hematoma can be similar in echogenicity to amniotic fluid, in which case the only abnormality detected by sonography may be an intrauterine membrane representing the elevated amniochorionic membrane.

7. Subchorionic hematoma that bulges toward amniotic cavity can give false impression of an intrauterine mass. Differential includes fibroid, uterine contraction, chorioangioma, and succenturiate (accessory) lobe of placenta. If the "mass" is due to a subchorionic hematoma, a follow-up ultrasound will show evolution in ultrasound appearance of the hematoma, which will become less echogenic and more complicated.

References

McGahan JP, Phillips HE, Reid MH (1980). The anechoic retroplacental area. Radiology 134:475–478.

Nyberg DA, Cyr DR, Mack LA et al (1987). Sonographic spectrum of placental abruption. AJR 148:161–164.

Nyberg DA, Mack LA, Benedetti TJ (1987). Placental abruption and placental hemorrhage: Correlation of sonographic findings with fetal outcome. Radiology 164:357–361.

FEVER AND PELVIC PAIN
(SUSPECTED PELVIC INFLAMMATORY DISEASE)

A. Clinical Findings

1. Negative β-HCG (β-HCG should be obtained because pelvic pain in a patient of childbearing age should be presumed to be due to a complication of pregnancy until proven otherwise).
2. Abdominal pain. Adnexal and cervical motion tenderness.
3. Fever.
4. Leukocytosis.
5. Purulent cervical discharge.
6. Sequelae: Chronic abdominal pain, infertility, ectopic pregnancy.

B. Imaging Modalities

1. Imaging not necessary in many patients: Women with mild disease receive ambulatory therapy and may not require any imaging study.
2. Ultrasound: Indicated when there is a need to rule out tubovarian abscess or evaluate for diseases causing symptoms that simulate PID.
3. MRI: Not usually necessary. Rarely may be useful in sorting out difficult to interpret ultrasound findings.
4. Plain films
    a. Flat and upright abdominal films to look for free air if perforation of a hollow viscus is suspected.
    b. Cone-down view of right lower quadrant to evaluate for an appendicolith if appendicitis is suspected.
5. CT: If an intraabdominal abscess is suspected.

C. Recommended Imaging Approach

1. Transabdominal ultrasound, endovaginal ultrasound, or both can be used. Transabdominal ultrasound provides a better overview of pelvic anatomy and is usually sufficient to demonstrate tubovarian

abscesses and pelvic fluid collections of significant size. Endovaginal ultrasound better resolves details of pelvic anatomy and pathology.

2. Serial ultrasound exams can be useful in following response to antibiotic therapy.

D. Differential Diagnostic Considerations

1. Many other disease processes can result in clinical picture suggesting PID: Clinical diagnosis of PID is incorrect in up to 35% of women. Other diagnostic considerations include endometriosis, hemorrhagic ovarian cyst, torsed ovary, appendicitis, ectopic pregnancy, torsed or degenerating fibroid, diverticulitis, and normal pelvis. Laparoscopy is occasionally necessary to make diagnosis.

2. If appendicitis is considered in differential diagnosis, this should be communicated to ultrasound physician. Scanning technique to image inflamed appendix (directed high-resolution graded compression scans of right lower quadrant) is different from standard pelvic sonography.

3. Ultrasound is frequently negative in mild cases of PID. Endovaginal ultrasound occasionally shows subtle findings not identified by transabdominal imaging, such as small collections of pus in the fallopian tubes or cul-de-sac.

4. Even in patients with positive findings by sonography, ultrasound appearance of PID is rarely specific. Other entities such as endometriomas or ectopic pregnancy can give identical ultrasound findings. Clinical correlation is necessary to interpret significance of ultrasound changes.

References

McCormack WM (1994). Pelvic inflammatory disease. N Engl J Med 330:115–119.

Moore Lori, Wilson SR (1994). Ultrasonography in obstetric and gynecologic emergencies. Radiol Clin North Am 32:1005–1022.

Swayne LC, Love MB, Karasick SR (1984). Pelvic inflammatory disease: Sonographic-pathologic correlation. Radiology 151:751–755.

ENLARGED UTERUS (SUSPECTED FIBROIDS)

A. Clinical Findings

1. Negative β-HCG (β-HCG should be obtained because pregnancy should be considered in differential diagnosis of pelvic mass in a woman of childbearing age).
2. Pelvic mass on bimanual exam.
3. Menorrhagia (excessive menstrual bleeding) and/or dysmenorrhea (painful menses).
4. Anemia.
5. Infertility.
6. Pelvic pressure.
7. Frequently asymptomatic.

B. Imaging Modalities

1. Ultrasound: Useful in localizing and measuring fibroids and distinguishing them from uterine fluid collections and adnexal masses.
2. Plain films of abdomen: Not usually necessary, although some calcified fibroids can have a diagnostic whorled calcification pattern termed *popcorn* calcification.
3. MRI: Not usually necessary but can be helpful in determining origin of a pelvic mass (i.e., from uterus or ovaries) when not clear by ultrasound. Also useful in distinguishing adenomyosis from small fibroids.
4. CT, radionuclide studies: Not indicated.

C. Recommended Imaging Approach

1. Transabdominal ultrasound: For overall impression of uterine size. Transabdominal ultrasound is necessary in patient with a markedly enlarged uterus, as very large fibroids or fibroids located high in the pelvis may be beyond field of view by endovaginal sonography.
2. Endovaginal ultrasound: When it is desirable to identify small fibroids and determine their relationship to endometrial cavity, as in the patient with unexplained vaginal bleeding. Improved resolution

afforded by endovaginal sonography will detect many smaller fibroids not seen by transabdominal approach.

3. When large fibroids are seen, ultrasound evaluation should include views of kidneys to evaluate for obstruction of collecting system.

D. Differential Diagnostic Considerations

1. Fibroids are also called *leiomyomas, myomas,* and *fibromyomas.*

2. Locations include submucous (immediately adjacent to endometrial cavity), intramural, and subserosal (protruding from outer surface of uterus).

3. An exophytic or pedunculated subserosal fibroid can be difficult to distinguish from adnexal mass by ultrasound. As a general rule, fibroid should be considered whenever ultrasound identifies a solid adnexal mass.

4. Necrotic change in a degenerating fibroid can mimic appearance of fluid in uterine cavity.

5. Differential diagnosis of enlarged uterus

   a. Adenomyosis: Ectopic location of endometrial tissue in myometrium. Ultrasound findings are nonspecific, although uterus usually enlarged, particularly in AP dimension.

   b. Retropositioned uterus: Can look remarkably similar to exophytic posterior fibroid. Distinguished by demonstrating uterine cavity in apparent mass.

   c. Endometrial carcinoma or hyperplasia: Echogenic or heterogeneous mass in uterine cavity.

   d. Hydrometrium, hematometrium (blood), or pyometrium (pus): Fluid collection enlarging uterine cavity. Occurs when there is obstruction to outflow, either congenital (vaginal anomaly or imperforate hymen), neoplastic (cervical or endometrial carcinoma), or iatrogenic (radiation therapy or cervical conization procedure).

   e. Sarcomatous degeneration of fibroid: Short of seeing metastases, ultrasound cannot distinguish between leiomyosarcoma and benign leiomyoma. Benign leiomyomas are by far the more common, however. Malignant degeneration is very rare.

References

Baltarowich OH, Kurtz AB, Pennell RG et al (1988). Pitfalls in the sonographic diagnosis of uterine fibroids. AJR 151:725–728.

Gross BH, Silver TM, Jaffe MH (1983). Sonographic features of uterine leiomyomas: Analysis of 41 proven cases. J Ultrasound Med 2:401–406.

Seidler D, Laing FC, Jeffrey R Jr, Wing VW (1987). Uterine adenomyosis: A difficult sonographic diagnosis. J Ultrasound Med 6:345–349.

PALPABLE ADNEXAL MASS (SUSPECTED OVARIAN NEOPLASM)

A. Clinical Findings

1. Negative β-HCG: Ectopic pregnancy should be considered whenever an adnexal mass is palpated in a woman of childbearing age. Negative serum β-HCG effectively excludes this diagnosis.
2. Palpable pelvic mass, separate from uterus.
3. If mass ruptures, torses, bleeds, or expands rapidly: Pelvic pain.

B. Imaging Modalities

1. Ultrasound: Imaging modality of choice to evaluate an adnexal mass. Accurately identifies uterus, ovaries, and adnexal masses.
2. MRI: Useful when ultrasound does not definitively identify origin of pelvic mass or to characterize components of a mass (e.g., can distinguish between blood and fat in a mass).
3. Abdominal radiographs: Not usually indicated, but can show calcification pattern characteristic of a dermoid or an exophytic fibroid.
4. CT, radionuclide studies: Not indicated.

C. Recommended Imaging Approach

1. Examination can begin with either transabdominal or endovaginal ultrasound. Transabdominal ultrasound gives a better overview of pelvic anatomy, but endovaginal ultrasound better resolves details of mass characteristics.

2. If available, endovaginal color Doppler and spectral Doppler analysis can be performed. Malignant masses frequently contain neovascularization, resulting in low-resistance, high diastolic flow waveform, but there is considerable overlap between waveforms obtained from benign and malignant masses.

3. In a woman of childbearing age, a follow-up study should be performed approximately 6 weeks after initial exam if there is significant chance mass could be due to a physiologic process such as a hemorrhagic corpus luteal cyst.

4. MRI can be performed if additional imaging information is needed after ultrasound has been done.

D. Differential Diagnostic Considerations

1. Most common cause of adnexal mass in women of childbearing age is physiologic cyst such as a follicle, follicular cyst, or corpus luteal cyst.

2. Hemorrhage into a corpus luteal cyst can cause a complex ultrasound appearance suggestive of neoplasm, but a hemorrhagic cyst will resolve or decrease in size if follow-up sonography is done in approximately 6 weeks.

3. Ultrasound appearance is frequently nonspecific, although sonography can help define mass, determine size and origin, and limit the differential diagnosis. Final diagnosis is usually made surgically. A multitude of different processes that cause palpable adnexal masses need to be considered, including functional cysts, benign and malignant ovarian neoplasms, endometriomas, ectopic pregnancy, exophytic fibroid, tubovarian abscess, torsion, polycystic ovary, paraovarian cyst, nongynecologic inflammatory mass (appendiceal or diverticular abscess), metastasis, lymph node, and pelvic kidney.

4. Cystic teratoma (dermoid) frequently has characteristic ultrasound appearance consisting of highly echogenic component ("dermoid plug") due to fat and sebaceous material. Occasionally a tooth is seen.

5. A postmenopausal adnexal mass is generally more worrisome for malignancy than premenopausal because functional cysts, en-

dometriomas, and tubovarian abscesses are less common and ovarian carcinoma is more common. A small, simple cyst without blood flow demonstrated by color Doppler will usually be benign, however, and is generally followed with serial ultrasound.

6. Most ovarian neoplasms are predominantly cystic by ultrasound, often with multiseptated appearance. Ultrasound cannot distinguish between benign and malignant ovarian neoplasms, although likelihood of malignancy increases with larger proportion of solid components.

7. Ovarian torsion can be very difficult to diagnose preoperatively. Clinically can mimic appendicitis, ectopic pregnancy, PID, endometriosis, diverticulitis, or urinary tract stone. Ultrasound appearance also nonspecific, although typically the ovary is enlarged with increased number of peripheral follicles. Potential role of endovaginal color Doppler is under investigation.

References

DiSantis DJ, Scatarige JC, Kemp G, Given FT et al (1993). A prospective evaluation of transvaginal sonography for detection of ovarian disease. AJR 161:91–94.

Moyle JW, Rochester D, Sider L, Shrock K, Krause P (1983). Sonography of ovarian tumors: Predictability of tumor types. AJR 141:985–991.

Sheth S, Fishman EK, Buck JL, Hamper UM, Sanders RC (1988). The variable sonographic appearances of ovarian teratomas: Correlation with CT. AJR 151:331–334.

POSTMENOPAUSAL BLEEDING (SUSPECTED ENDOMETRIAL CARCINOMA)

A. Clinical Findings

1. Vaginal bleeding, occurring more than 1 year after cessation of menses.
2. Anemia (if bleeding is excessive).
3. Enlarged uterus (in some women with endometrial carcinoma).

B. Imaging Modalities

1. Standard investigation of postmenopausal bleeding includes endometrial biopsy and/or fractional dilatation and curettage. Imaging studies are often not necessary.

2. Ultrasound: Helpful in identifying submucous fibroids and endometrial thickening due to hyperplasia, polyps, or carcinoma. Does not obviate need for histologic evaluation of endometrium.

3. Sonohysterography: New technique under investigation. Endovaginal ultrasound performed after fluid has been instilled into uterine cavity can provide a more detailed picture of endometrial pathology.

4. MRI: Not considered useful in detecting endometrial carcinoma, but can be helpful in evaluating depth of myometrial invasion and extension into cervix and in detecting extrauterine disease.

5. CT: Not considered useful in diagnosing endometrial carcinoma but can be useful in detecting spread of endometrial cancer to pelvic and abdominal lymph nodes.

6. Abdominal radiographs, radionuclide studies: Not indicated.

C. Recommended Imaging Approach

1. Imaging is frequently not necessary because endometrial sampling needs to be done in patient with postmenopausal bleeding regardless of imaging findings.

2. Ultrasound can be performed to evaluate thickness and heterogeneity of endometrium and search for adjacent lesions that may be source of bleeding.

3. MRI or CT may be helpful to evaluate depth of extension and image for distant metastases in some patients with histologically proven endometrial carcinoma.

D. Differential Diagnostic Considerations

1. Differential diagnosis for postmenopausal bleeding: Endometrial carcinoma, endometrial polyp, endometrial hyperplasia, atrophic change, submucous fibroid, coagulation disorder, cervical lesion,

or vaginal source. Underlying malignancy is present in approximately 25% of patients with postmenopausal bleeding.

2. Major considerations when ultrasound shows endometrial thickening: Endometrial carcinoma, polyp, hyperplasia. Usually cannot be distinguished from each other by ultrasound.

3. Endovaginal color Doppler and spectral analysis of endometrial contents: Under investigation as a potential method to improve sonographic detection of malignancy.

4. Endometrial carcinoma can extend to cervix and obstruct outflow from uterus, resulting in a fluid collection in uterine cavity by sonography.

5. Under investigation: Concept that endometrial sampling can be avoided if ultrasound reveals a normal, nonthickened uterine cavity in a postmenopausal woman with vaginal bleeding. Although this is currently controversial, if further investigations prove this to be safe, ultrasound would become routinely indicated in initial workup of postmenopausal bleeding.

References

Goldstein SR, Nachtigall M, Snyder JR, Nachtigall L (1990). Endometrial assessment by vaginal ultrasonography before endometrial sampling in patients with postmenopausal bleeding. Am J Obstet Gynecol 163:119–123.

Lin MC, Gosink BB, Wolf SI, Feldesman MR et al (1991). Endometrial thickness after menopause: Effect of hormone replacement. Radiology 180:427–432.

Sheth S, Hamper UM, Kurman RJ (1993). Thickened endometrium in the postmenopausal woman: Sonographic-pathologic correlation. Radiology 187:135–139.

INFERTILITY

A. Clinical Findings

1. Inability to achieve pregnancy after 1 year of unprotected intercourse.

B. Imaging Modalities

1. Majority of the workup for infertility (e.g., semen analysis, post-coital test, basal body temperature record, laparoscopy) does not include imaging procedures. Imaging is done at predetermined points in workup to evaluate for specific causes of infertility.

2. Hysterosalpingography (HSG): Injection of radiopaque contrast into the uterus to evaluate for uterine abnormalities and tubal disease.

3. Ultrasound: Not part of routine diagnostic workup, but can be helpful in identifying congenital anomalies, submucous fibroids, and adnexal masses such as endometriomas. Is routinely used to monitor folliculogenesis and guide interventions in patients undergoing ovulation induction, in vitro fertilization, and other therapeutic procedures.

4. MRI: Not routinely used but can be helpful in classifying congenital abnormalities of uterine fusion.

5. CT, radionuclide studies: Not indicated.

C. Recommended Imaging Approach

1. HSG is generally done before diagnostic laparoscopy is considered. Water-soluble radiopaque dye is injected into cervix under fluoroscopic observation to evaluate configuration of uterine cavity, patency of fallopian tubes, presence of rugations in ampullary portion of tube, and whether there is free flow of dye from fallopian tubes into peritoneal cavity.

2. HSG should be performed after menstruation has ceased but before ovulation could have taken place. It is very important to be certain the patient is not pregnant.

D. Differential Diagnostic Considerations

1. A wide variety of factors can contribute to infertility. Both male and female partners should be evaluated.

2. HSG can reveal a variety of abnormalities that contribute to infertility:

    a. Fallopian tube obstruction (usually a sequelae of PID or prior ectopic pregnancy).

    b. Absence of rugae in fallopian tubes.

    c. Congenital uterine anomaly.

    d. Intrauterine synechiae (Asherman's syndrome).

    e. Submucous fibroids distorting uterine cavity.

    f. Endometrial polyps.

3. The most common source of false-positive result for genital tract obstruction is apparent cornual or tubal occlusion due to myometrial or tubal spasm.

4. False-negative results can occur when fallopian tubes are patent but peritubal adhesions are missed because of lack of loculation of dye.

References

1. Friedman H, Vogelzang RL, Mendelson EB, Neiman HL, Cohen M (1985). Endometriosis detection by US with laparoscopic correlation. Radiology 157:217–220.

Mais V, Angiolucci M, Guerriero S, Paoletti AM et al (1993). The efficiency of transvaginal ultrasonography in the diagnosis of endometrioma. Fertil Steril 60:776–780.

Mintz MC, Grumbach K (1988). Imaging of congenital uterine anomalies. Semin Ultrasound CT MR 9:167–174.

▶ C H A P T E R 5

Pediatrics

Marilyn J. Siegel, MD
Mallinckrodt Institute of Radiology

Allen E. Schlesinger, MD
Baylor University

Michael DiPietro, MD
University of Michigan Medical Center

Imaging Handbook for House Officers, Edited by Paul M. Silverman and Douglas J. Quint.
ISBN 0-471-13767-7 © 1997 Wiley-Liss, Inc.

PREMATURITY (SUSPECTED INTRACRANIAL HEMORRHAGE)

A. Clinical Findings

1. Subependymal hemorrhage (SEH) is most common intracranial lesion of premature infant.

2. Risk factors: <1,500 g birth weight or <32 weeks gestation.

3. Etiology: Rupture of subependymal germinal matrix, located in caudothalamic groove (i.e., anterosuperior to third ventricle).

4. Acute complications of SEH: Intraventricular extension (80%), parenchymal hemorrhage or infarct (15%).

5. Symptoms: Hypotonia, seizures, apnea, coma. Occasionally asymptomatic and detected on screening examination.

6. Grading scheme: Grade 1, SEH; grade 2, SEH and intraventricular hemorrhage (IVH) without ventricular dilatation; grade 3, same as grade 2 with ventricular dilatation; grade 4, same as grade 3 with intraparenchymal hemorrhage (IPH).

7. Approximately 90% occur in first week of life.

8. Long-term morbidity: Hydrocephalus (70% patients with IVH), encephalomalacia (cystic lesions).

9. Mortality: Grade 1, <1%; grade 2, 10%; grade 3, 20%; grade 4, >50%.

B. Imaging Modalities

1. Cranial ultrasonography (ultrasound)
   a. Echogenic focus: Caudothalamic groove (SEH), ventricle (IVH), parenchyma (IPH).
   b. Ventricular dilatation.
   c. Acute hematoma hyperechoic; becomes hypoechoic within several days.
   d. Sequelae: Hydrocephalus, encephalomalacia, porencephaly (focal ventricular dilatation).
2. CT: Not indicated; premature infants are unstable, too risky to move to CT suite. (CT indicated in term infants because bleeds often extraaxial, difficult to image with ultrasound).
3. MRI: Not indicated (see above).

C. Recommended Imaging Approach

1. Ultrasound study of choice for detecting acute hemorrhage; sensitivity, >95%. Portability is advantage over CT and MRI.
2. CT or MRI study of choice to follow parenchymal changes or ventriculomegaly after anterior fontanelle has closed. Ultrasound depends on an open anterior fontanelle (normally closes about 12 months of age).

D. Differential Diagnostic Considerations

1. Choroid plexus hemorrhage.
   a. Occurs in term infants.
   b. Risk factors: Coagulopathy, heparin therapy, ECMO.
   c. Most common site is occipital horn. In contrast, germinal matrix hemorrhage involves caudothalamic groove.
   d. Ultrasound: Enlarged choroid plexus with irregular margins.
   3. CT: Hyperdense lesion.
2. Intraparenchymal hemorrhage.
   a. Affects term infants.
   b. Risk factors: Arteriovenous malformations, trauma, coagulopathy, heparin therapy, ECMO, sepsis.

      c. Ultrasound: Echogenic lesion.

      d. CT: Hyperdense lesion.

  3. Epidural hemorrhage.

      a. Older children.

      b. Etiology: Traumatic, tear of middle meningeal artery.

      c. Ultrasound/CT: Biconvex, lesion between brain and skull.

      d. Commonly associated with skull fracture.

  4. Subdural hemorrhage.

      a. Term neonate or older infant.

      b. Etiology: Trauma, tearing of falx or tentorial veins.

      c. Ultrasound/CT: Extraaxial crescentic lesion.

  5. Periventricular leukomalacia.

      a. Ischemic lesion of premature infant.

      b. Etiology: Hypoxia, resultant periventricular white matter necrosis.

      c. Clinical findings: Spastic diplegia.

      d. Ultrasound: Acute findings, increased periventricular echogenicity; chronic findings, periventricular cysts (Swiss cheese appearance).

      e. CT: decreased white matter density; cysts.

      f. MRI: T1 image, low signal; T2 image, high signal; cysts.

References

Herman TE, Siegel MJ (1992). Intracranial hemorrhage in the neonate.

Neuroimaging Clin North Am 2:107–117.

Volpe J (1989). Current concepts of brain injury in the premature infant. AJR 153:243–251.

NECK MASS (SUSPECTED CYSTIC HYGROMA)

A. Clinical Findings

  1. Cystic hygroma (lymphangioma) arises from sequestered embryonic lymph sacs.

2. Painless, compressible neck mass.
3. Almost always in posterior triangle of the neck behind sternocleidomastoid muscle; <10% extend into mediastinum.
4. Peak incidence <2 years.

B. Imaging Modalities

1. Plain films: Limited value.
2. Sonography
   1. Multilocular mass (multiple cysts surrounded by septa of variable thickness).
   b. Rarely solitary cyst.
3. CT
   a. Thin-walled, multiloculated mass, density near water.
   b. Thick walls, increased density imply hemorrhage or infection.
4. MRI
   a. Cystic areas: Low signal on T1-weighted images and high signal on T2-weighted images. Septations, low intensity both sequences.
   b. Increased signal intensity on T1-weighted images indicates hemorrhage, infection, or high lipid content.

C. Recommended Imaging Approach

1. Sonography is initial study. In small lesions no further imaging may be required.
2. MRI indicated when lesion is large and infiltrating to determine full extent (especially mediastinal and chest wall involvement) prior to surgical excision.
3. MRI preferable to CT if available, although CT is diagnostic. MRI > CT for detecting invasion of tissue planes and vessel encasement.

D. Differential Diagnostic Considerations

1. Branchial cleft cysts.
   a. Most arise from second branchial cleft.
   b. Usually painless; tender if infected.

    c. Occur near angle of mandible, along anterior border of sternocleidomastoid muscle.

    d. Imaging findings: Noninfected: thin-walled, unilocular mass; infected: thick walled, internal debris/septations. Density and signal intensity close to water.

2. Cervical abscess.

    a. Tender, enlarged cervical nodes.

    b. Submandibular and deep cervical nodes near angle of mandible most often involved.

    c. Imaging findings: Fluid-filled mass with thick enhancing rim; associated soft tissue inflammatory changes.

3. Ranula.

    a. Obstructed sublingual mucous gland.

    b. Most located in floor of mouth; occasionally descend into neck; midline location.

    c. Noninfected: Unilocular, thin-walled mass; infected: septated, thick-walled mass.

4. Teratoma.

    a. Composed of tissues from all three germ layers.

    b. Midline location, region of thyroid gland.

    c. Peak incidence: Infants.

    d. Imaging findings: Heterogeneous mass; contains calcifications, fat, fluid.

5. Dermoid cyst.

    a. Contains tissues from two germ layers.

    b. Location: Upper neck near midline.

    c. Peak incidence:<3 years.

    d. Imaging findings: Cystic mass; contains fluid, occasionally calcifications.

6. Thyroglossal duct cyst.

    a. Occurs anywhere from base of tongue to pyramidal lobe of thyroid.

    b. Most (65%) infrahyoid in location, midline.

    c. Imaging findings: Thin-walled cystic mass.

7. Cervical thymic cyst.
   a. Arises from thymopharyngeal duct.
   b. Peak incidence: 2–13 years
   c. Location: Off midline, anterior/lower neck.
   d. Imaging findings: Thin-walled, cystic mass; attached to thymus.
8. Neoplasms.
   a. Rhabdomyosarcoma: Soft tissue mass, lateral neck.
   b. Neuroblastoma: Soft tissue mass, posterior neck, paraspinal location.

References

Siegel MJ, St. Amour TE (1988). Neck. In Siegel MJ (ed); Pediatric Body CT. New York: Churchill Livingstone, pp. 293–312.

Som PM, Sacher M, Lanzieri CF et al (1985). Parenchymal cysts of the lower neck. Radiology 157:399–406.

STRIDOR (SUSPECTED EPIGLOTTITIS)

A. Clinical Findings

1. Difficulty swallowing (dysphagia), stridor, drooling, rigid neck.
2. High fever; acutely ill patient; life-threatening disease.
3. Peak incidence: 3–6 years.
4. Most frequent organism: *Haemophilus influenzae* type B.
5. Treatment: Intubation, antibiotics.

B. Imaging Modalities

1. Plain films
   a. Large, thick epiglottis ("thumb" sign).
   b. Swollen aryepiglottic folds.
   c. Effaced, small valleculae.
   d. Enlarged hypopharynx.
   e. Subglottic narrowing, 25% of cases.

C. Recommended Imaging Approach

1. Plain films are only radiographic study needed to diagnose epiglottitis. If diagnosis is suspected clinically, the examination is limited to cross-table lateral radiograph. Likelihood of airway compromise increases with movement of neck.
2. Other types of imaging studies are not needed and contraindicated because of possibility of apnea.

D. Differential Diagnostic Considerations

1. Hereditary angioneurotic edema.
   a. Allergic reaction.
   b. Autosomal dominant disease, deficiency of C1 esterase inhibitor.
   c. Swollen epiglottis and prevertebral soft tissues (latter rare in infectious epiglottis).
2. Laryngomalacia (soft larynx).
   a. Immature cartilage, resultant airway collapse (hypermobility syndrome).
   b. Peak age: Neonate.
   c. Imaging findings: Infolding (collapse) of larynx during inspiration.
   d. Self-limiting; disappears by 6–12 months.
3. Laryngocele.
   a. Rare in childhood.
   b. Imaging findings: Air-filled cyst arising from laryngeal ventricle.
4. Prevertebral cellulitis or abscess.
   a. Risk factors: Upper airway infection, penetrating injury, recent dental work.
   b. Radiographic findings: Prevertebral soft tissue thickening or air collections (suggest abscess); extrinsic compression displacement of hypopharynx; reversed cervical spine lordosis.
   c. Intrinsically normal epiglottis and subglottic area.
5. Croup (acute laryngotracheobronchitis).
   a. Peak age: 6 months to 3 years.

    b. Organisms: Parainfluenza, respiratory syncytial virus.

    c. Radiography: Symmetric subglottic narrowing (steeple sign), overdistended hypopharynx.

    d. Normal epiglottis and prevertebral soft tissues.

    e. Self-limited disease; conservative management.

6. Membranous croup.

    a. Peak age: 3 years to 3 months.

    b. Inciting organism: *Staphylococcus aureus*.

    c. Radiography: Long segment subglottic narrowing; intraluminal soft tissue densities (membranes).

    d. Normal epiglottis.

7. Neoplasms.

    a. Papilloma and hemangioma most common tumors.

    b. Papilloma, laryngeal location; hemangioma, subglottic location.

    c. Less frequent tumors: Neurofibroma, chondroma.

    d. Radiography: Soft Tissue mass.

8. Airway foreign body.

    a. Ages: 1–5 years

    b. 85% nonopaque (often peanuts; 15% opaque (toys).

    c. Radiography: Soft tissue mass in pyriform sinuses, larynx.

    d. Diagnosis occasionally made because of pulmonary findings: Obstructive emphysema (80%); atelectasis (20%).

9. Esophageal foreign body.

    a. Dysphagia and stridor, mimicking epiglottitis.

    b. Intrinsically normal upper airway.

    c. Radiography: Extrinsic displacement/compression of airway; foreign body (usually level of cricopharyngeus).

    d. Barium swallow: Intraluminal mass.

References

Macpherson RI (1985). Upper airway obstruction in children: An update. Radio-Graphics 5:339–376.

Strife JL (1988). Upper airway and tracheal obstruction in infants and children. Radiol Clin North Am 26:309–322.

NEONATAL RESPIRATORY DISTRESS (GENERAL DISCUSSION)

A. Clinical Findings

The neonatal period traditionally extends from birth to 1 month of age during which time respiratory distress can occur from several causes. These causes can be categorized according to various parameters, including the gestational age of the patient at birth, the postnatal age of the patient (minutes, hours, or days since birth), physical signs (stridor, tachypnea, grunting, cyanosis, nasal flaring, retractions) that might suggest the anatomic site of the problem, the acuteness or chronicity of the distress, perinatal history, and previous surgery.

B. Imaging Modalities

1. Plain Radiographs

Disadvantages
- Performed at bedside.
- Readily available.
- Low cost.
- Often diagnostic and all that is needed.

Disadvantages
- Ionizing radiation, which is cumulative in babies having many radiographs over long hospital stays.
- Sometimes difficult to get optimal exposures.

2. Ultrasonography

Disadvantages
- No ionizing radiation.
- Can be performed at bedside.
- Diaphragm motion, pleural effusion, and heart well-visualized.

Disadvantages
- Not useful to diagnose lung disease since it cannot see through air.
- Use limited to specific anatomy and to answer specific questions

C. Recommended Imaging Approach

Plain radiography is the initial and usually the only imaging method needed. Various projections are sometimes helpful. Since the neonate is usually supine, a pneumothorax will usually accumulate anteriorly, next to the heart. If pneumothorax is suspected but not definitely evident, a horizontal beam radiograph (cross-table lateral or lateral decubitus) will show the layered air more clearly. Patent ductus anteriosus, congenital heart disease, and extracardiac left to right shunt can be diagnosed with ultrasonography, which can also be performed at the bedside. Diaphragmatic paraly-

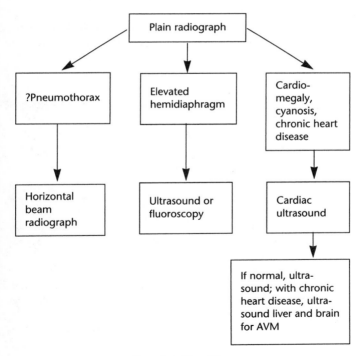

Imaging Algorithm

sis is rare and often accompanies Erb's palsy. Paradoxical motion of the involved hemidiaphragm is diagnostic as noted with ultrasonography (at the bedside) or fluoroscopy (in the radiology department). Tracheoesophageal fistula usually accompanies esophageal atresia that is obvious. Bowel gas indicates that a tracheoesophageal fistula accompanies the esophageal atresia. An H type tracheoesophageal fistula (i.e., without esophageal atresia) is diagnosed with a fluoroscopically monitored contrast esophagogram with nonionic water-soluble contrast or barium (performed carefully).

D. Differential Diagnostic Considerations

1. More common
   a. Retained fetal lung liquid (transient tachypnea of the newborn).
   b. Infant respiratory distress syndrome (hyaline membrane disease).
   c. Pneumonia (especially group B *Streptococcus*).
   d. Meconium aspiration syndrome.
   e. Persistent pulmonary hypertension in the newborn (persistent fetal circulation).
   f. Endotracheal tube malposition.
   g. Atelectasis.
   h. Pneumothorax, pneumomediastinum, pulmonary interstitial emphysema.
   i. Congestive heart failure.
2. Less common
   a. Congenital heart disease (both cyanotic and acyanotic lesions).
   b. Extracardiac (e.g., brain, liver) vascular malformations causing congestive heart failure.
   c. Diaphragmatic hernia.
   d. Congenital cystic lung lesion (congenital adenomatoid malformation, pulmonary sequestration, congenital lobar emphysema, bronchogenic cyst).
   e. Diaphragmatic paralysis or paresis.
   f. Tracheoesophageal fistula.
   g. Hypoplastic lungs.

h. Pleural effusion, chylothorax.
i. Pulmonary lymphangiectasia.
j. Choanal atresia.
k. Macroglossia.
l. Micrognathia, Pierre-Robin syndrome.

NEONATAL RESPIRATORY DISTRESS (SUSPECTED HYALINE MEMBRANE DISEASE)

A. Clinical Findings

1. Hyaline membrane disease is most common cause of neonatal respiratory distress.
2. Risk factors: Prematurity; infants of diabetic mothers.
3. Incidence: 50% at 27 weeks vs. 1% at 36 gestational weeks.
4. Etiology: Surfactant deficiency leading to decreased compliance. (Surfactant normally lowers alveolar surface tension and increases compliance.)
5. Symptoms within first 6–8 hours of life.
6. Treatment: Intubation, mechanical ventilation, supplemental oxygen, exogenous surfactant.

B. Imaging Modalities

1. Plain films
   a. Symmetric reticulogranular (ground-glass) infiltrates.
   b. Low lung volumes; air-bronchograms (hyperinflation excludes diagnosis).
   c. Absence of pleural effusions.
   d. Complications of ventilatory support: Pulmonary interstitial air, pneumothorax, pneumomediastinum, pneumopericardium.
   e. Diffusely increased lung opacity (white-out) implies superimposed atelectasis, pneumonia, pulmonary hemorrhage, or congestive heart failure.
2. Additional imaging studies: None indicated.

C. Recommended Imaging Approach

Plain radiographs are diagnostic; additional chest imaging not required.

D. Differential Diagnostic Considerations

1. Meconium aspiration.
   a. Postterm infant, meconium stained.
   b. Related to in utero fetal distress and gasping, resultant aspiration.
   c. Radiography: Hyperinflation, bilateral asymmetric coarse infiltrates.
   d. Complications of barotrauma (25%): Pneumothorax, pneumomediastinum.
   e. Treatment: Antibiotics, clearing in 3–5 days.
2. Neonatal pneumonia.
   a. Acquired in utero (transplacental spread) or perinatally, related to premature rupture of membranes or passage through infected vaginal canal.
   b. Gram-negative organisms most common: Group B *Streptococcus, E. coli, Enterococcus.*
   c. Radiography: Coarse asymmetric infiltrates, hyperinflation, pleural effusions. Rarely appearance mimicks hyaline membrane disease.
3. Transient tachypnea of newborn ("wet lung").
   a. Result of retained intrauterine fluid.
   b. Associated with cesarean section or precipitous delivery. Resultant absence of "birth canal squeeze," which normally clears lung fluid.
   c. Radiography: Well-expanded lungs, increased interstitial markings (edema), pleural effusions, fluid in fissures.
   d. Lungs clear in 24–48 hours.
4. Pulmonary lymphangiectasis.
   a. Congenital dilatation of lymphatic channels.

    b. Radiography: Well-expanded lungs, diffuse interstitial infiltrates, pleural effusions.

    c. Often fatal early in life.

5. Congestive heart failure.

    a. Result of cardiac anomalies, coarctation, extrathoracic arteriovenous malformation.

    b. Radiography: Cardiomegaly, large pulmonary vessels, interstitial/alveolar infiltrates (edema), pleural effusions.

6. Persistent fetal circulation.

    a. Increased pulmonary vascular resistance; resultant right-to-left shunting postnatally.

    b. Usually idiopathic.

    c. Radiography: Hyperinflated, clear lungs.

7. Bronchopulmonary dysplasia.

    a. Chronic pulmonary syndrome occurring in premature infants.

    b. Consequence of supplemental oxygen and barotrauma.

    c. Radiography: Hyperinflation, interstitial infiltrates, cysts (emphysematous changes), cardiomegaly (result of pulmonary hypertension).

    d. Residual pulmonary dysfunction and radiographic changes common for several years.

8. Wilson-Mikity syndrome.

    a. Onset of respiratory symptoms at 2–4 weeks of age.

    b. Etiology: Probably viral infection.

    c. Radiography: Normal chest at birth: Bronchopulmonary disease appearance by 6 weeks.

    d. Chest films usually normal by 1 year.

References

Dennehy PH (1987). Respiratory infections in the newborn. Clin Perinatol 14:667–682.

Wood BP (1993). Newborn chest. Radiol Clin North Am 31:667–676.

RECURRENT PNEUMONIA
(SUSPECTED PULMONARY SEQUESTRATION)

A. Clinical Findings

1. Sequestration is congenital mass of anomalous pulmonary tissue; fed by systemic artery from aorta; lacks normal communication with airway.
2. Symptoms: Recurrent or persistent pneumonia.
3. Occasionally asymptomatic: Incidental detection on chest films.
4. Two variants. Intralobar: Venous drainage through pulmonary veins, no separate pleural covering; extralobar: drainage through inferior vena cava, azygous vein or portal vein; own pleural covering.

B. Imaging Modalities

1. Plain radiographs
   a. Focal lower lobe infiltrate or mass near diaphragm; usually occurs in posterior basal segment of lower lobe.
   b. Cystic changes or air–fluid levels if infected.
2. Ultrasonography
   a. Lower lobe echogenic mass.
   b. Anomalous vessel arising from aorta and extending to mass.
3. CT
   a. Lower lobe infiltrate or solid mass, near diaphragm.
   b. Cystic changes or air–fluid levels if infected.
   c. Anomalous artery enhancing at same time as the aorta and extending to mass/infiltrate.
4. MRI
   a. Low signal on T1-weighted images and high signal on T2-weighted images, reflecting infection/edema.
   b. Anomalous vessel arising from the aorta.

C. Recommended Imaging Approach

1. Chest radiography is initial examination of choice to confirm presence of an infiltrate or mass.

2. Ultrasound should follow chest radiography in neonates to demonstrate anomalous artery.

3. CT or MRI should be performed after chest radiography in infants and older children, due to limitations of ultrasound (aerated lung).

4. Angiography not indicated.

D. Differential Diagnostic Considerations

1. Congenital cystic adenomatoid malformation.
   a. Result of overgrowth of terminal respiratory bronchioles.
   b. Path: Multicystic mass, communicates with airway, normal vascular supply.
   c. Symptoms: Respiratory distress in neonate; recurrent pneumonia in older infant.
   d. Upper lobes > lower lobes.
   e. Radiography/CT: Three types—single or multiple large air-filled cysts (>1 cm); multiple small cysts (<1 cm); solid mass (rare).

2. Bronchogenic cyst.
   a. Intraparenchymal masses caused by ectopic bronchial budding; no normal communication with airway; normal vascularity.
   b. Radiography/CT: Oval or round lesion; fluid density; air–fluid level if infected.

3. Foreign body.
   a. Usually nonopaque (85%).
   b. Radiography/CT: Early, hyperinflated lobe; late, atelectasis/infiltrate. Rarely, opaque foreign body seen.

4. Cystic fibrosis.
   a. Autosomal recessive disease; whites > blacks.
   b. Radiography: Hyperinflation, diffuse infiltrates, bronchiectasis, hilar lymph node enlargement; pneumothorax.
   c. Associated findings: Fatty pancreas; hepatic fibrosis/cirrhosis; meconium ileus.

5. Aspiration pneumonia.
   a. Usually neurologically impaired.

b. Radiography/CT: Lower lobe infiltrates, bronchiectasis, hilar lymph node enlargement.

6. Immunodeficiency diseases.

a. Rare cause of recurrent infection or pneumonia.

b. Bruton's disease (hypogammaglobulinemia): No adenoids or hilar lymph nodes (diagnostic clue); bronchiectasis; air-space consolidation.

c. Kartegener's syndrome (immotile cilia syndrome): Thoracic and abdominal situs inversus; air-space consolidation

d. Chronic granulomatous disease (X-linked recessive disorder; defect of intracellular killing of bacteria): Recurrent infiltrates, hilar lymph node enlargement, hepatosplenomegaly, antral narrowing on barium study.

References

Felker RE, Tonkin ILD (1990). Imaging of pulmonary sequestration. AJR 154:241–249.

Panicek DM, Heitzman ER, Randall PA et al. (1987). The continuum of pulmonary developmental anomalies. RadioGraphics 7:747–772.

ANTERIOR MEDIASTINAL MASS (SUSPECTED HODGKIN'S DISEASE)

A. Clinical Findings

1. Hodgkin's disease: Most common anterior mediastinal mass.

2. Patient age: Second decade.

3. Variable symptoms: Nontender, enlarged cervical or axillary lymph nodes; fever; cough; wheezing from tracheobronchial compression.

B. Imaging Modalities

1. Plain films

a. Superior mediastinal widening.

    b. Tracheal displacement.

    c. Pleural effusions, 15%.

    d. Lung involvement, 10%; large parenchymal mass or multiple nodules.

2. CT

    a. Enlarged mediastinal lymph nodes (prevascular/paratracheal nodes).

    b. Thymic enlargement, 40%; occasional cystic changes.

    c. Parenchymal disease, pleural effusions.

3. MRI

    a. Mediastinal lymph node enlargement.

    b. Thymic enlargement. Signal intensity equal to muscle on T1-weighted images; equal to fat on T2-weighted images. Homogeneous or heterogeneous (i.e., cystic changes).

4. Nuclear medicine: Gallium-67 imaging—active nodal and thymic disease are gallium avid. Inactive disease fails to demonstrate activity.

C. Recommended Imaging Approach

1. Chest radiography is initial study in patients with suspected Hodgkin's disease. Can detect and localize mass to a mediastinal compartment and guide subsequent studies.

2. CT is next examination to characterize mass further and determine extent.

3. ^{67}G imaging follows CT. Useful to confirm disease extent and assess response to therapy. Positive predictive value for active disease: CT, 45%; ^{67}Ga, 75%. Negative predictive value: CT and ^{67}Ga, 80%–90%.

4. MRI has no advantage over CT in evaluation of anterior mediastinum.

D. Differential Diagnostic Considerations

1. Germ cell tumors.

    a. Arise from rests of primitive cells.

       b. Benign, 90%; malignant, 10%.

       c. Imaging findings: Thick-walled cystic mass containing fluid calcification, fat, soft tissue.

       d. Local invasion, soft tissue elements >50% suggest malignancy.

  2. Thymolipoma.

       a. Benign tumor containing both thymic and adipose tissues.

       b. Age incidence: Adolescents and young adults.

       c. Imaging findings: Large mass containing soft tissue and fat.

  3. Thymoma.

       a. Very rare in children.

       b. Usually sporadic, rarely associated with myasthenia gravis, red cell aplasia.

       c. Benign, 90%; Malignant, 10%.

       d. Homogeneous CT density and signal intensity; asymmetric, focal mass in one thymic lobe.

       e. Malignant (invasive) thymomas grow through capsule; invade adjacent lung or mediastinum; spread to diaphragm by drop metastases.

  4. Benign thymic hyperplasia.

       a. Usually result of chemotherapy ("rebound" hyperplasia); rarely associated with myasthenia gravis, Grave's disease, red cell hypoplasia.

       b. Imaging: Diffusely enlarged thymus, normal density and signal intensity; no other signs of disease.

       c. Complete regression within 6 months.

  5. Thyroid masses.

       a. Extremely rare in childhood.

       b. Most represent ectopic thyroid tissue rather than direct extension of thyroid gland.

       c. Imaging features: Intensely enhancing mass.

References

Merten DF 1992. Diagnostic imaging of mediastinal masses in children. AJR 158:825–832.

Siegel MJ (1993). Diseases of the thymus in children and adolescents. Postgrad Radiol 13:106–132.

MIDDLE MEDIASTINAL MASS (SUSPECTED FOREGUT MALFORMATION)

A. Clinical Findings

1. Bronchopulmonary foregut malformations include enteric, bronchogenic, and neurenteric cysts.
2. Enteric cysts lined by gastrointestinal mucosa; bronchogenic cysts contain respiratory epithelium; neurenteric cysts contain neural and intestinal tissue.
3. Symptoms: Respiratory distress (tracheal compression) or dysphagia; occasionally asymptomatic and incidental detection on chest radiographs.

B. Imaging Modalities

1. Chest films
   a. Bronchogenic cysts: Subcarinal, paratracheal, or hilar location.
   b. Enteric duplication cysts: Middle or posterior mediastinum.
   c. Neurenteric cyst: Identical to enteric cysts except associated vertebral anomalies (hemivertebra, spina bifida, block vertebrae).
2. CT
   a. Round, water density mass.
   b. Higher density implies hemorrhage, infection, mucoid material, or milk of calcium.
3. MRI
   a. Low signal intensity mass.
   b. Increased T1 signal due to blood, infection, debris, protein.
4. Sonography
   a. Hypoechoic mass.
   b. Technically limited by aerated lung.

5. ^{99m}Tc pertechnetate
   a. Tracer uptake in lesions containing gastric mucosa.
   b. Not routinely performed.

C. Recommended Imaging Approach

1. Chest radiography is screening procedure of choice, because it establishes the presence of a mass and can localize abnormality to the middle mediastinal compartment.
2. CT follows plain chest radiography for further evaluation of character and extent of mass. Demonstration of water density mass allows specific diagnosis.
3. MRI comparable with CT. Used to confirm cystic nature of lesion with equivocal CT findings.

D. Differential Diagnostic Considerations

1. Pericardial cysts.
   a. Lined by mesothelial or endothelial cells.
   b. Communication with pericardial sac rare.
   c. Most located at right anterior cardiophrenic angle; few located superior to heart.
   d. Imaging findings: Round or oval, thin-walled, fluid-filled mass.
2. Lymphadenopathy.
   a. Causes: Neoplastic (lymphoma or leukemia) or granulomatous disease (Tb, histoplasmosis); rarely metastatic (Wilms' tumor, Ewing's sarcoma, osteogenic sarcoma, rhabdomyosarcoma).
   b. Imaging: Discreetly enlarged nodes or one conglomerate mass on CT and MRI.
   c. Soft tissue density on CT; intermediate signal intensity on T1-weighted images, and high signal intensity on T2-weighted MRI images.
   d. Calcifications frequent in granulomatous disease.
3. Fibrosing mediastinitis.
   a. Response to granulomatous infection, usually histoplasmosis.

b. Imaging findings: Multiple nodal masses surrounding compressing airway and esophagus; frequently calcify.

c. Complications: Occlusion of pulmonary artery, veins, or bronchi.

4. Neoplasms: Teratomas or hamartomas are extremely rare causes of middle mediastinal masses.

5. Vascular lesions.

a. Most common are double aortic arch and right aortic arch. Less frequent, pulmonary sling (anomalous origin of left pulmonary artery from right pulmonary artery).

b. Double arch: Posterior arch larger than anterior arch; descending aorta usually on left (left, 75%; right, 25%).

c. Right aortic arch often associated with aberrant left subclavian artery.

d. Aortic arch anomalies and pulmonary sling focally compresses trachea and esophagus.

References

Haddon MJ, Bowen A (1991). Bronchopulmonary and neurenteric forms of foregut anomalies. Imaging for diagnosis and management. Radiol Clin North Am 29:241–254.

Merten DF (1991). Diagnostic imaging of mediastinal masses in children. AJR 158:825–832.

POSTERIOR MEDIASTINAL MASS (SUSPECTED NEUROBLASTOMA)

A. Clinical Findings

1. Neuroblastoma is part of spectrum of sympathetic ganglion (small blue cell) tumors; also includes ganglioneuroblastoma and ganglioneuroma.

2. Often incidental detection on chest radiograph.

3. Occasional clinical findings: Respiratory distress, Horner's syn-

drome, bone pain if there are skeletal metastases, and hepato-megaly if there are hepatic metastases.

4. Age incidence:<5 years of age (mean, 2 years).

B. Imaging Modalities

1. Chest films
   a. Posterior mediastinal mass, calcifications.
   b. Posterior rib erosions.
   c. Intraspinal extension (widened, eroded neural foramen).
2. CT
   a. Fusiform; soft tissue mass. Extends over length of several verte-bral bodies. Calcifications frequent.
   b. Intraspinal extension, spinal cord displacement, chest wall inva-sion; bone metastases.
3. MRI
   a. Intermediate signal intensity on T1-weighted images and high signal intensity on T2-weighted images; enhance with gadolini-um administration.
   b. Intraspinal extension, spinal cord displacement; chest wall inva-sion; bone marrow involvement.
4. Myelography: No longer performed since the advent of MRI.

C. Recommended Imaging Approach

1. Chest radiograph is the screening procedure of choice for suspected mediastinal mass. Plain films localize abnormality to a mediastinal compartment, assist in differential diagnosis, and aid in selection of subsequent imaging studies.
2. MRI is the next study when chest films show a posterior mediasti-nal mass. It is more sensitive than CT in defining intraspinal exten-sion, chest wall invasion, bone marrow disease. MRI ends the imaging workup.
3. CT has largely been replaced by MRI. CT better than MRI in de-tecting calcifications, but calcifications are not clinically signifi-cant.

4. Scintigraphy is performed in all patients with suspected neuroblastoma to detect skeletal metastases. Sensitivity: Scintigraphy, 90%; plain radiographs, 30%–60%.

D. Differential Diagnostic Considerations

1. Other ganglion cell tumors: Ganglioneuroblastoma, 5–10 years of age; ganglioneuroma >10 years. Differentiation between neuroblastoma, ganglioneuroblastoma, and ganglioneuroma not possible on imaging studies, requires biopsy.
2. Ganglioneuroma.
   a. Peripheral nerve root tumor.
   b. Age incidence: >10 years.
   c. Round or oval; one or two vertebral bodies long.
3. Rare causes of posterior mediastinal masses (<1%) include posterior extension of normal thymus, enteric or neurenteric duplication cysts, abscess, extramedullary hematopoiesis.
4. Posterior thymic extension.
   a. Contiguous with normal thymus in anterior mediastinum.
   b. No mass effect.
   c. Density and signal intensity similar to normal thymus.
5. Enteric and neurenteric duplication cysts: Round, well-circumscribed mass with fluid contents; neurenteric cyst also has vertebral anomalies because it communicates with spinal canal.
6. Abscess: Well-defined mass, thick enhancing walls, fluid contents; usually associated with vertebral osteomyelitis.
7. Extramedullary hematopoiesis: Seen in thalassemia; produces multiple posterior mediastinal masses; coarsened vertebral body trabeculae.

References

Merten DF (1992). Diagnostic imaging of mediastinal masses in children. AJR 158:825–832.

Meza MP, Benson M, Slovis TL (1993). Imaging of mediastinal masses in children. Radiol Clin North Am 31:583–604.

PROJECTILE VOMITING
(SUSPECTED PYLORIC STENOSIS)

A. Clinical Findings

1. Hypertrophic pylorus stenosis is characterized by hypertrophy of circular pyloric muscle.
2. Incidence: 1 in 1,000 births, male to female ratio is 4:1.
3. History: Projectile, nonbilious vomiting.
4. Age incidence: 2–6 weeks.
5. Physical findings: Palpable, midabdominal mass ("pyloric olive"), weight loss, dehydration.

B. Imaging Modalities

1. Plain films
   a. Gastric distension secondary to retained fluid; paucity of gas distally.
   b. Irregular gastric contour, reflecting hyperperistaltic waves ("caterpillar" sign).
2. Ultrasonography
   a. Elongated pyloric channel on longitudinal image.
   b. Donut or target lesion (hypoechoic wall surrounding echogenic mucosa) on transverse view.
   c. Size criteria: Pyloric muscle thickness ≥4 mm; pyloric length ≥15 mm (normal thickness<3.5 mm; length <14 mm).
3. Upper gastrointestinal (GI) series
   a. Elongated pyloric channel ("string" sign).
   b. Mass effect on gastric antrum ("shoulder" sign).
   c. Compressed duodenal bulb.
   d. Delayed or absent gastric emptying of barium.

C. Recommended Imaging Approach

1. Ultrasound is initial imaging procedure for suspected pyloric stenosis. Sensitivity, nearly 100%. If ultrasound is positive, imaging workup terminates.

    2. If ultrasound is equivocal and clinical suspicion remains high, upper GI series is performed.

D. Differential Diagnostic Considerations

1. Pylorospasm.
   a. Characterized by delayed gastric emptying; no anatomic abnormality.
   b. Plain film: Normal.
   c. Ultrasound: Normal pyloric muscle thickness and length; delayed gastric emptying.
   d. Barium: Narrowed antrum; delayed emptying.
2. Chronic granulomatous disease.
   a. Sex-linked recessive trait; inability to kill bacteria.
   b. Plain film: Normal.
   c. Ultrasound: Thickened antral wall.
   d. Barium: Narrowed gastric antrum; delayed emptying.
3. Gastroesophageal reflux.
   a. Etiology: Idiopathic, due to immature lower esophageal sphincter; usually ceases spontaneously.
   b. Plain film: Normal.
   c. Barium: Regurgitation of contrast into esophagus; occasionally hiatal hernia.
   d. Ultrasound: Not indicated.
4. Malrotation/midgut volvulus.
   a. Developmental anomaly characterized by malfixed ligament of Treitz and shortened mesentery, allows small bowel to twist around superior mesenteric artery.
   b. Bilious vomiting in first month of life.
   c. Plain films: Normal; occasionally, bowel obstruction.
   d. Upper GI series: Malpositioned duodenum, midline or to right of midline; partial or complete obstruction of second duodenum; corkscrew appearance of small bowel; high-riding cecum.
   e. Ultrasound: Superior mesenteric artery (SMA) to right of superior mesenteric vein (SMV). (Normally SMA left of SMV).

(sensitivity, 65%; specificity, 65%). Fluid-filled proximal duodenum; ascites.

    f. Barium enema: Unreliable, 15%–20% of healthy neonates have high-riding cecum.

5. Duodenal atresia/stenosis.

    a. Bilious vomiting in first 24 hours of life. Other lesions more common after first week of life.

    b. Plain film: Double-bubble appearance (air-filled stomach and proximal descending).

    c. Ultrasound: Dilated fluid-filled stomach; normal pylorus.

    d. Upper GI: Complete obstruction of descending duodenum.

References

Bowen A (1988). The vomiting infant: Recent advances and unsettled issues in imaging. Radiol Clin North Am 26:377–392.

Haller JO, Cohen HL (1986). Hypertrophic pyloric stenosis: Diagnosis using US. Radiology 161:335–339.

NEONATAL DISTAL BOWEL OBSTRUCTION (SUSPECTED HIRSCHSPRUNG'S DISEASE)

A. Clinical Findings

1. Hirschsprung's disease (congenital megacolon): Characterized by absence of ganglion cells in myenteric plexus.

2. Extent: Distal sigmoid colon/rectum (80%); left colon to rectum (15%); total colon including distal ileum (5%).

3. Constipation in first month of life; boys > girls, 4:1.

4. Diagnosis based on rectal biopsy.

B. Imaging Modalities

1. Plain films: Low bowel obstruction, abundant feces.

2. Enema

a. Rectum narrower than sigmoid colon, ration <0.9 (normal ratio ≥0.9);

b. Dilated proximal colon.

c. Barium retention on 24-hour postevacuation film.

d. Irregular spiculated contractions in aganglionic colon ("sawtooth" sign).

C. Recommended Imaging Approach

1. Plain films are first step to identify presence of obstruction.

2. Enema (water-soluble or barium) is next study to pinpoint level of obstruction.

3. Upper GI series not indicated in distal bowel obstruction.

D. Differential Diagnostic Considerations

1. Meconium ileus.

   a. Nearly always (>98%) occurs in patients with cystic fibrosis; tenacious meconium inspissates and obstructs terminal ileum.

   b. Complications: Antenatal bowel perforation, volvulus.

   c. Plain films: Low bowel obstruction, "soap-bubble" appearance (meconium mixed with air).

   d. Contrast enema: Microcolon, normal caliber terminal ileum containing meconium pellets.

2. Meconium plug syndrome.

   a. Premature infants; infants of diabetic mothers.

   b. Inspissation of normal neconium in distal colon, result of functional colon immaturity and suboptimal peristalsis.

   c. Plain films: Distended small bowel loops.

   d. Contrast enema: Small left colon or normal-sized colon with filling defects (meconium plugs); normal caliber transverse/right colon.

   e. Osmotic diarrhea after water-soluble enema causes expulsion of meconium, usually therapeutic.

3. Duplication cysts.

    a. Terminal ileum most common site; obstruction result of extrinsic bowel compression.

    b. Plain films: Distended small bowel loops; soft tissue mass.

    c. Contrast enema: Normal caliber colon, extrinsic mass effect on terminal ileum.

    d. Ultrasound: Cyst with echogenic mucosal lining.

4. Ileal atresia.

    a. Due to fetal vascular accident.

    b. Maternal polyhydramnios, 20%–40% of cases.

    c. Plain films: Dilated small bowel loops; calcification 15% (meconium peritonitis); loculated, extraluminal air collection (pseudocyst, due to walled-off in utero perforation).

    d. Contrast enema: Microcolon (small colon due to disuse); no reflux into bowel proximal to atresia.

5. Imperforate anus.

    a. Failure to pass meconium (clue: absent anus).

    b. Associated anomalies common: Vertebral anomalies; tracheoesophageal fistula, renal anomalies, radial hypoplasia or absence (VATER association).

    c. Plain films: Distended bowel loops; vertebral anomalies.

    d. Transperineal contrast injection: Blind-ending pouch (distal rectum); fistula between rectum and adjacent structure (fistula to urethra in boys, vagina in girls, or perineum in both).

6. Colonic atresia.

    a. Rare; 1:40,000 live births.

    b. Plain films: Low bowel obstruction.

    c. Contrast enema: Filling of distal colon; no reflux into proximal bowel.

References

Berdon WE, Baker DH (1965). Roentgenographic diagnosis of Hirschsprung's disease in infancy. AJR 93:432–446.

Pochaczevsky R, Leonidas JC (1974). Meconium plug syndrome—Roentgenographic evaluation and differentiation from Hirschsprung's disease and other pathologic states. AJR 120:342–352.

PAINLESS RECTAL BLEEDING (SUSPECTED MECKEL'S DIVERTICULUM)

A. Clinical Findings

1. Omphalomesenteric duct remnant; near distal ileum.
2. Epithelial lined; ectopic gastric mucosa, 10% (100% bleeding diverticula).
3. Age incidence: <2 years of age.
4. Symptoms: Rectal bleeding (ulcerating gastric mucosa); pain (bowel obstruction).

B. Imaging Modalities

1. Plain films: Usually normal, occasionally show obstruction.
2. Upper GI series/barium enema: Usually normal; rarely shows mass effect on terminal ileum or filling of blind-ending diverticulum.
3. Scintigraphy
   a. Tracer: ^{99m}Tc pertechnetate; sensitivity 95% (taken up by gastric mucosa).
   b. Findings: Focal tracer accumulation in right lower quadrant.
4. Sonography: Not indicated.
5. Angiography: Not indicated.

C. Recommended Imaging Approach

1. Scintigraphy is study of choice for suspected Meckel's diverticulum.
2. Barium examinations usually not needed for diagnosis. In equivocal cases may show extrinsic mass effect on bowel or intussusception.

D. Differential Diagnostic Considerations

1. Intussusception.
   a. Invagination of proximal bowel into distal bowel; ileocolic most common.

b. Age incidence: 3 months to 2 years.

c. Clinical findings: Abdominal pain (85%–90%), vomiting (80%–90%), red currant-jelly stools (60%–65%), palpable abdominal mass (55%—65%).

d. Plain films: Mass in right abdomen.

e. Barium or air enema findings: Soft tissue mass, usually within transverse or right colon.

2. Intestinal duplication.

a. Age incidence: 1 month to 2 years.

b. Symptoms: Mass, pain, GI bleed due to ulcerating gastric mucosa (15% of duplications).

c. Plain x-rays: Soft tissue mass, bowel obstruction.

d. Ultrasound: Round, hypoechoic or anechoic mass with echogenic mucosal lining.

e. Scintigraphy (^{99m}Tc pertechnetate): Focal tracer accumulation in diverticula containing gastric mucosa (10%).

3. Juvenile polyps.

a. Age incidence: 1–10 years.

b. Painless, bright red rectal bleeding.

c. Pathology: Inflammatory or retention polyps.

d. Location: 75% rectosigmoid or descending colon; 15% transverse colon; 10% right colon.

e. Air contrast enema: Round or oval, polypoid mass.

4. Crohn's disease.

a. Age incidence: >10 years.

b. Clinical findings: Abdominal pain, diarrhea, rectal bleeding, perirectal fistulas.

c. Contrast studies: Ulcerated terminal ileum or colon, fistulas, mass (abscess); skip areas (normal bowel alternating with involved bowel).

d. Ultrasound: Thickened ileal wall.

5. Ulcerative colitis.

a. Age incidence: >10 years.

b. Symptoms: Diarrhea, abdominal pain, rectal bleeding.

   c. Contrast enema: Early, mild mucosal edema/granularity; late, large ulcers; shortened colon; loss of haustration.

   d. Disease sites: Rectosigmoid, 25%; transverse/left colon, 50%; entire colon, 25%.

6. Infectious colitis.
   a. *E. coli, Salmonella, Shigella, Yersinia* common pathogens.
   b. Symptoms: Diarrhea, abdominal pain, GI bleeding.
   c. Contrast studies: Nodular, thickened folds.

7. Typhlitis.
   a. Affects neutropenic children.
   b. *Pseudomonas,* cytomegalovirus common pathogens, resultant necrotizing colitis.
   c. Plain films: Thickened cecal wall, pneumatosis.
   d. Ultrasound: Thickened, avascular cecal wall.

References

Bisset GS III, Kirks DR (1988). Intussusception in infants and children: Diagnosis and therapy. Radiology 168:141–145.

Treem WR (1994). Gastrointestinal bleeding in children. Gastrointest Endosc Clin North Am 4:75–97.

ACUTE RIGHT LOWER QUADRANT PAIN (SUSPECTED APPENDICITIS)

A. Clinical Findings

1. Age: >10 years.
2. Acute right lower quadrant (RLQ) pain, fever, nausea, anorexia, leukocytosis.
3. Right flank pain when appendix is in retrocecal location.
4. Perforation: 30%–40%.

B. Imaging Modalities

1. Plain films
   a. Localized ileus RLQ (70%).

    b. Mass in RLQ or pelvis (25%).

    c. Obliterated properitoneal fat stripe (15%).

    d. Appendicolith (10%).

    e. Obstructed small bowel loops.

2. Ultrasonography

    a. Blind-ending, fluid-filled, noncompressible tube, >6 mm in outer diameter; hypervascular wall.

    b. RLQ or pelvic abscess, indicates perforation.

    c. Enlarged mesenteric lymph nodes.

3. Barium enema

    a. Nonfilling of appendix; extrinsic mass effect on cecum or terminal ileum.

    b. Complete appendiceal filling excludes diagnosis.

    c. Pitfall: 50% of normal appendices do not fill on barium enema.

C. Recommended Imaging Approach

1. Plain abdominal radiograph performed first to identify presence of an appendicolith or small bowel obstruction. If these findings present, no additional imaging needed.

2. In patients with normal radiographs or atypical clinical findings (35%), ultrasound performed next. If ultrasound diagnostic, surgery indicated. If ultrasound demonstrates walled-off abscess, CT performed to guide percutaneous drainage.

3. Barium enema: Not indicated.

D. Differential Diagnostic Considerations

1. Normal appendix.

    a. Identified in 5%–10% of healthy children on ultrasound.

    b. Ultrasound: <6 mm in diameter, compressible, no adjacent inflammatory changes. Size and compressibility help to differentiate between normal and abnormal appendix.

2. Meckel's diverticulum.

    a. Age incidence: <10 years.

    b. Symptoms: Pain, with or without bleeding.

    c. Ultrasound: Usually normal; rarely, blind-ending tube, mimics appendicitis. Differentiation requires surgery.

3. Crohn's disease.
    a. Age incidence: >10 years.
    b. Acute onset mimics appendicitis.
    c. Plain films: Normal or RLQ mass.
    d. Ultrasound: Thick-walled ileum, hypervascular.
    e. Barium enema: Ulcerated ileum/colon.

4. Mesenteric adenitis.
    a. Viral etiology common; rarely *Yersinia*.
    b. Age incidence: >5 years.
    c. Symptoms: Pain, fever.
    d. Sonography: Enlarged RLQ mesenteric nodes; normal bowel.

5. Hemorrhagic ovarian cyst.
    a. Age incidence: Adolescent girl.
    b. Acute pelvic pain, but no fever or leukocytosis.
    c. Plain radiographs: Normal
    d. Sonography: Ovarian cyst with internal debris.

6. Adnexal torsion.
    a. Age incidence: Prepubertal or adolescent girl.
    b. Symptoms: Pain, fever, leukocytosis.
    c. May be idiopathic or associated with tumor or cyst.
    d. Plain films: normal.
    e. Ultrasound: Enlarged ovary with dilated peripheral follicles; cul-de-sac fluid; no flow on color Doppler ultrasound.

7. Pelvic inflammatory disease.
    a. Age incidence: Adolescent girls.
    b. Symptoms: Acute pelvic pain, tender cervix, vaginal discharge.
    c. Ultrasound: Swollen uterus; dilated fallopian tube (pyosalpinx); ovarian or peritoneal abscesses.

References

Siegel MJ, Carel C, Surratt S (1991). Ultrasonography of acute abdominal pain in children. JAMA 14:1987–1989.

Winsey HS (1967). Acute abdominal pain in childhood: Analysis of a year's admissions. BMJ 1:653–655.

NEONATAL JAUNDICE (SUSPECTED BILIARY ATRESIA)

A. Clinical Findings

1. Age incidence: Infant <4 weeks of age.
2. Most likely sequelae of in utero hepatitis with sclerosing cholangitis.
3. Signs: Cholestatic jaundice, hepatomegaly, hyperbilirubinemia.
4. Complication: Cirrhosis in patients diagnosed after 3 months of age.

B. Imaging Modalities

1. Ultrasonography
   a. Early, normal hepatic parenchyma; late, cirrhosis (small, heterogeneous liver, irregular margins).
   b. Gallbladder: Absent, 80%; normal or small, 20%.
   c. Nonvisualized common bile duct (CBD).
2. Scintigraphy
   a. Tracer: ^{99m}Tc iminodiacetic acid (IDA) derivatives.
   b. IDA scan; sensitivity, 97%; specificity, 82%.
   c. Good hepatic extraction unless cirrhosis develops.
   d. No bowel excretion at 24 hours.
   e. Increased renal excretion.
3. Cholangiography: Absent or hypoplastic intrahepatic ducts; with or without atresia.

C. Recommended Imaging Approach

1. Ultrasound is initial study in jaundiced neonates. Cannot provide specific diagnosis of biliary atresia because findings are nonspecific, but is useful to exclude other causes of jaundice (choledochal cysts, perforated bile ducts).

2. Scintigraphy is next examination. If scintigraphy is positive, intra-operative cholangiogram is performed to identify anatomy. Primary anastomosis feasible if proximal common hepatic duct patent (15% cases); portoenterostomy (Kasai procedure) used with total ductal atresia (>85% cases).

D. Differential Diagnostic Considerations

1. Neonatal hepatitis.
   a. Symptoms similar to biliary atresia.
   b. Ultrasound: Normal or heterogeneous hepatic parenchyma; visualized gallbladder in nearly all patients.
   c. Scintigraphy: Delayed hepatic uptake of tracer, bowel activity at 24 hours, frequent gallbladder visualization.
2. Spontaneous perforation of the bile ducts.
   a. Clinical history: Jaundice.
   b. Normal hepatic enzymes; in contrast, abnormal liver function tests in biliary atresia and neonatal hepatitis.
   c. Ultrasound: Ascites, normal hepatic parenchyma, gallbladder, and distal common bile duct calculi.
   d. Scintigraphy: Leakage of tracer into peritoneal cavity; good hepatic extraction and duodenal emptying.
   e. Treatment: Spontaneous closure after simple drainage of ascitic fluid; direct ductal repair not required.
3. Choledochal cyst.
   a. Congenital dilatation of common bile duct.
   b. Age incidence: None.
   c. Symptoms: Jaundice (80%), palpable right upper quadrant mass (50%), abdominal pain (50%).
   d. Ultrasound: Cystic mass in hepatic hilum (i.e., dilated common bile duct); dilated proximal right and left hepatic ducts.
   e. ^{99m}Tc IDA scintigraphy: Normal hepatic uptake; tracer accumulation in cyst; delayed bowel excretion.
   f. Treatment: Total excision, enteric drainage of residual duct.
4. Syndromic causes of neonatal cholestasis.

   a. Arteriohepatic dysplasia (Alagille syndrome): Decreased inter-lobular ducts; vertebral anomalies.
   b. α_1-Antitrypsin deficiency.
5. Nonsyndromic disorders.
   a. Metabolic disorders: Tyrosinemia, galactosemia, glycogen storage disease, cystic fibrosis, hemochromatosis.
   b. Infection: Toxoplasmosis, rubella virus, herpes virus, cytomegalovirus, Coxsackie virus.
   c. Parenteral nutrition.
   d. Sepsis.
   e. Congenital bile duct hypoplasia.
   f. Imaging findings (nonsyndromic and syndromic disorders): Similar to neonatal hepatitis.

References

Balistreri WF (1985). Neonatal cholestasis. J Pediatr 106:171–184.

Haller JO (1991). Sonography of the biliary tract in infants and children. AJR 157:1051–1058.

URINARY TRACT INFECTION (SUSPECTED ACUTE PYELONEPHRITIS)

A. Clinical Findings

1. Urinary tract infection defined as >100,000 bacterial organisms/ml in a sterilely collected urine specimen.
2. Risk factors: Vesicoureteral reflux; sepsis, urinary obstruction.
3. Most common pathogens: *E. coli, Proteus* species, *Staphylococcus aureus.*
4. Symptoms: Flank pain, dysuria, fever, hematuria.
5. Complications: Abscess, renal scarring, renal failure.
6. Imaging indicated for first urinary tract infection in both boys and girls.
7. Role of imaging: Detect anatomic abnormality (vesicoureteral reflux, obstruction), abscess, scarring.

B. Imaging Modalities

1. Voiding cystourethrogram (VCUG)
   a. Radiographic VCUG: Iodinated contrast used to detect urine reflux from bladder into ureter and/or kidney.
   b. Nuclear VCUG: Performed with ^{99m}Tc pertechnetate. Tracer in ureter or collecting system diagnostic of reflux.
   c. Anatomic resolution: Radiographic > nuclear VCUG.
   d. Radiation dose: Nuclear < radiographic VCUG (5% of dose from radiographic VCUG).

2. Excretory urogram
   a. Renal enlargement, attenuated collecting system, delayed excretion (edema).
   b. Cortical irregularity, thinning (scarring).
   c. Pelvocalyceal dilatation (obstruction or reflux).

3. Ultrasonography
   a. Focal or diffuse increased echogenicity (edema), nephromegaly.
   b. Pelvocalyceal dilatation (obstruction or reflux).
   c. Cortical irregularity, thinning (scarring).
   d. Well-defined, hypoechoic mass (abscess).
   e. Sensitivity: Grayscale, 25%; color Doppler, 50%.

4. Renal scintigraphy (radionuclide scan)
   a. Performed with cortical agents: ^{99m}Tc glucoheptonate or ^{99m}Tc dimercaptosuccinic acid (DMSA).
   b. Acute infection: Focal decreased cortical activity.
   c. Sensitivity, 65%–90%; specificity, >95%.

5. CT
   a. Nephromegaly, delayed contrast excretion (edema).
   b. Patchy enhancement or hypodense areas (edema).
   c. Hypodense mass with enhancing wall (abscess).

C. Recommended Imaging Approach

1. Child <5 years of age with well-documented urinary tract infection: Radiographic VCUG performed first to diagnose reflux, followed

by ultrasound and renal scan. Ultrasound to diagnose anatomic abnormality; renal scan to detect parenchymal damage. CT performed if renal abscess suspected on ultrasound.

2. Older child/adolescent: Ultrasound is screening study of choice. If normal, imaging terminated. Abnormal ultrasound followed by VCUG and renal scan.
3. Treated reflux is followed with nuclear VCUG (lower radiation dose).

D. Differential Diagnostic Considerations

1. Focal cortical (junctional) defect.
   a. Developmental variant; represents junction line between embryonic renal lobules.
   b. Imaging features: Cortex irregular, but not thinned; normal-sized kidney. (In contrast, scarring produces parenchymal thinning, small kidney).
2. Other "medical" renal diseases.
   a. Acute glomerulonephritis, nephrotic syndrome, Henoch-Schonlein purpura, hemolytic uremic syndrome; renal vein thrombosis.
   b. Symptoms: Abdominal pain, hematuria, renal failure, body wall edema.
   c. Ultrasound: Increased cortical echogenicity; nephromegaly; no cortical thinning.
   d. Differentiation based on clinical findings.
3. Fungal pyelonephritis.
   a. Most common pathogen: *Candida albicans*.
   b. Risk factors: Indwelling catheters, immunodeficiency diseases, prolonged antibiotic therapy.
   c. Ultrasound: Nephromegaly; increased echogenicity; hydronephrosis; echogenic mobile masses in renal pelvis or calyces (fungal balls).

References

Bjorgvinsson E, Majd M, Eggli KD (1991). Diagnosis of acute pyelonephritis in children: Comparison of sonography and ^{99m}Tc-DMSA scintigraphy. AJR 157:539–543.

Lebowitz RL, Mandell J (1987). Urinary tract infection in children: Putting radiology in its place. Radiology 165:1–9.

ABDOMINAL MASS IN A CHILD (SUSPECTED WILMS' TUMOR)

A. Clinical Findings

1. Wilms' tumor, most common renal neoplasm of childhood.
2. Mean patient age: 2 years.
3. Abdominal mass (90%); fever, anorexia, hematuria (5%–15%); hypertension (90%).
4. Common anomalies: Aniridia, hemihypertrophy, Beckwith-Wiedemann syndrome (macroglossia, omphalocele, visceromegaly).

B. Imaging Modalities

1. Plain films: Large soft tissue mass displacing bowel.
2. Ultrasonography
   a. Echogenic mass, 12 cm mean diameter, necrotic.
   b. Associated findings: Lymph node enlargement, bilateral tumors, hepatic metastases, tumor extension into renal vein and/or inferior vena cava.
3. CT
   a. Large soft tissue mass, minimal contrast enhancement.
   b. Central necrosis, 80%; calcification, 10%.
   c. Associated findings, same as on ultrasound.
   d. Extraabdominal findings: Pulmonary metastases.
4. MRI
   a. Low signal intensity on T1-weighted images, high signal intensity on T2-weighted images, enhancement with gadolinium administration.
   b. Associated findings, same as in with ultrasound.
5. Excretory urography: No longer performed.

C. Recommended Imaging Approach

1. Plain radiograph is initial study in evaluation of abdominal mass. It can indicate general location of the mass, demonstrate calcifications, and assess GI tract for obstruction or fecal contents. Obstructed bowel loops and feces can simulate mass.

2. In absence of obstruction, ultrasound is next study. If ultrasound demonstrates cystic mass (i.e., hydronephrosis), scintigraphy is indicated to evaluate renal function. If ultrasound shows solid mass suggesting Wilms' tumor, CT is performed. CT > ultrasound in determining local extension and pulmonary metastases.

3. MRI is not performed unless there is inferior vena caval extension of tumor. MRI > CT for determining extent of vascular invasion for surgical planning.

D. Differential Diagnostic Considerations

1. Mesoblastic nephroma.
   a. Most common neonatal renal mass; benign.
   b. Imaging findings: Large, solid intrarenal mass. Mimics Wilms' tumor, but patient age (under 1 year) is diagnostic clue.

2. Nephroblastomatosis.
   a. Represents persistence of primitive nephrogenic blastema.
   b. Not malignant per se, but it precursor to Wilms' tumor.
   c. Imaging findings: Nephromegaly, peripheral cortical or subcapsular masses.

3. Multilocular cystic nephroma.
   a. Boys > girls; <4 years of age.
   b. Most benign; rarely Wilms' tumor found in cyst wall.
   c. Imaging findings: Multilocular mass containing fluid-filled cysts and soft tissue septations.

4. Rare renal tumors.
   a. Renal cell carcinoma: Appearance mimics Wilms' tumor, but patient age (9–10 years) is clue.
   b. Clear cell sarcoma: Intrarenal mass, subcapsular fluid, bone metastases.

    c. Rhabdoid tumor: Intrarenal mass, subcapsular fluid, brain tumors.

    d. Lymphoma: Multiple masses, splenomegaly, retroperitoneal adenopathy.

5. Angiomyolipoma.

    a. Almost always associated with tuberous sclerosis.

    b. Fatty mass.

6. Neuroblastoma.

    a. Arises in adrenal medulla or sympathetic ganglia.

    b. Mean patient age: 2 years.

    c. Imaging findings: Large, solid, extrarenal, tumor; calcifications, 85%; midline extension; vessel encasement, intraspinal tumor.

    d. Metastases to skeleton, liver, lymph nodes.

References

Donaldson JS, Shkolnik A (1988). Pediatric renal masses. Semin Roentgenol 23:194–204.

Mahaffey SM, Ryckman FC, Martin LW (1988). Clinical aspects of abdominal masses in children. Semin Roentgenol 23:161–174.

UNILATERAL FLANK MASS IN A NEONATE (SUSPECTED HYDRONEPHROSIS)

A. Clinical Findings

1. Hydronephrosis is most common cause of neonatal abdominal mass.

2. Most neonatal hydronephrosis diagnosed prenatally.

3. Postnatally, patients present with palpable mass abdominal distention, or urinary tract infection.

B. Imaging Modalities

1. Plain films: Soft tissue mass displacing bowel loops.

2. Ultrasonography

       a. Pelvocalyceal dilatation, thin parenchyma.

       b. Ureteral dilatation suggests distal obstruction (normal ureter not seen on ultrasound).

3. Renal scintigraphy

       a. Tracer: DTPA (filtered) or Mag 3 (tubular excretion).

       b. Delayed tracer accumulation in collecting system.

4. Voiding cystourethrography (VCUG)

       a. Vesicoureteral reflux.

       b. Bladder/urethral anomalies (i.e., ureteral ectopia, posterior urethral valves, prune-belly syndrome).

5. Excretory urography: Not indicated; replaced by scintigraphy.

C. Recommended Imaging Approach

1. Ultrasound is first examination when neonatal hydronephrosis suspected. Normal ultrasound virtually excludes obstructed hydronephrosis.

2. VCUG and renal scan performed if ultrasound abnormal. VCUG used to diagnose reflux, which can cause urinary tract dilatation. Renal scan, especially with furosemide (loads collecting system with extra urine) is helpful in assessing severity of obstruction.

D. Differential Diagnostic Considerations

1. Ureteropelvic junction and ureterovesical junction obstruction comprise 65% of hydronephrosis. Reflux, duplication anomalies, posterior urethral valves, and prune-belly syndrome comprise remainder.

2. Ureteropelvic junction obstruction.

       a. Imaging findings: Calyceal/renal pelvic dilatation, thin parenchyma, normal caliber ureter.

       b. Extrarenal pelvis may mimic obstruction. Diuretic renal scintigraphy helpful in differentiating between prominent pelvis and hydronephrosis.

3. Ureterovesical junction obstruction.

       a. Functional or mechanical distal ureteral obstruction.

    b. Imaging findings: Calyceal/renal pelvic dilatation, ureteral dilatation to level of obstruction.

4. Duplicated collecting system.

    a. Kidney drained by two ureters. Upper pole ureter inserts into bladder inferomedially to trigone (ectopic) or into uterus, vagina, epididymis or urethra. Lower pole ureter inserts into normal trigonal position (orthotopic). Ectopic ureter often obstructed and associated with a ureterocele (dilated distal ureter herniating into bladder).

    b. Imaging findings: Dilated (obstructed) upper pole, parenchymal thinning, dilated tortuous ureter, ureterocele. Lower pole may reflux.

5. Posterior urethral valves.

    a. Most common cause of bilateral hydronephrosis in newborn boys.

    b. Imaging findings: Bilateral dilated calyces, renal pelvis, ureters; thin parenchyma; thick bladder wall; dilated prostatic urethra; normal anterior urethra. Vesicoureteral reflux often present.

6. Prune-belly (Eagle-Barrett) syndrome.

    a. Triad of absent abdominal musculature, urinary tract anomalies, undescended testes.

    b. Imaging findings: Dilated calyces, renal pelvis, ureters; thin-walled bladder; dilated proximal and/or anterior urethra. Clinical findings of wrinkled abdomen and undescended testes separate prune-belly syndrome from posterior valves.

7. Multicystic dysplastic kidney.

    a. Second most common neonatal abdominal mass.

    b. Multiple cysts of varying size; absent renal pelvis; no normal parenchyma; nonfunctioning on scintigraphy.

    c. Contralateral renal anomaly (20%).

    d. Majority (65%) regress or involute spontaneously.

References

Brown T, Mandell J, Lebowitz RL (1987). Neonatal hydronephrosis in the era of sonography. AJR 148:959–963.

Strife JL, Souza AS, Kirks DR et al (1993). Multicystic dysplastic kidney in children: US follow-up. Radiology 186:785–788.

SCROTAL PAIN (SUSPECTED TORSION)

A. Clinical Findings

1. Acute onset of testicular pain and swelling.
2. Affects adolescent patients.
3. Etiology believed to be malfixation of testis: Tunica vaginalis completely surrounds testis and spermatic cord, allowing testis to twist on its vascular pedicle.
4. Physical exam: Tender testis with transverse lie (bell-clapper deformity); swollen, erythematous hemiscrotum.
5. Prompt diagnosis important because testicular viability declines abruptly after 6 hours.

B. Imaging Modalities

1. Ultrasonography
   a. Normal testicular echogenicity first 4–6 hours of symptoms; absent flow.
   b. Enlarged, hypoechoic testis after 4–6 hours; absent flow.
   c. Heterogeneous testis after 24 hours; soft tissue hyperemia.
   d. Other findings: Enlarged epididymis, hydrocele.
   f. Sensitivity: Pubertal boys, 90%–100%; prepubertal, unknown.
2. Scintigraphy
   a. Decreased perfusion in first 24 hours ("cold" testis).
   b. Hypervascular peripheral soft tissues after 24 hours (rim sign).
   c. Sensitivity; 90%–100%.

C. Recommended Imaging Approach

1. When clinical suspicion of torsion is high, emergency surgery is indicated. Diagnostic imaging not warranted because any delay in surgical treatment reduces likelihood of testicular salvage.

2. Imaging is performed in patients with an acute scrotum in whom clinical diagnosis is equivocal and to confirm torsion in patients with prolonged symptoms (>24–36 hours) when surgical salvage of the testis unlikely. Ultrasound preferred in adolescent patients. In prepubertal boys, scintigraphy preferred, because testicular arteries are small and detection of flow can be difficult on ultrasound.

D. Differential Diagnostic Considerations

1. Acute epididymitis.
   a. More common in pubertal than prepubertal boys.
   b. Pubertal boys: Sexually transmitted.
   c. Prepubertal boys: Idiopathic or associated with genitourinary abnormalities.
   d. Clinical findings: Scrotal edema, pain, tenderness, fever.
   e. Ultrasound findings: Enlarged, hypervascular epididymis. Associated findings: Reactive hydrocele; testicular enlargement due to orchitis; testicular abscess; thickened scrotal skin.
   f. Scintigraphy: Increased epididymal/testicular flow.
2. Torsion of appendix testis.
   a. Age incidence: 6–12 years.
   b. Physical findings: Small, firm, paratesticular nodule in upper scrotum.
   c. Ultrasound: Small, hyper- or hypoechoic mass adjacent to testis or epididymis, hypervascular on color-flow images.
   d. Scintigraphy: Increased perfusion.
3. Henoch-Schonlein purpura.
   a. Testis and scrotum involved in 15%–40% of cases.
   b. Ultrasound: Normal testis, enlarged epididymis, reactive hydrocele, scrotal skin swelling. Epididymal hyperperfusion on color-flow imaging; normal testicular flow.
4. Idiopathic scrotal edema.
   a. Age incidence: <10 years.
   b. Ultrasound: Thickened scrotal skin; hypervascular on color-flow imaging; normal epididymis and testis.

References

Atkinson GO Jr, Patrick LE, Ball TI, Stephenson CA, Broecker BH, Woodard JR (1992). The normal and abnormal scrotum in children: Evaluation with color Doppler sonography. AJR 158:613–617.

Luker GD, Siegel MJ (1994). Color Doppler sonography of the scrotum in children. AJR 163:649–655.

LIMP AND FEVER (SUSPECTED SEPTIC ARTHRITIS)

A. Clinical Findings

1. Irritability, lack of lower extremity movement, fever, leukocytosis.
2. Hip held in flexion, abduction, and external rotation.
3. Etiology: Hematogenous infection; direct implantation related to penetrating injury; contiguous extension from focus of osteomyelitis.
4. Common organisms: <2 years, group B *Streptococcus/Haemophilus influenzae*; >2 years, *Staphylococcus aureus*.

B. Imaging Modalities

1. Plain films
   a. Normal early in disease.
   b. Late changes: Asymmetric fat planes around obturator, psoas, gluteal muscles; laterally displaced femoral head.
2. Bone scintigraphy (radionuclide scan)
   a. Tracer: ^{99m}Tc methylene diphosphonate (MDP).
   b. Absence of tracer in femoral head (photopenic), result of compressed vascular supply by joint fluid.
   c. Associated osteomyelitis: Focally increased skeletal activity ("hot" spot).
3. Ultrasonography
   a. Joint effusion: Distended joint capsule (>3 mm) with convex margin (normal margin is concave).

　　　b. Transudate often hypoechoic; hemorrhage/exudate often echo-
　　　　genic.
　　4. CT: Not indicated in acute septic arthritis.

C. Recommended Imaging Approach

　　1. Plain radiograph is first examination for suspected septic arthritis.
　　　Plain radiographs can demonstrate hip displacement and changes
　　　of osteomyelitis. If films are diagnostic, no further imaging need-
　　　ed. If films are normal, ultrasound performed. More sensitive than
　　　plain radiographs for detecting joint fluid (sensitivity, >90%).
　　2. Scintigraphy performed after ultrasound to determine presence or
　　　absence of osteomyelitis.

D. Differential Diagnostic Considerations

　　1. Toxic (transient) synovitis.
　　　a. Age incidence <10 years.
　　　b. Etiology: Probable recent viral infection or allergic reaction.
　　　c. Clinical findings: Acute hip pain or limp; low grade fever; mild
　　　　leukocytosis.
　　　d. Plain films: Normal or subluxed femoral head.
　　　e. Ultrasound: Joint fluid. Joint aspiration required to exclude sep-
　　　　tic arthritis.
　　　f. Spontaneous improvement within 24–48 hours.
　　2. Acute osteomyelitis.
　　　a. Primarily affects metaphysis of long bones.
　　　b. Plain films: Early (<7–10 days), normal or soft tissue swelling;
　　　　late (>10 days), bone destruction.
　　　c. Scintigraphy: Focus of increased bone activity.
　　3. Legg-Calvé-Perthes disease.
　　　a. Avascular necrosis of femoral head.
　　　b. Age incidence: Boys, 5–8 years.
　　　c. Bilateral 15% of cases.
　　　d. Films: Fragmented, flattened, sclerotic femoral epiphyses.

4. Slipped capital femoral epiphyses.
   a. Fracture of proximal femoral growth plate.
   b. Cause: Unknown.
   c. Age incidence: Overweight teenagers.
   d. Clinical findings: Pain, often history of trauma.
   e. Films: Displaced femoral epiphysis, widened growth plate; bilateral 20%–25% of cases.
5. Juvenile rheumatoid arthritis.
   a. Joint findings (100%): Soft tissue swelling, epiphyseal overgrowth, osteopenia, periosteal new bone formation, bony erosions.
   b. Occasional splenomegaly, lymphadenopathy (Still's disease).

References

Majd M, Frankel RS (1976). Radionuclide imaging in skeletal inflammatory and ischemic disease in children. Radiology 126:832–841.

Miralles M, Gonzalez G, Pulpeiro JR et al. (1989). Sonography of the painful hip in children: 500 consecutive cases. AJR 152:579–582.

BACK PAIN AND FEVER (SUSPECTED DISCITIS)

A. Clinical Findings

1. Discitis: Inflammatory lesion of vertebral disc spaces.
2. Age incidence: Two peaks, 6 months to 4 years and 10–14 years.
3. Symptoms: Back pain and tenderness, limp, fever.
4. Etiology: *Staphylococcus aureus*; low-grade viral infection.

B. Imaging Modalities

1. Plain films
   a. Normal in first 10 days of infection.
   b. Narrowed disc space (10–14 days after onset of infection).

    c. Late changes: Destruction of vertebral endplates; disc space calcification.

    d. Complications: Vertebral osteomyelitis (destroyed vertebral bodies).

2. Bone scintigraphy

    a. Increased uptake in vertebral bodies on either side of involved disc space.

    b. Positive as early as 2 days after onset of infection.

3. CT

    a. Narrowed disc space.

    b. Vertebral body destruction.

    c. Paraspinal soft tissue mass.

4. MRI

    a. Narrowed disc space.

    b. Abnormal signal in vertebral bodies on either side of disc, reflecting edema or infection.

    c. Paraspinal mass.

C. Recommended Imaging Approach

1. Plain radiographs are always obtained first. Despite their insensitivity for discitis early, they can exclude other lesions (tumors or fractures).

2. Scintigraphy is next examination. Scans are more sensitive and abnormal earlier than radiographs. Negative bone scan usually terminates workup for discitis.

3. If scintigraphy abnormal, MRI performed to determine disease extent, especially intraspinal extension.

D. Differential Diagnostic Considerations

1. Osteoid osteoma.

    a. Benign tumor containing osteoid and connective tissue.

    b. Age incidence: 10–12 years.

    c. Most involve neural arches.

    d. Symptoms: Back pain, worse at night, relieved by aspirin.

    e. Radiography/CT: Sclerotic lesion with lucent center (nidus); calcification in nidus.

    f. Scintigraphy: Avid uptake of tracer.

2. Spondylolysis (stress fracture).

    a. Age incidence: 5–7 years.

    b. Involves pars interarticularis

    c. Radiography/CT: Defect in neural arch.

    d. Scintigraphy: Increased uptake of tracer.

3. Herniated disc.

    a. Extremely rare in childhood.

    b. Age incidence: 12–16 years.

    c. Radiography/CT: Disc space narrowing; normal vertebral bodies.

    d. Scintigraphy usually normal.

4. Scheuermann's disease.

    a. Age incidence: Adolescents.

    b. Radiography/CT: Vertebral endplate irregularity, anterior wedging of involved vertebrae, kyphosis.

    c. Bone scintigraphy usually normal.

5. Metastases.

    a. Most common: Neuroblastoma, leukemia, histocytosis.

    b. Age incidence: <5 years.

    c. Radiography/CT: Vertebral body destruction, paraspinal mass.

    d. Scintigraphy: Increased tracer uptake.

    e. MRI: Intraspinal extension, tumor in vertebral marrow.

References

du Lac P, Panuel M, Devred P, Bollini G, Padovani J (1990). MRI of disc space infection in infants and children. Report of 12 cases. Pediatr Radiol 20:175–178.

Wenger DR, Bobechko WP, Gilday DL (1978). The spectrum of intervertebral disc-space infection in children. J Bone Joint Surg 60A:100–108.

MULTIPLE BRUISES
(SUSPECTED NONACCIDENTAL TRAUMA)

A. Clinical Findings

1. Nonaccidental trauma (or child abuse): 1.5 million cases/year.
2. Characterized by intracranial and skeletal injuries.
3. Head trauma in 10% of child abuse victims; usually result of severe acceleration–deceleration injury with rotation of brain.
4. Age incidence: Usually <2 year.
5. Clinical findings: Seizures, lethargy, coma, retinal hemorrhage, shallow respirations, bruises.
6. Injuries result of either direct blunt blows or shaking.
7. Direct injuries: Subdural hematoma, cerebral contusion, skeletal/calvarial fractures.
8. Shaking injuries: Subdural hematoma, cerebral contusion, subarachnoid hemorrhage, shearing injury (gray–white junction laceration).

B. Imaging Modalities

1. Plain films
   a. Diagnosis based on presence of multiple fractures of varying age or unusual fractures.
   b. Highly specific fractures: Posterior rib; sternal, scapular, spinous process; metaphyseal (i.e., corner fractures).
   c. Moderately specific fractures: Vertebral body, metacarpal, metatarsal, skull (complex), epiphyseal separation.
   d. Low specificity (but common) fractures: Skull (linear), clavicular, shafts of long bones.
2. Head sonography (ultrasound)
   a. Asymmetric, extraaxial fluid collections.
   b. Parenchymal mass (hematoma).
3. Bone scintigraphy

       a. Multiple "hot" spots, representing fractures.

       b. Shortcoming: Inability to define type and age of fracture.

   4. Head CT

       a. Subdural > contusion > shearing injury > subarachnoid.

       b. Acute hemorrhage (<3 days): Hyperdense relative to brain.

       c. Subacute blood (3–14 days): Hypointense.

       d. Chronic blood (>2 weeks): Hypodense.

       e. Sensitivity: Shearing injury, 20%; hemorrhage, 90%.

   5. Head MRI

       a. Acute: Bright on T1, dark on T2.

       b. Subacute: Dark on both T1 and T2.

       c. Chronic: Dark on T1; bright with dark rim on T2.

       d. Sensitivity: Shearing injury, 70%–95%; hemorrhage, >90%.

C. Recommended Imaging Approach

   1. Skeletal survey performed first to identify fractures.

   2. If abnormal neurologic exam or radiographic findings, CT performed to detect acute hematomas and identify surgically correctable lesion. CT > MRI for detecting acute subarachnoid hemorrhage and skull fractures.

   3. Head MRI performed if CT normal or equivocal and there is still high suspicion of abuse based on clinical or radiographic findings. MRI > CT for detecting shearing injury, interhemispheric and tentorial subdural hematomas, and cortical contusions.

   4. Ultrasound not applicable: Depends on patent anterior fontanelle; cannot characterize age of blood; poorly depicts brain periphery and extraaxial spaces.

   5. Scintigraphy comparable to skeletal survey, not routinely used.

D. Differential Diagnostic Considerations

   1. Infantile hydrocephalus.

       a. Infants between 2 and 7 months of age.

       b. No underlying brain anomalies.

       c. Normal neurologic development.

    d. Symmetric extra-axial collections on ultrasound, CT, or MRI.

    e. Resolves by second year of life.

2. Syndromic disorders: Osteogenesis imperfecta—multiple fractures, blue sclerae.

3. Nonsyndromic systemic diseases: Lesions producing periosteal reaction (congenital syphilis, leukemia, multifocal osteomyelitis, scurvy, hypervitaminosis A) may mimic fractures. History, clinical findings, laboratory data help in diagnosis.

4. Accidental trauma.

References

Kleinman PK (1990). Diagnostic imaging of infant abuse. AJR 155:703–712.

Sato Y, Yuh WT, Smith WL, Alexander RC et al (1989). Head injury in child abuse: Evaluation with MR imaging. Radiology 173:653–657.

► CHAPTER **6**

Breast Disease

Jacquelyn P. Hogge, MD
Rebecca A. Zuurbier, MD
Georgetown University Medical Center

Deborah J. Crowe, MD
Henry Ford Hospital

Todd E. Wilson, MD
University of Michigan Medical Center

Imaging Handbook for House Officers, Edited by Paul M. Silverman and Douglas J. Quint.
ISBN 0-471-13767-7 © 1997 Wiley-Liss, Inc.

TENDER, SWOLLEN, ERYTHEMATOUS BREAST (SUSPECTED INFLAMMATORY CARCINOMA)

A. Clinical Findings

1. Palpable focal or diffuse breast mass.
2. Diffusely enlarged or edematous breast.
3. Skin thickening (peau d'orange).
4. Erythema with increased breast temperature; palpable ridge at the margin of induration.
5. Diffuse or focal breast pain.
6. Nipple retraction.
7. Axillary adenopathy.

B. Imaging Modalities

1. Mammography: Mammography is generally the only imaging modality needed in the evaluation of the patient with a tender, swollen, erythematous breast.
2. Sonography: Ultrasound may aid in the evaluation of a focal mass lesion.

C. Recommended Imaging Approach

1. Mammography should be the initial imaging modality in a patient with suspected inflammatory carcinoma. Mammography findings mirror the clinical features and include diffusely increased stromal

density, skin thickening, focal mass or microcalcifications, nipple inversion, and axillary adenopathy.

2. As the diagnosis of inflammatory carcinoma is usually made clinically, the importance of mammography is in excluding occult abnormalities in the contralateral breast prior to institution of treatment.

3. Special views to demonstrate the ipsilateral axilla are recommended, as the rate of axillary nodal involvement has been reported to be as high as 91%.

4. Mammography is indicated in patients with puerperal mastitis or breast abscess who fail conventional therapy.

5. Ultrasound may be used to differentiate cystic from solid masses or to guide biopsy of nonpalpable masses seen mammographically.

D. Differential Diagnostic Considerations

1. Inflammatory carcinoma of the breast represents 1%–4% of all breast cancer. It is a form of locally advanced carcinoma with a poor prognosis, classified as a T4 tumor by the TNM system and is stage IIIB. Inflammatory carcinoma may be diagnosed clinically or pathologically and has characteristic findings on mammography. Pathologic diagnosis depends on identification of tumor emboli in dermal lymphatics. Any histologic subtype of primary breast carcinoma may develop into inflammatory carcinoma.

2. Mastitis with or without breast abscess is usually seen in relation to lactation in the puerperium and typically occurs in the first few weeks of breastfeeding. The patient usually presents with an inflamed breast, fever, and leukocytosis. Mammography is usually not indicated unless the patient fails to respond to conventional therapy.

3. Differential diagnosis also includes postlumpectomy radiation therapy, recent breast surgery, venous outflow obstruction (dialysis patients, SVC syndrome, central venous thrombosis), lymphatic outflow obstruction in the ipsilateral axilla (lymphoma, other metastases), and rare chronic inflammatory processes of the breast (sarcoidosis, tuberculosis).

References

Bozzetti F, Saccozzi R, De Lena M, Salvadori B (1981). Inflammatory cancer of the breast: Analysis of 114 cases. J Surg Oncol 18:355–361.

Dershaw DD, Moore MP, Liberman L, Deutch BM (1994). Inflammatory breast carcinoma: Mammographic findings. Radiology 190:831–834.

SUPERFICIAL THROMBOPHLEBITIS OF THE BREAST (MONDOR'S DISEASE)

A. Clinical Findings

1. Acute pain in the lateral breast.
2. Tender cordlike mass that follows the distribution of one of three major superficial veins of the chest.
3. Skin retraction or furrowing over a tubular mass.
4. Evidence of thrombophlebitis in other anatomic sites.
5. Erythema.

B. Imaging Modalities

1. Mammography
   a. Mammography is indicated to exclude breast pathology, as Mondor's disease is associated with breast cancer in 4%–12% of cases.
   b. Tangential views are used to demonstrate the superficial location of the abnormality.
2. Sonography: Sonography shows the thrombosed vein as a superficial hypoechoic, noncompressible tubular structure.

C. Recommended Imaging Approach

1. Sonography may be the initial examination in younger patients with a palpable mass.
2. Mammography with a tangential view shows a beaded or tubular superficial opacity that corresponds to the palpable painful mass.
3. Biopsy is not necessary in the absence of mammographic signs of malignancy.

    4. Follow-up mammography shows regression of the cordlike mass with a return to a narrower vascular structure.

D. Differential Diagnostic Considerations

1. A tubular mass must be differentiated from a dilated duct, which may indicate malignancy or an intraductal papilloma. A thrombosed vein should be located superficially, while a dilated duct is characteristically located in the retroareolar region. A dilated duct may have associated calcification, which is unlikely in Mondor's disease.
2. The clinical symptoms of Mondor's disease last from 2 to 8 weeks. Resolution can be confirmed clinically or with follow-up mammography.
3. Veins most commonly involved in superficial thrombophlebitis of the breast include the thoracoepigastric vein, the superficial epigastric vein, the lateral thoracic vein, and, rarely, tributaries of the external jugular or internal mammary veins.
4. Mondor's disease has been associated with direct trauma, breast surgery, excessive physical activity, infection, malignant ipsilateral axillary adenopathy, and primary breast cancer.

References

Catania S, Zurrida S, Veronesi P, Galimberti V, Bono A, Pluchinotta A (1992). Mondor's disease and breast cancer. Cancer 69:2267–2270.

Conant EF, Wilkes AN, Mendelson EB, Feig SA (1993). Superficial thrombophlebitis of the breast (Mondor's disease): Mammographic findings. AJR 160:1201–1203.

PAGET'S DISEASE OF THE NIPPLE

A. Clinical Findings

1. Scaly, eczematous changes in the nipple–areolar complex.
2. Itching.
3. Erythema.
4. Nipple discharge (bloody, clear).

  5. Breast mass.
  6. Nipple retraction.
  7. Ulceration.

B. Imaging Modalities

1. Mammography: Mammography should always be obtained in a patient with pagetoid changes of the nipple.
2. Sonography: Ultrasound may be indicated to evaluate the cystic or solid nature of any mass seen on mammography.
3. Galactography: Galactography may be indicated in the presence of bloody nipple discharge.

C. Recommended Imaging Approach

1. Mammography is imperative in these patients as an initial step to exclude an underlying in situ or invasive breast cancer.
2. Ultrasound may be used to evaluate any masses detected by mammography. Biopsy is indicated for all solid masses.
3. Galactography may be helpful in identifying the abnormal ductal system in patients with pagetoid changes, bloody nipple discharge, and nonconclusive mammographic findings.

D. Differential Diagnostic Considerations

1. Paget's disease of the nipple nearly always indicates underlying in situ or invasive breast cancer. Up to 2% of patients with primary breast cancer have Paget's disease of the nipple. All histologic subsets of primary breast cancer have been described in association with Paget's disease.
2. Mammographic findings include no abnormality (in up to 50% of cases), thickening or retraction of the nipple–areolar complex, calcifications, architectural distortion, and mass.

References

Ashikari R, Park K, Huros AG, Urban JA (1970). Paget's disease of the breast. Cancer 26:680–685.

Ikeda DM, Helvie MA, Frank TS, Chapel KL, Anderson IT (1993). Paget disease of the nipple: Radiologic–pathologic correlation. Radiology 189:89–94.

AXILLARY ADENOPATHY

A. Clinical Findings

1. Axillary mass.
   a. unilateral.
   b. bilateral.
2. Breast mass.
3. Systemic symptoms: Fever, pruritus, night sweats, weight loss.

B. Imaging Modalities

1. Mammography
   a. Indicated as the initial imaging study in a patient with a unilateral axillary mass.
   b. Not necessarily indicated for the initial workup of a patient with bilateral axillary masses.
2. Sonography
   a. May be indicated for evaluation of a unilateral axillary mass.
   b. Usually not indicated.
3. MRI: If available, gadolinium-enhanced breast MRI is indicated if mammography, physical examination, and ultrasound are inconclusive.

C. Recommended Imaging Approach

1. Mammography is indicated in a patient with unilateral axillary adenopathy to identify an occult primary breast cancer. If mammography is negative, fine-needle aspiration of the palpable axillary mass should be performed.
2. MRI of the breast with gadolinium enhancement may identify a breast carcinoma that is not visible mammographically. Technology is being developed that will permit MRI-guided breast needle lo-

calizations and biopsies, although this is currently limited to research centers.

3. ^{99m}Tc Sestamibi breast scintigraphy is also currently being studied as a method for identifying and localizing mammographically occult breast cancers.

D. Differential Diagnostic Considerations

1. From 0.3% to 1.0% of breast carcinomas present as axillary metastases with no palpable breast mass, representing an uncommon form of stage II disease. Mammograms are negative in 53%–76% of cases. In 45% of cases where mammograms are negative, pathologic examination reveals a primary breast cancer, including intraductal and invasive histologies.

2. Differential diagnosis for unilateral axillary adenopathy includes lymphoma; metastases from other primary sites including melanoma, thyroid, lung, GI tract, ovary, renal; a breast primary occurring in ectopic axillary breast tissue; and infectious etiologies: cat scratch fever, streptococcal disease, TB, sarcoidosis (usually bilateral), mononucleosis (usually generalized).

References

Patel J, Nemoto T, Rosner D, Das TL, Pickren JW (1991). Axillary lymph node metastases from an occult breast cancer. Cancer 47:2923–2927.

Rosen PP, Kimmel M (1990). Occult breast carcinoma presenting with axillary lymph node metastases. Hum Pathol 21:518–523.

MASTALGIA

A. Clinical Findings

1. Mastalgia.
   a. Cyclical: With pain increasing in the premenstrual period; unilateral or bilateral; usually diffuse, but may be localized.
   b. Noncyclical: Usually chronic and nonfluctuating; localized to a distinct area in the breast.

2. Breast lump.
3. Diffuse breast nodularity.

B. Imaging Modalities

1. Mammography: Mammography is indicated in patients presenting with a complaint of mastalgia.
2. Sonography.
   a. May be used to evaluate masses detected mammographically or a palpable mass.
   b. Should be performed as a directed exam. Full-breast ultrasound as a screening study is not indicated.

C. Recommended Imaging Approach

1. Generally, a patient presenting with mastalgia of any type should have a mammogram to screen for underlying breast pathology.
2. Additional views, such as spot compression or tangential views, may be used to evaluate localized areas of concern.
3. Ultrasound should be used to evaluate the cystic or solid nature of any dominant mass detected by physical examination or mammography.
4. Solid masses are an indication for biopsy.

D. Differential Diagnostic Considerations

1. Mastalgia is the most common breast symptom. Many women experience cyclical premenstrual breast pain. Although the exact etiology of the cyclical breast pain is not fully understood, the changes are physiologic and should not be labeled as a breast disorder.
2. Noncyclical mastalgia is breast pain with no relationship to the menstrual cycle.
3. From 5% to 17% of cancers initially present with breast pain, with up to 7% presenting with mastalgia.
4. Tietze's syndrome: Painful costochondral junction syndrome, may be mistaken for breast pain and should be considered as an etiology in patients with medially located breast pain.

References

Preece PE, Baum M, Mansel RE, Webster DJT, Fortt RW, Gravelle IH, Hughes LE (1982). Importance of mastalgia in operable breast cancer. BMJ 284:1299–1300.

BREAST MASS IN PREGNANT PATIENT

A. Clinical Findings

1. Breast mass.
2. Nipple discharge.
3. Diffuse breast enlargement with skin thickening.
4. Nipple retraction.
5. Axillary adenopathy.

B. Imaging Modalities

1. Sonography: Ultrasound should be the initial imaging study in a pregnant or lactating patient with a breast mass.
2. Mammography
   a. Not routinely performed as a screening study in the age group most likely to be pregnant.
   b. May be performed as a diagnostic study in a symptomatic pregnant or lactating patient. There is minimal risk of radiation exposure to the fetus with current mammographic technology and abdominopelvic lead shielding.

C. Recommended Imaging Approach

1. Sonography
   a. Should be the initial imaging study obtained.
   b. Differentiates cystic (galactocele, cysts) from solid masses.
   c. No ionizing radiation.
2. Mammography
   a. Mammography may be useful in evaluation of palpable masses, for assessing the presence of calcifications and extent of disease, and screening the remaining breast parenchyma.

  b. The sensitivity of mammography is diminished in pregnant and lactating patients because of the increased glandularity and water content of the breast tissue.

  c. The sensitivity of mammography in palpable or otherwise clinically evident pregnancy-associated breast cancer is approximately 80%.

D. Differential Diagnostic Considerations

1. Breast cancer is the most common cancer to occur in women during pregnancy or lactation, accounting for 1%–2% of all breast cancer. Pregnancy-associated breast cancer is breast cancer occurring within 1 year of pregnancy.

2. There is often a delay in diagnosis of pregnancy-associated breast cancer of 5–15 months. This is a reflection of the difficulty in breast evaluation both clinically and mammographically during pregnancy and lactation.

3. From 53% to 89% of patients diagnosed with pregnancy-associated breast cancer will have positive ipsilateral axillary lymph nodes.

4. Other diagnostic possibilities include galactocele, fibroadenoma, abscess, mastitis, cysts.

5. A dominant mass in a pregnant or lactating patient should be managed aggressively.

References

Hoover HC (1990). Breast cancer during pregnancy and lactation. Surg Clin North Am 70:1151–1163.

Liberman L, Giess CS, Dershaw DD, Deutsch BM, Petrick JA (1994). Imaging of pregnancy-associated breast cancer. Radiology 191:245–248.

BREAST MASS IN AN ADULT MALE PATIENT

A. Clinical Findings

1. Breast mass: Painless or tender.
2. Breast enlargement: May be unilateral or bilateral.

3. Nipple discharge: Clear, milky, sanguineous.
4. Nipple or areolar abnormality
   a. Itching of eczema.
   b. Inversion.
   c. Fixation.
   d. Ulceration.
5. Enlarged axillary nodes.
6. Breast pain.
7. Erythema.

B. Imaging Modalities

1. Mammography
   a. Mammography is generally the only imaging modality necessary in males presenting with a breast mass.
   b. A complete bilateral mammogram with craniocaudal and mediolateral oblique views should be obtained.
2. Sonography
   a. May be helpful to confirm a discrete mass if mammographic findings are inconclusive.
   b. Has not been as helpful in males as in evaluation of breast masses in females.
3. Galactography: May aid in localization of the abnormal duct when no mass is palpable and mammographic findings are inconclusive in a patient with nipple discharge.

C. Recommended Imaging Approach

1. Initially, mammography should be obtained in adult males with breast symptoms.
2. The false-negative rate of detection of breast cancer in men mammographically is similar to that in women (6%–15%). Sonography and galactography may aid in detection of a localized abnormality when physical exam and mammographic findings are inconclusive.

3. Gynecomastia may hide an underlying breast cancer. The presence of a mass in a male breast should be approached aggressively.

D. Differential Diagnostic Considerations

1. Breast cancer is uncommon in men, representing less than 0.5% of all breast cancers and less than 1.0% of all cancers in males. Early signs are often misinterpreted by both patient and clinician, resulting in delay in diagnosis. Carcinoma classically presents clinically as an eccentrically located painless hard mass.

2. Gynecomastia is the most common cause of a benign breast mass in males (one-third bilaterally symmetric, one-third bilaterally asymmetric, one-third unilateral). It presents as a tender, discoid subareolar enlargement of breast tissue produced by benign ductal and stromal proliferation. True acinar lobules are absent in males. A number of disease states, hormonal factors, drugs, and syndromes are associated with gynecomastia.

3. Benign breast neoplasms are rare in males: Cystosarcoma phylloides, papillomas, papillomatosis, lipomas, epidermal inclusion cysts, neurofibromas.

4. Metastases to the breast are rare: Prostate, lung, renal.

References

Dershaw DD, Borgen PI, Deutch BM, Liberman L (1993). Mammographic findings in men with breast cancer. AJR 160:267–270.

Jaiyesimi IA, Buzdav AU, Sahin AA, Ross MA (1992). Carcinoma of the male breast. Ann Intern Med 117:771–777.

BREAST MASS IN A PEDIATRIC OR ADOLESCENT FEMALE

A. Clinical Findings

1. Breast mass.
2. Unilateral breast enlargement.

3. Prominent veins.
4. Axillary adenopathy.
5. Erythema.

B. Imaging Modalities

1. Sonography: Ultrasound should be the primary imaging modality for breast masses in the pediatric age group.
2. Mammography: Mammography is not indicated in the pediatric age group.

C. Recommended Imaging Approach

1. The primary differential is between developmental breast abnormalities and true breast masses. Imaging is usually not necessary in developmental abnormalities of the breast unless the diagnosis is uncertain.
2. Ultrasound is useful in evaluating palpable masses, in aiding differentiation of developmental asymmetric breast hypertrophy from breast enlargement due to underlying mass lesion, and in guiding biopsy or aspiration (e.g., abscess drainage).
3. Mammography is not indicated in the pediatric age group due to
   a. The low incidence of breast carcinoma.
   b. Limited imaging due to dense glandular tissues.
   c. The low risk of radiation-induced malignancy in the immature breast.

D. Differential Diagnostic Considerations

1. The most common breast abnormalities in females in the pediatric age group are asymmetric breast hypertrophy, fibroadenomas, and cystosarcoma phylloides. Less common are abscess, cysts, metastases to the breast, primary breast carcinoma, primary involvement of the breast by sarcoma, lymphoma, or leukemia, neurofibromas,

lipoma, intraductal papilloma, fat necrosis, and, rarely, extra-medullary hematopoiesis.

2. A malignant breast mass in the pediatric age group is more commonly due to metastases from a nonbreast malignancy (such as lymphoma) or nonbreast primary malignancy (such as rhabdomyosarcoma) than a primary breast carcinoma.

3. Developmental breast abnormalities that do not require imaging include polythelia, premature thelarche, juvenile hypertrophy, gigantomastia, symmastia, polymastia, or ectopic breast tissue.

References

Boothroyd A, Carty H (1994). Breast masses in childhood and adolescence. Pediatr Radiol 24:81–84.

Bower R, Bell MJ, Ternberg JL (1976). Management of breast lesions in children and adolescents. J Pediatr Surg 11:337–346.

BREAST MASS IN A PEDIATRIC OR ADOLESCENT MALE

A. Clinical Findings

1. Breast mass.
   a. Tender versus painless.
   b. Discrete mass versus diffuse enlargement.
   c. Subareolar versus eccentric.
   d. Unilateral versus bilateral.
2. Axillary adenopathy.

B. Imaging Modalities

1. Usually no imaging is indicated for pediatric male breast abnormalities.
2. Sonography: Ultrasound may be helpful in selected cases for evaluation of a discrete mass.

3. Mammography: Mammography is not indicated for pediatric male breast abnormalities.

C. Recommended Imaging Approach

1. Usually no imaging is indicated in the evaluation of pediatric male breast abnormalities, as most cases represent gynecomastia.
2. Ultrasound examination may aid in the characterization of a focal mass lesion or in the case of suspected abscess. Sonography may be used to guide aspiration or drainage of breast abscess.
3. Mammography is not indicated in the pediatric male patient.

D. Differential Diagnostic Considerations

1. Gynecomastia is any visible or palpable development of the breast in males most commonly in puberty (39% incidence in males aged 10–16 years). It is believed to be a transient physiologic event and is usually self-limited, regressing spontaneously in 6 months to 2 years. It manifests most frequently as a unilateral or bilateral, tender, discoid subareolar mass.
2. Prepubertal development of gynecomastia is unusual and has been associated with exogenous hormones or drugs, hermaphroditism, Klinefelter's syndrome, adrenal feminizing tumor, testicular tumor, hepatoblastoma, neurofibromatosis, and thyroid disease.
3. Rare etiologies of breast masses in pediatric or adolescent males include metastasis (rhabdomyosarcoma, neuroblastoma, lymphoma), abscess, primary breast carcinoma, intraductal papilloma. Discrete masses require biopsy.

References

Bower R, Bell MJ, Ternberg JL (1976). Management of breast lesions in children and adolescents. J Pediatr Surg 11:337–346.

Greydanus DE, Parks DS, Farrell EG (1989). Breast Disorders in Children and Adolescents. Pediatr Clin North Am 36:601–638.

ASYMMETRIC BREAST SIZE

A. Clinical Findings

1. Marked asymmetry of breast size.
2. Breast mass.

B. Imaging Modalities

1. Mammography: Mammography is indicated as the initial imaging study in a patient with breast asymmetry.
2. Sonography: Ultrasound is indicated in the evaluation of any discrete mass detected by physical examination or mammographically.

C. Recommended Imaging Approach

1. Mammography should be obtained as the initial imaging study in a patient with asymmetric breast size to assess for an underlying mass lesion as the cause of the breast asymmetry.
2. Ultrasound should be used to evaluate discrete masses that are detected by physical exam or mammography.

D. Differential Diagnostic Considerations

1. The primary differential is between normal variation in breast size versus an underlying mass lesion or inflammatory process as the etiology of breast asymmetry.
2. Mild asymmetry of breast size is a common normal variant, occurring in 25% of adult females. Amastia, absence of the breast, is rare and may be associated with other congenital anomalies (Poland syndrome).
3. Marked asymmetry of breast size may be due to hypoplasia secondary to injury to the prepubertal breast bud (infection, trauma, prior surgery), underlying tumor, inflammatory process (mastitis, inflammatory carcinoma), drug therapy (D-penicillamine), or congenital hypoplasia.

4. Inflammatory causes can be excluded by systemic signs and secondary changes in the skin.
5. Tumors that commonly cause unilateral breast enlargement include lipoma, fibroadenoma, cystosarcoma phylloides.

References

Greydanus DE, Parks DS, Farrell EG (1989). Breast disorders in children and adolescents. Pediatr Clin North Am 36:601–638.

FEMALE PREMENOPAUSAL BREAST LUMP— UNILATERAL (RULE OUT BREAST CANCER)

A. Clinical Finding

1. Focal palpable mass.
2. Usually nontender.
3. Usually hard, not rubbery or fluctuant.
4. Occasionally, thickening fullness without discrete mass.
5. Generally does not fluctuate in size with menses.
6. Size is not a distinguishing feature.

B. Imaging Modalities

1. Mammography
   a. Helpful to identify nature of lesion (size, location) and possible association with microcalcifications.
   b. Helpful in excluding benign etiologies as cause of lump (e.g., lipoma, lymph node).
   c. Helps identify synchronous lesions that are not clinically apparent.
   d. Identifies areas that may represent cysts, for subsequent sonographic evaluation.
2. Sonography
   a. Should never be used to screen for breast cancer because of un-

acceptably high false-negative and false-positive rates.

b. The sonogram should be performed by the radiologist in a directed fashion after careful review of the mammogram.

c. In general, a breast sonogram can be ordered as first-line evaluation of a palpable lump in a woman <30 years old.

3. Breast MRI

a. Considered investigational in breast cancer detection and diagnosis.

b. Enroll patient in clinical trial if available.

4. Stereotactic–guided core biopsy

a. Used more often in cases where the lesion is nonpalpable but helpful when lesion is more definitively identified by mammography than by physical examination.

b. 14-Gauge core samples are obtained using precise radiologic guidance and a biopsy gun to provide histologic diagnosis of a lesion.

c. Accuracy is equal to open surgical biopsy.

d. Approximately one-third the cost of excisional biopsy.

e. Minimal mammographic or cosmetic disfigurement.

5. Ultrasound–guided core biopsy

a. Used in cases where the lesion is more definitively identified by ultrasound.

b. 14-Gauge core samples are obtained using real-time ultrasound guidance and a biopsy gun to provide histologic diagnosis of a lesion.

c. Accuracy is equal to open surgical biopsy.

d. Usually less expensive than stereotactic core biopsy.

e. Less expensive than excisional biopsy.

f. Minimal mammographic or cosmetic disfigurement.

6. Stereotactic- or ultrasound-guided fine-needle aspiration

a. Can only provide a cytologic diagnosis that is less definitive than histologic diagnosis.

b. Significant insufficient sampling rate.

c. Need for trained cytopathologist.

C. Recommended Imaging Approach

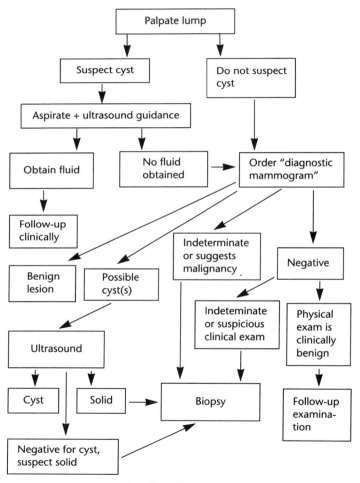

Imaging Algorithm

D. Differential Diagnostic Considerations

1. Always exclude malignancy: Up to 30% of malignancies occur in premenopausal women, though cysts and fibroadenomas are more common.
2. Pseudolumps: The convexity of an underlying rib may produce "lump."
3. Cysts are more common than fibroadenomas among women 40–50 years old.
4. Fibroadenomas are more common in women <35 years old.
5. Clearly mark the area of concern (preferably with stickers designated for this purpose, but felt pen will do) or at least indicate the lesion location and size on a diagram. Patients cannot always be relied on to describe the area accurately.
6. A negative imaging workup should not delay biopsy of a suspicious palpable abnormality.

References

Feig SA (1992). Breast masses: Mammographic and sonographic evaluation. Radiol Clin North Am 30:67–92.

NIPPLE DISCHARGE (GENERAL)

A. Clinical Findings

Nipple discharge is fluid that is released from the milk ducts either spontaneously or with stimulation or compression of the nipple/breast.

B. Imaging Modalities

1. Mammography: Useful in excluding an associated mass or other suspicious findings. Mammography is most frequently normal, but it may show a dilated duct.
2. Ductogram: The discharging duct is cannulated with a blunt-tipped needle, and contrast is injected, followed by a mammogram. May demonstrate a papilloma or a carcinoma in duct lu-

men. Surgical removal of the duct often still necessary to distinguish the two. The patient must be having the discharge at the time of the ductogram in order to localize the appropriate duct for cannulation.

C. Recommended Imaging Approach

1. Bloody nipple discharge should be referred to a breast specialist (see Nipple Discharge—Unilateral).
2. Bilateral mammograms should be obtained in women over the age of 35 years if they have not recently had a mammogram. Patients should be referred to a breast specialist if they have suspicious mammographic findings.
3. Bilateral nipple discharge from multiple ducts is almost always benign. If the discharge is milky, check serum prolactin levels. See the appropriate section in Chapter 8 for hypothalamic/pituitary imaging if a tumor (i.e., prolactinoma) is suspected.
4. If there is skin breakdown involving the nipple or areola, refer to a breast specialist.
5. Ductography (galactography) is usually only obtained in patients who have a clinically suspicious discharge.

D. Differential Diagnostic Considerations

1. Physiologic: Lactation is the most common cause. Milk may continue to be secreted years after cessation of breastfeeding, especially in multiparous women. Secretions may be expressed with squeezing of the nipple (which is a part of breast self-examination) or even with vigorous breast stimulation in women who have never been pregnant.
2. Galactorrhea: Milky white, bilateral discharge, not related to lactation or breast stimulation.
   a. Central causes
      Prolactinoma: Most common tumor causing galactorrhea. Causes the highest serum prolactin levels.
      Other CNS hypothalamic and hypophyseal lesions (i.e., craniopharyngioma).

Drugs: Phenothiazines, antihypertensives, oral contraceptives, etc.

Idiopathic/other

b. Peripheral

Target organ failure: Hypothyroidism, Addison's disease.

Feminizing adrenal carcinoma, polycystic ovary syndrome.

Decreased prolactin clearance: Renal, liver, thyroid failure.

Breast conditions: Thoracic/breast trauma or inflammation.

3. Serous or serosanguineous discharge.

a. Frequently associated with fibrocystic breast disease. Usually green, yellow, or brown discharge.

b. Bloody or blood-tinged discharged may indicate an intraductal papilloma or carcinoma. A guaiac test may help to distinguish bloody discharge from the brown discharge of fibrocystic disease.

4. Purulent discharge.

a. Subareolar infection: May be associated with nipple erythema and tenderness.

b. Nipple infection must be distinguished from Paget's disease, which is a breast cancer that produces a weeping, crusty lesion involving the nipple, which may be associated with erythema and swelling. Mammography is most frequently normal. Diagnosed by nipple biopsy.

5. A mammogram may be obtained in patients aged 30–35 years if they are judged to be at increased risk due to historical or clinical factors.

NIPPLE DISCHARGE—UNILATERAL (RULE OUT BREAST CANCER)

A. Clinical Findings

1. Bloody
2. Clear or watery

3. Spontaneous
4. Usually unilateral, arising from one orifice on the nipple.

B. Imaging Modalities

1. Mammography: To evaluate for a clinically occult malignancy that may be causing the discharge.
2. Ductography (galactography): To provide the surgeon with a "road map" of the duct system.
3. Directed ultrasound: If ductography fails, high-resolution ultrasound may help identify a dilated duct system and intrinsic lesion.

C. Recommended Imaging Approach

1. Diagnostic mammogram.
2. Ductogram: Virtually painless procedure.
   a. Insert blunt-tipped 30-g cannula into duct orifice and inject water-soluble contrast, then obtain mammographic images with magnification.
   b. Can add blue dye when performed preoperatively to guide the surgeon's duct dissection.

D. Differential Diagnostic Considerations

1. Benign papilloma: Most common cause of bloody nipple discharge.
2. Least ominous nipple discharges (but not definitely excluding malignancy) are nonbloody, opaque, straw-colored, light to dark green, brown, gray or blue, from multiple orifices.
3. Papillomas are typically central (nearer to the nipple) and solitary but may be multiple and peripheral.
4. Clinically occult cancer presenting with nipple discharge is usually ductal carcinoma in situ or papillary carcinoma. If the discharge is associated with cancer, it usually is associated with a palpable mass.
5. From 10% to 12% of cases of nipple discharge are associated with carcinoma.

References

Schuh ME, Takuma N, Penetrante RB, Rosner D, Dao TL (1986). Intraductal carcinoma. Analysis of presentation, pathologic findings, and outcome of disease. Arch Surg 121:1303–1307.

NIPPLE DISCHARGE—BILATERAL (RULE OUT BREAST CANCER)

A. Clinical Findings

Bilateral nipple discharge is rarely associated with breast cancer. Typically hormones, medications, or chronic disease account for this finding.

Careful review of the patient's history and physical exam and evaluation for possible adrenal and pituitary tumors may be indicated if the patient is not on a medication that may exacerbate cystic disease (e.g., some cardiovascular medications, antihypertensive agents, tranquilizers, antidepressants, antihistamines, oral contraceptive agents).

If the discharge is in any way ominous (spontaneous episode, bloody, or watery) evaluation is indicated.

B. Imaging Modalities

1. Mammography: To exclude clinically occult lesions.
2. Ductography (galactography).
3. Ultrasound: If ductography fails.

C. Recommended Imaging Approach

1. Diagnostic mammography.
2. Ductography (galactography).
3. Ultrasound: If ductography fails.

D. Differential Diagnostic Considerations

Breast cancer rarely presents with bilateral nipple discharge. Consider hormone- or drug-related etiologies as discussed above.

BREAST LUMPS—BILATERAL (RULE OUT BILATERAL BREAST CANCER)

A. Clinical Findings

1. Firm palpable masses, usually nontender.
2. Usually hard, not rubbery or fluctuant.
3. Occasionally thickening or fullness bilaterally without discrete masses.
4. Generally does not fluctuate in size with menses.
5. Size is not a distinguishing feature.

B. Imaging Modalities

1. Mammography
   a. Helpful to identify nature of lesion (size, location) and possible association with microcalcifications.
   b. Helpful in excluding benign etiologies as cause of lump (e.g., lipoma, lymph node).
   c. Helps identify synchronous lesions that are not clinically apparent.
   d. Identifies areas that may represent cysts, for subsequent sonographic evaluations.

C. Recommended Imaging Approach

See Female Premenopausal Breast Lump—Unilateral.

D. Differential Diagnostic Considerations

1. Malignancy must always be excluded, though synchronous breast cancer is rare.
2. The convexity of an underlying rib may produce a "lump."
3. Cysts and fibroadenomas are typically multiple and bilateral and are more common than bilateral breast cancers.
4. Be wary that malignancy can coexist with benign lesions.

5. Distinguish "lumps" from "lumpiness"—consult an examiner trained in breast physical examination if uncertain.
6. A negative imaging workup should not delay biopsy of a clinically suspicious lesion.

IMPLANTS (RULE OUT IMPLANT RUPTURE)

A. Clinical Findings

1. Scar in inframammary fold.
2. Capsular contracture may cause hardening of the implants.
3. An implant rupture may present with pain, lump(s), abrupt or gradual contour change, or volume decrease. Frequently asymptomatic.

B. Imaging Modalities

1. Breast MRI: Considered the gold standard for implant imaging because of ability to image in multiple planes and posterior to implant. The test is not operator dependent (unlike ultrasound) but is more expensive than ultrasound. Breast MRI is more sensitive and specific for implant rupture than breast ultrasound or mammography.
2. Breast ultrasound: Operator dependent. May not see posterior to implant. Less sensitive and specific than MRI (but usually less expensive).
3. Mammography
   a. Not useful in reliably excluding implant rupture.
   b. Useful to screen the breast for malignancy by using standard and "implant-displaced" views.
   c. Implants obscure variable amounts of native glandular tissue, which may impair cancer detection and diagnosis.
4. CT
   a. Radiation dose to the breast relatively high and may not accurately detect free silicone in breast tissues.

    b. Not routinely used when MRI or ultrasound is available.

    c. Can detect intracapsular rupture.

C. Recommended Imaging Approach

MRI, if available; ultrasound or CT if MRI is not available.

D. Differential Diagnostic Considerations

1. Must always exclude malignancy. A lump in a patient with implants is just as easily breast cancer.

2. Approximately 50% of implants may rupture at 12 years.

3. Implant rupture may be "intracapsular" or "extracapsular," the "capsule" being the patient's fibrous tissue that forms around the implant itself.

References

de Camera DL, Sheridan JM Kammer BA (1991). Rupture and aging of silicone gel breast implants, abstracted. Plastic Surgery Forum: 60th Annual Scientific Meeting, Seattle, WA, 1991. Arlington Heights, IL: American Society of Plastic and Reconstructive Surgeons, p. 244.

AFTER MASTECTOMY—WITHOUT RECONSTRUCTION (RULE OUT RECURRENCE)

A. Clinical Findings

1. Absent breast tissue.

2. Surgical scars.

3. Palpable lump.

B. Imaging Modalities

1. Mammography.

2. CT.

3. MRI experimental.

C. Recommended Imaging Approach

There is no consensus on the appropriateness of imaging modalities for screening or diagnosing cancer in the postmastectomy breast that has not been reconstructed. Typically the lump will be biopsied. Some argue that recurrences are easily palpable on the chest wall. One study concluded that mammography of the mastectomy site does not increase the detection of local recurrences.

But, CT is helpful in evaluating extent of disease in the chest wall when symptoms are present. Mammography may sometimes reassure the patient that lumpiness is attributable to normal residual fatty tissue.

D. Differential Diagnostic Considerations

1. Modified radical mastectomy usually preferred over radical mastectomy since this preserves the pectoralis major muscle, allowing better cosmetic results with equivalent disease-free survival.
2. Mammographically screen the contralateral intact breast.
3. Mastectomy theoretically removes all breast tissue, but foci of glandular tissue or malignancy can remain. Local–regional recurrence as the first sign of relapse occurs in 10%–20% of postmastectomy patients.

References

Fajardo LL, Roberts CC, Hunt KR (1993). Mammographic surveillance of breast cancer patients: Should the mastectomy site be imaged? AJR 161:953–955.

Valagussa P, Bonadonna G, Veronesi U (1978). Patterns of relapse and survival following radical mastectomy: Analysis of 716 consecutive patients. Cancer 41:1179–1178.

AFTER MASTECTOMY—WITH IMPLANT (RULE OUT RECURRENCE)

A. Clinical Finding

1. Absent breast tissue.
2. Surgical scar.

    3. Palpable implant.

    4. Palpable lump.

B. Imaging Modalities

    1. MRI.

    2. CT.

    3. Mammography.

C. Recommended Imaging Approach

There is no consensus on the appropriateness of imaging modalities for screening or diagnosing cancer in the postmastectomy breast that has been reconstructed with an implant. Breast MRI can discriminate implant rupture or herniation from local recurrence. Free silicone droplets or bulging areas of the implant may account for palpable abnormalities. CT may be helpful in evaluating the extent of disease present and visualizing the tissue posterior to the implant. Mammography can only image the thin rim of tissue seen in tangent at the edges of the implant. The implant obscures significant amounts of residual native tissue, and mammography is not typically helpful in recurrent cancer diagnosis in these cases, but may be performed.

D. Differential Diagnostic Considerations

    1. Implants may be prepectoral or retropectoral.

    2. Retropectoral implants minimize fibrous contraction and are less likely to compromise physical and mammographic examinations.

AFTER MASTECTOMY—AUTOGENOUS RECONSTRUCTION (RULE OUT RECURRENCE)

A. Clinical Findings

    1. Breast mound absent native glandular tissues.

    2. Surgical scars (breast and donor sites, e.g., abdomen).

    3. With or without palpable lump.

B. Imaging Modalities

1. Mammography.
2. Imaging-guided core biopsy.

C. Recommended Imaging Approach

1. Mammography: Helpful in identifying areas of fat necrosis that may account for palpable lump. May also be used to screen the breast for nonpalpable recurrences, since the autogenous reconstruction is primarily fatty tissue, which is radiographically lucent, unlike silicone or saline implants.

   No definite consensus on need to image the reconstructed breast.

2. Imaging-guided core biopsy (ultrasound or stereotactic) can be used to provide definitive histologic diagnosis of a lesion seen better with imaging than by palpation.

D. Differential Diagnostic Considerations

1. Transverse rectus abdominis myocutaneous (TRAM) flaps are the most common form of autogenous reconstruction performed by isolating and transferring the patient's native tissue (including skin, fat, and muscle on a vascular pedicle) to form a breast mound.
2. Fat necrosis usually explains a palpable mass in the TRAM flap.

SKIN CHANGES OF THE BREAST

A. Clinical Findings

1. Retraction of skin/nipple.
2. Thickening or edema (peau d'orange [orange peel]).
3. Erythema.

B. Imaging Modalities

1. Mammography.
2. Ultrasound.

C. Recommended Imaging Approach

1. Diagnostic mammography to determine presence and extent of underlying lesion.
2. Directed ultrasound as suggested by mammography and physical examination.

D. Differential Diagnostic Considerations

1. Skin changes when associated with malignancy are considered an ominous secondary sign of breast cancer.
2. Skin/nipple retraction suggests an underlying lesion that produces fibrosis and tethering of the Cooper's ligaments.
3. Inflammatory breast cancer is a locally advanced (stage IIIB) form of breast cancer, presenting with skin thickening or edema that resembles an orange peel, hence "peau d'orange." This is secondary to dermal lymphatic invasion.
4. Skin thickening in the appropriate clinical context may reflect blocked axillary lumphatics in patients with metastatic lymph node disease or secondary to axillary node dissection.
5. Consider also postradiation change, infection, or edema (e.g., congestive heart failure).
6. Erythema: May be related to inflammation or infection, but inflammatory carcinoma must be excluded.

ASYMPTOMATIC PATIENT—BREAST CANCER SCREENING

A. Clinical Findings

Screening guidelines apply to women without signs or symptoms of breast cancer.

B. Imaging Modalities

1. Mammography is the *only* imaging modality at the present time that is indicated for breast cancer screening.

    a. Film-screen mammography (black and white image on a clear film) is the preferred method for screening and diagnostic (symptomatic) mammography.

    b. Xeromammography (blue and white image on paper) is considered to be inferior to film-screen mammography. Also has higher radiation dose than film-screen technique.

2. Clinical breast examination is an extremely important screening method. Mammography may not detect 10%–20% of clinically apparent breast cancers. Optimal detection rates will be achieved only when mammography is combined with thorough clinical breast examination.

3. Ultrasound: *Never* to be used for screening.

4. Other imaging modalities (i.e., MRI) are being investigated for potential usefulness in screening, but are currently only for experimental use.

C. Recommended Imaging Approach

1. Clinical examination of the breasts and mammography are the basic detection methods. Guidelines are from the American Cancer Society.

2. The screening process should begin by the age of 40 years and should consist of an annual clinical examination and mammography at 1 to 2 year intervals.

3. Beginning at age 50 years, both clinical examination and mammography should be performed on an annual basis.

4. Patients judged to be at higher risk of breast cancer due to factors such as family history, prior radiation exposure, or prior breast biopsy showing cancer or atypia may need to begin screening at an earlier age and may require different screening intervals. A breast specialist should be consulted for these patients.

D. Differential Diagnostic Considerations

1. Note that the previous recommendation for a baseline mammogram at age 35–40 years has been changed. The wording of the American Cancer Society now is that screening should begin by the age of 40.

2. Despite recent controversy over the value of screening women between the ages of 40 and 49 years, numerous medical associations, including the American Cancer Society and the American College of Radiology, continue to support strongly the guidelines described above. The National Cancer Institute recommends that women between the ages of 40 and 49 years consult their physicians regarding screening mammography.

► CHAPTER 7

Chest and Cardiac Disease

Ella Kazerooni, MD
Barry H. Gross, MD
James Meaney, MRCPI, FRCR
University of Michigan Medical Center

Imaging Handbook for House Officers, Edited by Paul M. Silverman and Douglas J. Quint.
ISBN 0-471-13767-7 © 1997 Wiley-Liss, Inc.

Most cardiothoracic pathologic processes present with cough, dyspnea, hemoptysis, or pain. Chest radiographs are the most commonly performed radiologic examination. Many chest radiographs are performed in asymptomatic individuals undergoing "screening" examinations (e.g., preemployment physicals, enlisting in the military); therefore, many findings, such as the solitary pulmonary nodule, may be first detected on the chest radiograph. In addition to presenting *algorithmic approaches* for the evaluation of the symptoms listed above, we have also included algorithms pertinent to the evaluation of abnormalities that are often identified initially on the chest radiograph in an attempt to avoid wasteful and inappropriate use of the more expensive "high-tech" imaging modalities (e.g., CT, MRI, nuclear medicine scans, and angiography). The last two topics, *Staging of Lung Cancer* and *Suspected Opportunistic Infection*, are presented as two specific common clinical problems.

SOLITARY PULMONARY NODULE (SUSPECTED LUNG CANCER)

A. Clinical Findings

1. A solitary pulmonary nodule in an adult must be considered to be malignant until proven otherwise.
2. This applies to asymptomatic patients and those with signs and symptoms of lung cancer, such as cough, hemoptysis, and weight loss.
3. Overall, the most common etiology is a benign granuloma.
4. A lung nodule or mass associated with vocal cord paralysis and hoarse voice implies mediastinal lymph node metastases in the aortopulmonary window due to involvement of the left recurrent laryngeal nerve.
5. Horner's syndrome may be associated with a superior sulcus or Pancoast tumor.

B. Imaging Modalities

1. Chest radiograph
   a. Method by which most solitary nodules are first detected.
   b. High spatial resolution and low cost.

    c. Detects gross hilar and mediastinal lymph node enlargement, pleural fluid, and chest wall invasion, but is not very sensitive for these findings with less extensive disease.

2. CT (from lung apex through the adrenal glands)

    a. Thin sections done to identify the 4 benign patterns of calcification: Solid and diffuse; central; concentric calcified rings; popcorn-like calcification of a hamartoma.

    b. For lung cancer staging. Detects enlarged lymph nodes not identified on the chest radiograph; demonstrates relationship of mass to contiguous structures, including the chest wall (pleura, ribs, spine), hilar vessels, aorta, mediastinum, and heart. Contrast enhancement important.

3. MRI

    a. More expensive than CT.

    b. Inferior to CT in detecting small lung nodules.

    c. Equal to CT in detecting lymph node enlargement.

    d. Superior to CT for detection and delineation of chest wall invasion.

    e. Multiplanar capability; coronal plane particularly useful for superior sulcus (Pancoast) tumors.

4. Percutaneous fine-needle aspiration

    a. For peripheral nodules not accessible to bronchoscopy.

    b. Fluoroscopic guidance for nodules identified on both PA and lateral chest radiographs; otherwise CT guidance (typically for smaller nodules).

C. Recommended Imaging Approach

1. Comparison with prior chest radiographs: A nodule stable in size for 2 or more years is usually considered benign. Some malignant tumors, such as a carcinoid, and some benign lesions, such as a granuloma or hamartoma, may grow very slowly.

2. CT for any new nodule or growth of an old nodule should be performed prior to bronchoscopy or thoracotomy for tumor staging. Lymph nodes identified with CT may be sampled with bronchoscopy or mediastinoscopy, which may change tumor stage and

treatment.

3. Tissue sampling with percutaneous fine-needle aspiration for peripheral lesions and bronchoscopy for central lesions. Remember, a positive fine-needle aspiration or bronchoscopy makes the diagnosis of malignancy, but a negative biopsy does not exclude it.

4. Unless there is suspicion for infection or metastasis from a known primary tumor, patients who are surgical candidates who have a new solitary nodule suspicious for lung cancer without enlarged contralateral mediastinal or hilar lymph node enlargement on CT may go directly to lobectomy without preoperative pathologic proof of malignancy.

D. Differential Diagnostic Considerations

1. *Old films are invaluable.* While it may take extra effort to dig up old films, this may enable the work up of a benign nodule to stop before expensive and interventional procedures are performed.

2. Identifying a benign pattern of calcification on chest radiographs or benign calcification and/or fat in a nodule indicate benign etiologies such as a granuloma or hamartoma and require no further investigation.

3. CT may detect an unsuspected adrenal nodule/mass in approximately 15% of patients, the majority being incidental adrenal adenomas. Proof of benignity must be obtained by biopsy. CT or newer techniques such as chemical-shift MRI may provide a confident diagnosis in many cases.

4. Most common differential diagnoses include
   a. Neoplasm.
      - Bronchogenic carcinoma.
      - Metastasis.
      - Lymphoma.
      - Carcinoid.
      - Hamartoma.
   b. Infection.
      - Fungus: Histoplasmosis (Ohio River Valley), coccidiomycosis (Southwest), nocardia.

- Tuberculosis ("tuberculoma").
- Abscess.
  c. Pseudonodule.
    - Chest wall lesions: Nipple shadow, rib lesion, pleural plaque.
    - Items outside the chest: Hair braids, clothing, buttons, etc.
    - Loculated fluid in a fissure, the so-called pseudotumor.
  d. Other.
    - Arteriovenous malformation: Look for large vein extending to the hilum.
    - Bronchogenic cyst.
    - Pulmonary infarct.
    - Round atelectasis: Associated with asbestos exposure; mimics bronchogenic carcinoma.
    - Pneumoconiosis with conglomerate masses: Upper lobes.
    - Rheumatoid nodule.

References

Webb WR (1990). Radiologic evaluation of the solitary pulmonary nodule. AJR 154:701–708.

Cummings SR, Lillington GA, Richard RJ (1986). Managing solitary pulmonary nodules. Am Rev Respir Dis 134:453–460.

Gurney JW (1993). Determining the likelihood of malignancy in solitary pulmonary nodules with Bayesian analysis. Part 2, application. Radiology 186:415–422.

RECURRENT/PERSISTENT PNEUMONIA OR LOBAR COLLAPSE

A. Clinical Findings

1. When pneumonia recurs within the same lobe, the first concern is to ensure that an appropriate antibiotic regimen has been followed for the treatment of the initial pneumonia.

2. If pneumonia persists or fails to resolve despite antibiotics, or when lobar collapse is encountered in any circumstance, a bronchial ob-

structing lesion, particularly bronchogenic carcinoma, should be suspected.

B. Imaging Modalities

1. Chest radiograph
   a. Pneumonia: Typically air-space (alveolar) disease, characterized by air-bronchograms, ill-defined margins, and a lobar or segmental distribution.
   b. Lobar collapse: In addition to seeing the opacity of the collapsed lobe itself, which is marginated by the pleural fissures, look for secondary signs of volume loss such as:
      - Shift of mediastinal structures (heart, trachea) toward the side of collapse.
      - Elevation of the ipsilateral hemidiaphragm.
      - Crowding of the ipsilateral ribs.
      - Hyperinflation of the contralateral lung.
   c. May see a central hilar mass with lung cancer or lymph node enlargement of any etiology
   d. Identifies level of bronchial obstruction by lobar/segmental distribution of the abnormality
   e. Limited ability in identifying the actual endobronchial/bronchial/peribronchial lesion
2. CT and MRI
   a. See discussion of staging of lung cancer and solitary pulmonary nodule.
   b. In addition to standard images, typically 1 cm in thickness, CT images of smaller thickness through the suspect lobar bronchus optimizes detection of endobronchial lesions.

C. Recommended Imaging Approach

1. *Persistent pneumonia or improvement without complete resolution* in 4–8 weeks despite an optimized antibiotic regimen and *any case of lobar collapse* indicates a bronchial obstructing lesion.
2. While a mass may be seen on chest films, a small central endo-

bronchial (typically squamous cell) lung cancer may be too small to detect on chest films or may be masked by the adjacent pneumonia. Proceed to CT.

3. *Chest CT* is the study of choice. By detecting calcium in an endobronchial lesion, the diagnosis is narrowed to broncholith or foreign body. Locating the endobronchial lesion guides bronchoscopy (see solitary pulmonary nodule and lung cancer staging discussion of CT).

D. Differential Diagnostic Considerations

1. Silhouette sign: Contiguous aerated and soft tissue structures normally create a sharp black–white interface of aerated lung (black) against the soft tissues of the mediastinum and diaphragm/upper abdomen (white). When abnormal lung, such as pneumonia or a collapsed lobe, is adjacent to the mediastinum or diaphragm, air in the lung (black) is replaced by disease (white) and the sharp black–white interface is absent or ill-defined. The right middle lobe is adjacent to the right heart margin; the lingula, the left heart margin; and the lower lobes, the diaphragm.

2. Location of bronchial obstruction portends the affected lobe; a right lower lobe bronchus lesion will have right lower lobe pneumonia or collapse, a bronchus intermedius lesion will have right middle and lower lobe pneumonia/collapse, and a lesion in the right mainstem bronchus will have pneumonia/collapse of the entire right lung. A single primary lung cancer does not usually obstruct the right upper and lower lobes without affecting the middle lobe.

3. Bronchoalveolar carcinoma: Do not forget this malignancy, which has many radiographic appearances, including a solitary nodule or mass (most common), multiple nodules, and "classically" persistent focal or diffuse air-space disease that mimics pneumonia.

4. Lobar collapse in a patient with an asthma exacerbation or occurring in an ICU patient is typically secondary to a mucous plug.

5. Lobar or whole lung collapse in children is most commonly due to an aspirated foreign body.

6. Dilated left atrium: May obstruct the left lower lobe bronchus by extrinsic compression.
7. Differential diagnoses (most common are italicized).
   a. Medical Regimen: Inadequate antibiotic therapy for initial pneumonia.
   b. Neoplasm: Endobronchial tumor or enlarged lymph nodes compressing the bronchus.
      - *Bronchogenic carcinoma.*
      - *Bronchoalveolar cell carcinoma.*
      - Carcinoid.
      - Adenoid cystic carcinoma, mucoepidermoid carcinoma—typically large central airway.
      - Lymphoma.
      - Metastases.
   c. *Foreign Body*: Particularly young children (aspirated pea/peanut) and mentally impaired.
   d. Airway Abnormality.
      - Bronchiectasis.
      - Bronchial stenosis: Congenital, posttraumatic, post-inflammatory.
   e. Inflammatory Conditions: *mucous plug*, asthma, cystic fibrosis—typically acute onset.
   f. Infection.
      - *Atypical organisms*: Fungus, tuberculosis.
      - Right middle lobe syndrome: Chronic, non-neoplastic condition secondary to quiescent granulomatous lymph node disease, usually histoplasmosis or tuberculosis.
      - Chronic organizing pneumonia.
   g. Less Common Etiologies.
      - Radiation pneumonitis and fibrosis.
      - Broncholith: A calcified lymph node from prior granulomatous infection, such as histoplasmosis or tuberculosis, erodes into a bronchus and may be coughed up (broncholithoptysis).

References

Woodring JH (1988). Determining the cause of pulmonary atelectasis: A comparison of plain radiography and CT. AJR 150:757–763.

Hill CA (1988). Bronchioloalveolar cell carcinoma: A review. Radiology 150:15–20.

Kantor HG (1981). The many radiographic faces of pneumococcal pneumonia. AJR 137:1213–1220.

HEMOPTYSIS

A. Clinical Findings

1. Hemoptysis more commonly arises from the lungs and bronchi than the nose, throat, or larynx.
2. Before an investigation of hemoptysis is started, distinguish hemoptysis from hematemesis.
3. Bright red blood indicates an arterial source, either the bronchial arteries as in bronchiectasis or the bronchial veins as in mitral stenosis. Expectorated clots indicate that blood has been in the airway for some time.
4. The most common causes of hemoptysis are acute and chronic bronchitis and pneumonia. These are typically evident from the history and physical examination, supported by the chest radiograph.
5. If hemoptysis is new, persistent, or changes in nature, further investigation should be pursued, particularly in smokers and patients over 40 years of age.
6. Even with investigation, the etiology of hemoptysis remains unexplained in 5%–10% of patients.

B. Imaging Modalities

1. Chest radiograph
   a. First radiologic test in the investigation of hemoptysis.
   b. May directly identify the source by specific diagnosis: Pneumonia, bronchiectasis, bronchogenic carcinoma, mitral stenosis, airway narrowing.

    c. May identify the location of pulmonary hemorrhage: Appears as air-space opacity, with ill-defined margins and air-bronchograms.

2. Planar tomography

    a. Largely replaced by CT. CT is considered superior especially with use of thin sections. However, the ability to image in the coronal and sagittal planes with good spatial resolution has some advantages compared with axial CT. CT reconstructions in the other planes are typically not satisfactory unless performed using helical (spiral) CT.

    b. Particularly useful to evaluate the airway after airway anastomoses or complicated reconstruction, as well as diseases that affect the trachea and mainstem bronchi such as Wegener granulomatosis.

3. CT

    a. Depending on the etiologies under consideration, CT or bronchoscopy is the next step.

    b. Particularly useful for evaluating abnormalities of the airway, such as endobronchial neoplasm and bronchiectasis, with thin-section technique.

    c. Also used for further evaluation of abnormalities identified on chest radiograph, such as a lung mass; little or no role in diffuse hemorrhage.

4. MRI: No primary role in diagnosis.

5. Ventilation/perfusion scan and/or pulmonary angiography. See Suspected Pulmonary Embolus.

C. Recommended Imaging Approach

1. Detailed history and physical examination are essential to reveal the etiology; while some causes are obvious, such as penetrating knife injury, others may require more in-depth investigation, such as Goodpasture's syndrome.

2. Chest radiograph is the first imaging modality to perform. At this point, most infectious, cardiac, and traumatic etiologies will be known and many causes of diffuse pulmonary hemorrhage isolated.

3. If the diagnosis remains in question, bronchoscopy or CT is per-

formed next depending on the suspected etiology. CT is recommended for suspected lung neoplasm or bronchiectasis, bronchoscopy for inflammatory airway disease such as Wegener granulomatosis.

4. Ventilation/perfusion scan and/or pulmonary angiography are reserved for suspected pulmonary embolus.

5. Bronchial arteriography with possible embolization may be used for both diagnosis and treatment of bright red persistent hemoptysis in patients with cystic fibrosis and aspergillosis.

D. Differential Diagnostic Considerations

1. While the chest radiograph is the initial imaging investigation of hemoptysis, some common etiologies may have an entirely normal chest radiograph. While no further investigation is needed when bronchitis is the diagnosis after careful history and physical examination, a negative chest radiograph raises the possibility of endobronchial neoplasm, pulmonary embolus, or bronchiectasis.

2. *Differential diagnoses*
   a. Neoplasm.
      - Bronchogenic carcinoma: Often accompanied by vague chest pain and cough; hemoptysis implies communication of the tumor with airway; this rarely occurs with metastases.
      - Carcinoid: Bleeding may be difficult to arrest, particularly after biopsy.
   b. Infection.
      - Pneumonia.
      - Tuberculosis: Acute pneumonia or active cavity.
      - Fungal: Hemoptysis occurs most commonly in the setting of a fungus ball (*Aspergillus, Nocardia*) in a residual lung cavity secondary to tuberculosis or sarcoidosis; may also occur with necrotizing and ulcerating inflammation or bronchiectasis.
      - Bronchiectasis: Brisk bleeding from bronchial artery; most stops spontaneously, but may recur; may be treated by bronchial artery embolization performed by interventional radiologists.

   c. Diffuse Pulmonary Hemorrhage.
- Goodpasture's syndrome.
- Anticoagulation.
- Bleeding dyscrasia: Idiopathic thrombocytopenic purpura, hemophilia.
- Scurvy.
- Idiopathic pulmonary hemosiderosis: May be life-threatening.

   d. Cardiac and Vascular.
- Mitral stenosis: Bleeding from submucosal bronchial veins, which proliferate as a response to elevated pressure in left atrium and pulmonary veins; may develop secondary hemosiderosis, which may be massive; in some circumstances hemoptysis may be the presenting complaint in a patient with mitral stenosis.
- Pulmonary embolus: See Suspected Pulmonary Embolus.
- Left ventricular failure with chronic pulmonary edema: Pink and frothy sputum, not bright red.

   e. Trauma.
- Penetrating lung trauma: Knife, rib fracture.
- Severe blunt injury: Lung contusion, pulmonary hematoma, lacerations due to shearing forces.
- Fractured bronchus: Associated with persistent pneumomediastinum with or without pneumothorax and collapse of the lung distal to the fractured bronchus.
- Toxic inhalation of fumes or smoke: Airway lining necrosis.
- Severe coughing with mucosal lacerations.
- After lobectomy or pneumonectomy

      Early: Spontaneous emptying of hemothorax; must oversew airway or evacuate hemothorax.

      Late: Recurrent neoplasm, granulation tissue, bronchial sutures; bronchoscopy to evaluate.

   f. Other.
- Vicarious hemoptysis with menstruation.

- Aspirated fractured bronchus, damaging adjacent airway mucosa with or without bronchiectasis.
- Right middle lobe syndrome—lymph node calcification erodes into airway; associated collapse.

References

Colice GL, Chappel GJ, Frenchman SM (1985). Comparison of computerized tomography with fiberoptic bronchoscopy in identifying endobronchial abnormalities in patients with known or suspected lung cancer. Am Rev Respir Dis 131:397–400.

Set PAK, Flower CDR, Smith IE et al (1993). Hemoptysis: Comparative study of the role of CT and fiberoptic bronchoscopy. Radiology 189:677–680.

Mauro MA, Jaques PF, Morris S (1992). Bronchial artery embolization for control of hemoptysis. Semin Intervent Radiol 9:45.

DYSPNEA—NONCARDIAC ETIOLOGIES (SUSPECTED INTERSTITIAL LUNG DISEASE OR PULMONARY VASCULAR DISEASE)

A. Clinical Findings

1. In a patient with clinical evidence of primary lung disease, including progressive shortness of breath, dyspnea on exertion, and cough, supported by pulmonary function tests, the differential diagnosis is vast.

2. Findings on the chest radiograph are used to narrow the differential diagnosis by combining the morphology of the findings with the distribution of the abnormality. The radiologic descriptors and differential diagnoses are used to come closer to a diagnosis; they do not imply that the pathology is entirely within the interstitial or alveolar compartment of the lungs.

3. Honeycombing and linear septal lines of interstitial disease tend to be sharply defined, whereas alveolar disease is typically ill-defined or fluffy.

4. The differential diagnoses below reflect chronic, indolent, or slow-

ly progressive disease, not diseases with an acute onset. In addition to the disease entities, a few clinical and radiologic clues that may favor one diagnosis over another are listed.

B. Imaging Modalities

1. Chest radiograph
   a. Narrows the differential diagnosis based on the findings and their distribution; see Differential diagnoses, below.
   b. May be normal in as many as 10% of patients with interstitial lung disease.
2. High-resolution chest CT
   a. Uses the same machines as standard CT, with the thinnest axial slices of the body possible, typically 1–2 mm.
   b. By using a data reconstruction algorithm that enhances the edges of small opacities and photographing images at a larger size than for standard CT, the detection of subtle abnormalities is enhanced.
   c. Used for the following
      • Better defines chest radiograph abnormalities and narrows differential diagnosis.
      • Normal chest radiograph, but still suspect lung disease.
      • Indicates best site for lung biopsy by identifying the most severely diseased areas.
      • Determines disease activity: Ground-glass appearance may represent reversible alveolitis, whereas honeycombing represents nonreversible fibrosis.
3. Ventilation/perfusion scan and pulmonary angiography: Performed when pulmonary embolus is suspected; refer to Suspected Pulmonary Embolus for further information; the chest radiograph may be entirely normal.
4. MRI: No role in primary diagnosis.

C. Recommended Imaging Approach

1. If interstitial lung disease is suspected and the chest radiograph is normal, high-resolution chest CT is the next step. Remember, the

chest radiograph may be normal in up to 10% of patients with interstitial lung disease. Abnormality on high-resolution CT may lend further support to performing an open or thoracoscopically guided lung biopsy to establish the presence of disease before proceeding to medical therapy, which may include corticosteroids or cytotoxic agents.

2. Rarely, high-resolution CT is normal when there is fibrosis at open lung biopsy. If the clinical picture strongly indicates interstitial fibrosis, a lung biopsy may still be indicated.

D. Differential Diagnostic Considerations

1. Begin with the chest radiograph. The diagnosis may be immediately apparent.

    Example 1: Honeycombing and interstitial opacities with a lower lobe predominance. This is pulmonary fibrosis. Is there a known etiology, such as connective tissue disease? Fibrosis with calcified pleural plaques of asbestos exposure indicate asbestosis. If no etiology can be gleaned from history, physical examination, and laboratory tests (including immunological workup), the diagnosis is idiopathic pulmonary fibrosis. High-resolution CT may further confirm this, but in cases of extensive disease the abnormality is usually well-defined with the chest radiograph.

    Example 2: Diffuse miliary nodules. The most common etiologies are tuberculosis (TB) and metastatic disease. With TB, the patients are typically symptomatic, if not very sick. This is not true with miliary metastases. In addition, a history of renal cell carcinoma, thyroid cancer, and some other tumors lends further support to the diagnosis of metastases. Miliary nodules with an upper lobe predominance together with an appropriate exposure history suggests silicosis.

    Example 3: Normal lungs. If disease is still suspected, consider etiologies such as chronic pulmonary embolus and primary pulmonary hyptertension or early interstitial lung disease.

2. When disease is diffuse, look to an area on the chest radiograph

that is relatively less involved to determine what the pattern is. In more diseased areas, the overlap of multiple lines or nodules may create confluent opacities that may be confused with alveolar disease.

3. Differential diagnoses (most common diagnoses are italicized)

   a. Interstitial disease

      - Honeycombing and/or linear opacities (Septal lines)-(*HIPS—RDS*)

        *H*istiocytosis X (also called eosinophilic granuloma): Upper lobe (UL) > lower lobe (LL), young males, smokers.

        Idiopathic pulmonary fibrosis: LL > UL.

        Pneumoconiosis: UL, silicosis, coal-workers; LL, asbestosis (look for pleural plaques).

        Sarcoidosis:UL > LL; enlarged lymph nodes in stages I and II disease, absent in stages III and IV.

        *R*heumatoid arthritis: LL > UL; history of arthritis; usually males.

        *D*ermatomyositis: LL > UL; soft tissue calcifications.

        *S*cleroderma: LL > UL; abnormal radiographs of hands with soft tissue calcification and acroosteolysis (eroded tips of distal phalanges); dilated esophagus.

        OTHER

        Drug toxicity: Bleomycin, methotrexate, busulfan, nitrofurantoin, amiodarone, gold.

        Inhalation injury: Smoke, chemicals.

        Desquamative interstitial pneumonitis, usual interstitial pneumonitis.

        Lymphangiomyomatosis (LAM): Actual disease is innumerable cysts, but overlapping cyst walls may be seen as faint linear opacities; only in women; hyperinflated lungs.

        Tuberous sclerosis: Same pathology, cysts and hyperinflation of LAM; males and females.

- Miliary Nodules (3–5 mm, tiny) (*TB-Fungus-SHRIMP*)

  *T*uberculosis.

  *F*ungal infections.

  *S*arcoidosis: UL > LL; enlarged lymph nodes in stages I and II disease, absent in stages III and IV.

  *H*istiocytosis X (also called eosinophilic granuloma): UL > LL; young males, smokers.

  *R*heumatoid arthritis: LL > UL.

  *I*diopathic pulmonary fibrosis: LL > UL.

  Metastases: Thyroid carcinoma, renal cell carcinoma.

  *P*neumoconiosis: UL, *silicosis* and coal-workers; LL, asbestosis (look for pleural plaques).

- Reticulonodular Opacities or Small Irregular Shadows (combination of HIPS—RDS and TB—fungus—SHRIMP)

  Lymphangitic spread of neoplasm: Lung, breast primary tumors, lymphoma.

  Sarcoidosis: UL > LL.

  Extrinsic allergic alveolitis (hypersensitivity pneumonitis): Farmer's lung, pigeon breeder's lung, etc.

b. Alveolar disease

- Chronic Alveolar Opacities (ill-defined, air-bronchograms) (*TB-Fungus-DALLAS*)

  *T*uberculosis.

  *F*ungal infections.

  *D*esquamative interstitial pneumonitis.

  *A*lveolar cell carcinoma: Most common finding is a solitary nodule; classic appearance is chronic air space opacity, one or multiple foci; looks like chronic focal pneumonia, but does not resolve with antibiotics.

  *L*ipoid pneumonia: Aspiration of fat-containing material such as cod liver oil; diagnostic fat attenuation on CT.

  *L*ymphoma: Lymph node enlargement; may not have large nodes with primary pulmonary form.

*A*lveolar proteinosis: M > F.

*S*arcoidosis: UL > LL; enlarged lymph nodes in stages I and II disease, absent in stages III and IV.

OTHER

Extrinsic allergic alveolitis (hypersensitivity pneumonitis): Farmer's lung, pigeon breeder's lung, etc.; etiology may be revealed from careful history.

Bronchiolitis obliterans organizing pneumonia.

Wegener granulomatosis: Also look for lung nodules, which may cavitate.

c. Normal chest radiograph
- No disease.
- False-negative chest radiograph in up to 10% of patients with interstitial lung disease.
- Chronic pulmonary emboli: Look for enlarged pulmonary arteries as evidence of pulmonary hyptertension secondary to the chronic emboli.
- Primary pulmonary arterial hypertension: Look for enlarged central pulmonary arteries, with rapid tapering of blood vessels as they extend from the hila to the periphery of the lungs; typically occurs in young women.

References

Bessis L, Callard P, Gotheil C et al (1992). High-resolution CT of parenchymal lung disease: Precise correlation with histologic findings. RadioGraphics 12:45–48.

Grenier P, Chevret S, Beigelman C et al (1994). Chronic diffuse interstitial lung disease: Determination of the diagnostic value of clinical data, chest radiography and CT with Bayesian analysis. Radiology 191:383–390.

Orens JB, Kazerooni EA, Martinez FJ, Curtis JL, Gross BH, Flint A, Lynch JP (1995). The sensitivity of high-resolution computed tomography in detecting biopsy-proven idiopathic pulmonary fibrosis. Chest 108:109–115.

SUSPECTED AORTIC DISSECTION

A. Clinical Findings

1. Acute aortic dissection is a medical emergency; without early diagnosis and treatment, mortality is 25% in the first 24 hours and 90% at 1 year.

2. Diagnosis is suspected with classic presentation of acute-onset interscapular back pain or chest pain, associated with hypertension.

3. Increased incidence of dissection with Marfan syndrome, bicuspid aortic valve, aortic coarctation, and pregnancy.

4. Symptoms often confusing. Approximately 5%–25% of patients do not experience chest pain. Symptoms may be secondary to extension of the dissection into aortic branch vessel and include stroke, myocardial infarction, hemiparesis, bowel ischemia, limb ischemia, and renal failure.

B. Imaging Modalities

1. Chest radiograph
   a. First examination performed.
   b. Findings
      - Wide mediastinum (up to 80%).
      - Double contour of the aorta (40%).
      - Irregular or indistinct aortic margin.
      - Pleural fluid: Hemothorax (27%).
      - Enlarged cardiac silhouette: Hemopericardium.
      - Inward displacement of intimal calcification by greater than 1 cm (7%).
   c. If there is a comparison chest radiograph, look for interval enlargement of the aorta.
   d. Normal in up to 25% of cases.

2. Transesophageal echocardiography (TEE)
   a. Study of choice for diagnosis of acute aortic dissection.

    b. Sensitivity and specificity of 97%–100%.

    c. Rapid examination performed at bedside in 15–30 minutes.

    d. Semi-invasive compared with angiography.

    e. Useful for detecting aortic regurgitation and hemopericardium.

    f. May visualize the proximal coronary arteries and detect myocardial wall motion abnormalities as evidence of ischemia.

    g. Excellent by experienced operators; user-dependent modality with steep learning curve.

3. Aortography

    a. Long held as gold standard for diagnosis.

    b. Invasive catheter procedure in patients at risk for aortic rupture.

    c. Requires large volume of intravenous contrast in patients at risk for renal failure.

    d. Direct finding: Opacification of two lumens separated by an intimal flap, "double barrel aorta."

    e. Limitations of aortography have been better defined with the advent of CT, MRI and TEE; may miss a thin false lumen that is thrombosed and does not deform the true lumen.

    f. Indirect findings, particularly important for diagnosis when the false lumen is thrombosed.

       • Narrow, irregular, or distorted true lumen.

       • Abnormal catheter position, displaced inward from the outer opacity of the aortic margin.

       • Increased aortic wall thickness, greater than 1 cm.

       • Branch vessel involvement: Occlusion by intimal flap or extension of flap into the vessel.

    g. Sensitivity, 80%–85%; specificity, 95%.

4. CT

    a. Noninvasive; requires optimal intravenous contrast bolus.

    b. Findings

       • Intimal flap (linear; calcified in 20%–30%) separates contrast-enhanced true and false lumens.

       • Contrast-enhanced true lumen with an adjacent parallel rim

of low-attenuation material representing thrombus in false
lumen.

- Mediastinal, pleural, pericardial, retroperitoneal blood.
- Asymmetric renal enhancement indicating impaired blood
  flow to the kidney.

c. Standard contrast-enhanced CT: Sensitivity, 80%–83%; specificity, 100%.

d. Currently inadequate for detection of branch vessel involvement (especially coronary arteries) and cannot detect aortic
valve incompetence; newer scanners, specifically spiral CT
with 2D and 3D reconstruction abilities, and rapid scan times
may increase sensitivity and allow better delineation of branch
vessel involvement.

5. MRI

a. Non-invasive; no intravenous contrast; multiplanar capability.

b. Less readily available than CT and TEE; often in remote sites;
difficult to monitor unstable patients; cannot yet directly identify coronary artery involvement.

c. Sensitivity, 91%–100%; specificity, 95%–100%.

d. Perhaps best used in patients when suspicion for acute dissection is low, for evaluation of chronic dissection, and for follow-
up of aortic dissection. Limited in sick patients on support devices.

C. Recommended Imaging Approach

1. Begin with chest radiograph to identify findings to support the diagnosis of dissection and identify other reasons for the patient's
symptoms, such as pneumonia and pulmonary edema.

2. If the clinical suspicion is strong, the next step is less certain and
may depend on the expertise with the various imaging modalities
available, and on the thoracic surgeon. To make the diagnosis of
aortic dissection, proceed to transesophageal echocardiography or
CT. If evaluation of the aorta is complete with TEE, and the coronary arteries are well visualized, some surgeons will proceed directly to surgery for dissection involving the ascending aorta. If

dissection is diagnosed and spares the ascending aorta, medical therapy for control of pain and hypertension is indicated; however, if the patient is hemodynamically unstable or if pain persists, surgery may be warranted.

3. If transesophageal echocardiography is not readily available, is inconclusive, or cannot be completed due to difficulty passing the intraesophageal probe, CT is recommended as the imaging modality for diagnosis. CT is readily available, is more sensitive and less invasive than aortography, and can be performed in 30–60 minutes. CT is widely used as a primary diagnostic procedure.

4. Aortography is reserved for the delineation of the dissection and branch vessel involvement when surgery is planned or contemplated. When a dissection is complicated by bowel, renal, or extremity ischemia, indicating reduced blood flow to these structures, a fenestration procedure may be performed at the time of aortography (a hole is created in the flap) to increase blood flow in the lumen responsible for ischemia. Lastly, investigational work is being performed with aortic stents, placed percutaneously into the aorta or branch vessels, for treatment of ischemic complications.

D. Differential Diagnostic Considerations

1. A normal chest radiograph does not exclude the diagnosis of aortic dissection.

2. Helical (spiral) CT can now effectively evaluate for dissection with conservative doses of contrast. Helical CT also has the ability in some cases to demonstrate dissection involving the great vessels and display this in 3D form.

References

Cigarroa JE, Isselbacher EM, DiSanctis RW et al (1993). Medical progress: Diagnostic imaging in the evaluation of suspected aortic dissection: old standards and new directions. AJR 161:485.

Fisher ER, Stern EJ, Godwin JD et al (1994). Acute aortic dissection: Typical and atypical imaging features. RadioGraphics 14:1263–1271.

Spittell PC, Spittell JA, Joyce JW et al (1993). Clinical features and differential diagnosis of aortic dissection: Experience with 236 cases (1980–1990). Mayo Clin Proc 68:643–651.

SUSPECTED PULMONARY EMBOLUS

A. Clinical Findings

1. Dyspnea, pleuritic chest pain, tachypnea and, less commonly, hemoptysis are the common signs and symptoms of pulmonary embolus (PE).

2. Many patients are asymptomatic or have nonspecific complaints, which delays the diagnosis.

3. Oral contraceptive use, lower extremity deep venous thrombosis (DVT), prolonged bedrest, recent myocardial infarction, or congestive heart failure should heighten the suspicion for PE.

4. With prompt diagnosis and treatment, mortality can be reduced from 30% to less than 10%.

B. Imaging Modalities

1. Chest radiograph
   a. Usually normal; may see atelectasis or pleural effusion.
   b. Less common findings include
      - Westermark's sign: Lung supplied by vessel containing embolism is oligemic and more lucent in comparison to the rest of the lung; difficult to appreciate, even in retrospect.
      - Hampton's hump: Peripheral wedge-shaped opacity with broad surface of contact against the pleural surface and apex pointing toward hilum; this is a pulmonary infarct.

2. Ventilation/perfusion (V/Q) scan
   a. Noninvasive means of diagnosing PE.
   b. Careful correlation with chest radiograph obtained within 24 hours is essential.
   c. Normal perfusion scan completely excludes the diagnosis of PE.
   d. Low-probability scan has a <10% incidence of PE.

    e. Intermediate-probability scan has a <20%–40% incidence of PE.

    f. High-probability scan has a >85% incidence of PE.

    g. These figures are from the widely quoted PIOPED study.

3. Pulmonary angiography

    a. Gold standard for the diagnosis of PE.

    b. As an invasive catheter procedure, there are associated complications.

    c. It is important to know several things before a pulmonary angiogram is performed.

- Is there known pulmonary hypertension? If yes, the rate and total amount of contrast injected is reduced to minimize the occurrence of sudden death.

- Is there a left bundle branch block? If yes, strong consideration should be given to the placement of a transvenous pacemaker in the event that a right bundle branch block develops during the procedure.

- If the study is positive, is there a contraindication to anticoagulation? If yes, an inferior vena cava filter can be placed as part of the same procedure.

4. Noninvasive studies for DVT

    a. Have largely replaced intravenous contrast venography for the diagnosis of DVT.

    b. The combination of V/Q scan and results of noninvasive studies may strengthen or weaken the suspicion for PE and the conviction with which to proceed to angiography.

5. CT

    a. Filling defects in large, central pulmonary arteries may be incidentally detected on contrast-enhanced CT; however, this is not used for the routine diagnosis of PE.

    b. Newer CT technology—helical (spiral) CT—allows faster imaging with excellent enhancement of the pulmonary arteries; images may be reconstructed in three dimensions, yielding images similar to conventional angiography; there may be a larger role for this noninvasive modality for the detection of PE in the future for central clots; however, distal to the segmental arteries, helical CT is not yet reliable.

6. MRI
   a. Like CT, MRI is not currently a modality used for the diagnosis of acute pulmonary embolism.
   b. MR angiography produces images similar to pulmonary angiography and is currently being investigated as a noninvasive means of diagnosis.

C. Recommended Imaging Approach

1. The chest radiograph is the first examination in a patient with suspected PE.
2. The next test to perform is the V/Q scan. A normal perfusion scan excludes PE, and a high-probability V/Q scan is considered to represent PE, other factors should be considered.
   - Low-probability V/Q scan and low clinical suspicion: Terminate workup for PE.
   - Low-probability V/Q scan and high clinical suspicion for PE: Proceed to angiography.
   - Intermediate-probability V/Q scan: Again, the decision to proceed to angiography or end the investigation depends on the clinical suspicion for PE versus other etiologies of symptoms, including risk factors for PE and the presence of DVT, and the findings on chest radiograph; when in doubt, noninvasive studies of the lower extremities may be useful in looking for DVT, which strengthens the case for the possibility of PE.
3. Pulmonary angiography is the gold standard for diagnosis and may be performed after a V/Q scan if the diagnosis remains a question.
4. The V/Q scan may be bypassed in cases when there is clinical suspicion of acute life-threatening massive PE. Pulmonary embolectomy can be performed acutely in the angiography suite via suction catheters. The other alternative for massive PE with right heart strain is surgical embolectomy.

5. Noninvasive studies of the lower extremities may alter the clinical suspicion for PE. In particular, when positive noninvasive studies for DVT are encountered with an intermediate-probability V/Q scan, this increases the diagnostic certainty of the V/Q scan for PE, and a patient may be anticoagulated.

6. Developing technologies such as helical CT and MR angiography may play a role in the future. Using 3D techniques and image manipulation, data from these scans can be used to generate images similar to formal endovascular angiography. For the detection of emboli in large pulmonary vessels, helical CT may obviate the need for V/Q scanning. However, as these technologies are still relatively primitive, their respective roles are as yet not fully defined.

D. Differential Diagnostic Considerations

1. A normal chest radiograph does not exclude the diagnosis of PE. In fact, no chest radiograph excludes PE. The chest radiograph is important to exclude other etiologies that may have a similar clinical presentation, such as pneumonia or pneumothorax. In addition, the chest radiograph is essential in the interpretation of ventilation/perfusion scans, as the schemes for interpretation of V/Q scans include the chest radiograph.

2. Helical CT can confidently make the diagnosis of PE in larger vessels. Thus this technique can be used as a noninvasive method to document and follow such clot.

References

PIOPED Investigators (1990). Value of the ventilation-perfusion scan in acute pulmonary embolism. JAMA 263:2753–2759.

Quinn RJ, Butler SP (1991). A decision analysis approach to the treatment of patients with suspected pulmonary emboli and an intermediate probability lung scan. J Nuclear Med 32:2050–2056.

Webber MM, Gomes AS, Roes D et al (1990). Comparison of Biello, McNeil, and PIOPED criteria for the diagnosis of pulmonary emboli on lung scans. AJR 154:975–981.

CHEST PAIN—CARDIOGENIC (SUSPECTED MYOCARDIAL INFARCTION)

A. Clinical Findings

1. When a patient presents with chest pain, the first step is to decide whether the pain is cardiac, pleural, tracheobronchial, gastrointestinal, or related to the chest wall. Another etiology of chest pain to consider is aortic dissection. Careful history and physical examination should distinguish the organ of origin in patients with chest pain.

2. Classic crushing retrosternal chest pain described as "it feels like there's an elephant standing on my chest" that radiates to the left arm or neck in a diaphoretic patient should immediately raise the possibility of myocardial infarction.

3. Pleuritic pain is localized close to the chest wall in the lower half of the thorax, often exacerbated by coughing, laughing, or deep inspiration, with resultant rapid respiratory rate and small tidal volumes. Most often secondary to pleural effusion or inflammation, commonly infection, and therefore often accompanied by fever, malaise, and dyspnea.

4. Pain related to the large airways usually represents tracheobronchitis or tracheitis and is sharp or searing in nature, exacerbated by coughing, and localized to the large central airways.

5. Chest wall pain is focal, reproducible on direct palpation.

6. Chest pain of gastrointestinal abnormalities, particularly gastroesophageal reflux and esophagitis, may mimic myocardial infarction. This pain is often related to eating habits and may be more severe in the recumbent position or after a large meal.

7. Obtaining a history that is consistent with coronary artery disease, including previous angina pectoris, will strengthen conviction regarding the cardiac etiology of chest pain. The evaluation of suspected acute myocardial infarction centers on the careful history and physical examination and the electrocardiogram (ECG). Pain not relieved by nitroglycerin, severe and prolonged pain, hypotension, pulmonary edema, left ventricular failure and, ECG changes

of myocardial injury support acute myocardial infarction. Serial ECGs and cardiac enzymes can be used to strengthen diagnostic certainty. However, in the patient with an acute myocardial infarction, a decision must be made quickly in order to undertake measures to reduce or prevent further myocardial damage, including thrombolytic therapy or emergent cardiac catheterization and possible acute angioplasty.

B. Imaging Modalities

1. Chest radiograph.
2. Nuclear cardiology study.
3. Endocardiography.
4. Direct coronary angiography.

C. Recommended Imaging Approach

1. Chest radiograph
   a. Used to exclude other causes of chest pain.
   b. Look for pulmonary edema; this is a poor prognostic sign in the setting of acute myocardial infarction.
   c. New, massive pulmonary edema delayed by a few days from initial presentation should raise the possibility of papillary muscle rupture and acute myocardial infarction.
2. Nuclear imaging: Pyrophosphate scan (^{99m}Tc)
   a. 60%–90% sensitive, 66%–99% specific for myocardial infarction.
   b. "Hot spot" imaging; an infarct takes up tracer and appears as a focus of tracer deposition.
   c. Used to make the diagnosis of myocardial infarction when serial enzymes are equivocal or unreliable (after CPR, cardiac massage, open heart surgery) or when the window of opportunity to use cardiac enzymes has expired.
   d. Becomes positive 24–48 hours after the onset of injury, with greatest uptake at 48–96 hours.
   e. Returns to normal in 7–10 days.

3. Echocardiography
   a. Used in the setting of acute infarction to evaluate cardiac valve function, particularly if there is a new cardiac murmur; also looks at wall motion abnormalities, which may be evidence of acute myocardial injury.
   b. Used to look for pericardial effusion when there is a pericardial rub or evidence of cardiac tamponade; this may occur a few days after a large full-thickness infarct if there is cardiac rupture.
4. Coronary angiography and acute angioplasty. There is increasing evidence to support the use of angioplasty for the treatment of acute myocardial infarction, in an attempt to open the causative arterial blockage as soon as possible and reduce myocardial injury, instead of thrombolytic therapy (which is associated with bleeding complications—stroke, retroperitoneal hemorrhage); others believe in the use of thrombolytic therapy acutely, followed by cardiac catheterization and coronary angiography within several days; stay tuned to the cardiology literature for the final word.

D. Differential Diagnostic Considerations

Diagnosis can be difficult. Radiographic evaluation is limited to subspecialty areas.

References

Aisenberg J Castell DO (1994). Approach to the patient with unexplained chest pain. Mt. Sinai J Med 61:476–483.

Hackshaw BT (1992). Excluding heart disease in the patient with chest pain. Am J Med 92(5A):46S–51S.

Seager LH (1995). Diagnosis of chest pain. Pluses and minuses of stress tests. Postgrad Med 97:131–136, 139–140, 143–145.

MEDIASTINAL MASS

A. Clinical Findings

1. The radiologic diagnosis of a mediastinal mass is a two-step

process. First is recognition of a mass; second is localization of the abnormality to the mediastinum. The latter is generally accomplished by noting where the mass is centered and by demonstrating an obtuse or right angle at the margin of the mass (lesions originating in the lung are usually almost surrounded by lung, resulting in an acute angle at the margin of the lesion).

2. Mass detection is more challenging; in our experience, one-third of CT-detected mediastinal masses are missed by chest radiography, with more than half of middle mediastinal masses escaping detection.

3. Differential diagnosis is facilitated by separating anterior, middle, and posterior mediastinal masses a la Felson—on the lateral radiograph, draw a line down the front of the trachea and the back of the heart and a second line 1 cm behind the anterior margin of the thoracic spine, and you have three compartments.

B. Imaging Modalities

1. Plain chest radiograph
   a. Usual first tool.
   b. Low cost, low radiation.
   c. Poor sensitivity, poor specificity.

2. Barium swallow: Good tool for middle mediastinal masses, especially those of esophageal origin.

3. Computed tomography
   a. In reality, everyone goes to CT after chest radiograph.
   b. CT helpful even after negative chest film in high-risk patients (i.e., myasthenia gravis, rule out thymoma).
   c. CT contributes to differential diagnosis by demonstrating fat, water, or calcium in a lesion; by precisely localizing abnormality; by revealing extent of mass (single or multiple); and by showing concomitant abnormalities (axillary or neck nodes, lung nodules, upper abdominal disease).

4. MRI: A problem-solving tool, such as for patients allergic to iodinated contrast injection.

C. Recommended Imaging Approach

1. Careful correlation between clinical information and chest radiographic features (e.g., a teenager with a calcified anterior mediastinal mass has teratoma).
2. CT for further information (smooth water attenuation middle mediastinal mass is bronchogenic cyst).
3. Tissue sampling is usually a surgical procedure, now sometimes accomplished via thoracoscopy.

D. Differential Diagnostic Considerations

1. Lymphoma almost never a single middle mediastinal mass; patients with multiple masses do not have thymoma or teratoma.
2. CT demonstration of enhancing mediastinal mass strongly suggests thyroid (rarely extraadrenal pheochromocytoma or paraganglioma; rarely, Castleman's disease) and virtually eliminates lymphoma and metastases.
3. Lymphoma versus metastases: Enlarged axillary nodes favor lymphoma, while focal liver lesions, bone lesions, or a focal lung mass favor metastases.
4. Differential diagnoses
   a. Anterior Mediastinal Mass.
      - Thymoma.
      - Teratoma.
      - Thyroid.
      - Terrible lymphoma.
   b. Middle Mediastinal Mass.
      - Esophageal abnormality.
      - Bronchogenic cyst.
      - Lymph node disease (lymphoma, metastases, sarcoidosis, tuberculosis, fungus).
   c. Posterior Mediastinal Mass.
      - Neurogenic tumor.
      - Disc space infection.

    d. Any Mediastinal Mass.
- Metastases.
- Aneurysm.
- Trauma.
- Infection.

References

Rebner M, Gross BH, Robertson JM et al (1987). CT evaluation of mediastinal masses. Comput Radiol 11:103–110.

Spizarny DL, Renber M, Gross BH (1987). Enhancing mediastinal masses: CT evaluation. J Comput Assist Tomogr 11:990–993.

HILAR MASS

A. Clinical Findings

1. A hilar mass is an important presentation of bronchogenic carcinoma.
2. The first step is to confirm that there really is a hilar mass. A lesion in the lung parenchyma may overlie the hilum on one view (either frontal or lateral), but the other view will usually reveal that the lesion is not hilar.
3. A more difficult situation is enlargement of a pulmonary artery; masses tend to be lobular, while arterial enlargement tends to be smooth, but this is often hard to distinguish.

B. Imaging Modalities

1. Plain chest radiograph
   a. Usual means for detecting a hilar abnormality.
   b. Low cost, low radiation.
2. CT
   a. Very sensitive for detecting enlarged hilar lymph nodes.
   b. Also sensitive for detecting concurrent mediastinal lymph node enlargement.

    c. With the administration of bolus intravenous contrast, is excellent for distinguishing lymph nodes (do not enhance) from enlarged arteries (enhance).

  3. MRI

    a. May differentiate artery from lymph node or mass without administration of contrast.

    b. More expensive, slower, and less readily available than CT.

    c. Not currently advisable for concurrent evaluation of lung parenchyma, especially compared with CT.

C. Recommended Imaging Approach

1. Comparison with prior chest radiographs remains the first step! If hilar enlargement is stable for 2 or more years, no further workup is generally required.

2. CT is the preferred modality to differentiate artery from mass and to detect other thoracic abnormality; MRI used occasionally in patients with contrast allergy or for problem solving.

3. Clinical correlation may suffice—an asymptomatic young patient with bilateral hilar lymph node enlargement (often with right paratracheal lymph node enlargement) most commonly has sarcoidosis.

4. Tissue sampling is usually accomplished by transbronchial biopsy, less commonly with fluoroscopic or CT guidance.

D. Differential Diagnostic Considerations

1. Separate unilateral from bilateral hilar abnormality. Bilaterality favors sarcoidosis, lymphoma, or small cell lung carcinoma. Unilaterality suggests non-small cell bronchogenic carcinoma, lymphoma, or tuberculosis.

2. Look for other mediastinal lymph node abnormality. Significant mediastinal nodal abnormality favors lymphoma, small cell carcinoma, or metastatic disease, especially if there is significant enlargement of anterior mediastinal prevascular nodes (rare in sarcoidosis).

3. Differential diagnoses.

  a. Malignancy.
   - Bronchogenic carcinoma.
   - Lymphoma.
   - Metastasis.
  b. Infection.
   - Tuberculosis.
   - Fungal infection (especially histoplasmosis and coccidioidomycosis).
   - Mononucleosis.
  c. Miscellaneous.
   - Sarcoidosis.
   - Dilantin therapy.
  d. Arterial Abnormalities.
   - Pulmonary artery hypertension.
   - Central or chronic pulmonary embolus.
   - Pulmonic stenosis (left hilum only).

References

Glazer GM, Francis IR, Shorazi KK et al (1983). Evaluation of the pulmonary hilum: Comparison of conventional radiography, 55 posterior oblique tomography and dynamic computed tomography. J Comput Assist Tomogr 7:983–989.

Glazer GM, Gross BH, Aisen AM et al (1985). Imaging of the pulmonary hilum: A prospective comparison in patients with lung cancer. AJR 145:245–248.

PNEUMOTHORAX

A. Clinical Findings

  1. Radiologic detection of pneumothorax depends significantly on patient position and requires knowledge of the key diagnostic radiologic signs. Remember, whatever the patient's position, pleural air will collect in the most nondependent part of a hemithorax.
  2. Apical lucency and failure to demonstrate lung markings are not especially helpful signs of pneumothorax, particularly in the supine

patient; these findings may only indicate bullous emphysema. Paradoxically, many patients who have pneumothorax as a significant clinical concern are repeatedly radiographed in the supine position.

3. Upright chest radiography is far more sensitive than supine films; lateral decubitus radiography is a good alternative if the patient cannot sit up. The decubitus position differs from that used to diagnose pleural effusion; right lateral decubitus radiography is good for right pleural effusion or left pneumothorax.

4. The key finding is detection of the lung edge displaced from the chest wall by pleural air. In the supine position air accumulates at the base of the hemithorax; there may be a demonstrable lung edge caudally, or there may only be increased lucency.

5. A small pneumothorax is difficult to detect, no matter how experienced the interpreter is.

B. Imaging Modalities

1. Plain chest radiography
   a. Good first step.
   b. Upright frontal preferred.
   c. If there is a strong clinical suspicion for pneumothorax and the inspiratory view is negative, an expiratory view may reveal a small pneumothorax; even so, these pneumothoraces are typically small and do not usually require chest tube placement.

2. Lateral decubitus radiography: The best alternative if the patient cannot sit up.

3. Cross-table lateral chest radiography: Invariably useless.

4. CT
   a. Has detected numerous unsuspected pneumothoraces, particularly in supine trauma patients.
   b. Nevertheless, lateral decubitus radiography is far more cost-effective and is preferred.
   c. In every trauma patient who has a chest or abdominal CT, pneumothorax should specifically be looked for.

C. Differential Diagnostic Considerations

1. Any diffuse interstitial disease can cause pneumothorax from rupture of honeycomb cysts, but in young males this is especially likely to occur with pulmonary eosinophilic granuloma; in young females lymphangiomyomatosis is an important consideration, especially if there are Kerley lines, (chylous) pleural effusions, or enlarged low attenuation mediastinal and/or retroperitoneal lymph nodes.

2. Metastatic sarcoma (e.g., osteosarcoma) has a predilection for cavitation and may rupture into the pleura with resultant pneumothorax; metastatic squamous cell carcinoma cavitates less often, but is so much more common that most cavitary metastases are squamous.

3. Tuberculosis is well-known to cause pneumothorax with an otherwise near-normal chest radiograph because of cavitary subpleural foci of infection.

4. Pneumothorax does not cause subsequent pneumomediastinum, but pneumomediastinum may result in pneumothorax.

5. Differential diagnoses.

   a. Idiopathic: Ruptured blebs—by far the most common, usually in asthenic young males.

   b. Increased Intrathoracic Pressure.
      - Asthma.
      - Pregnancy.

   c. Diffuse Parenchymal Abnormality.
      - Emphysema.
      - Diffuse interstitial fibrosis.
      - Cystic fibrosis.
      - Diffuse cystic disease (eosinophilic granuloma, lymphangiomyomatosis, tuberous sclerosis).

   d. Miscellaneous.
      - Trauma (blunt, penetrating, or iatrogenic).
      - Cavitary metastases.
      - Cavitary infectious disease.

References

Carr JJ, Reed JC, Chopkin RH et al (1992). Plain and computed tomography for detecting experimentally induced pneumothorax in cadavers: Implications for detection in patients. Radiology 183:193–199.

Seow A, Kazerooni EA, Cascade PN, Pernicano P, Neary M (1996). Comparison of upright inspiratory and expiratory chest radiographs for the detection of pneumothorax. AJR (in press).

Tocino IM (1985). Pneumothorax in the supine patient: Radiographic anatomy. RadioGraphics 5:557–585.

PLEURAL EFFUSION

A. Clinical Findings

1. Imaging plays two important roles in patients with pleural effusion. The first is detection of the effusion; many patients with pleural effusion have no related symptoms, while many patients with pleural symptoms (pleuritic chest pain, referred shoulder pain) have no pleural effusion.

2. The second role (in some patients) is guidance for sampling of fluid. Pleural effusion is usually detected because it results in blunting of the costophrenic sulci. On the frontal radiograph this is seen laterally. A much earlier sign on the lateral radiograph is blunting of the posterior costophrenic sulci. Up to 75 ml of fluid can occupy the subpulmonic pleural space without blunting costophrenic sulci. At least 175 ml is needed to blunt the lateral sulci, and 150 ml is required to blunt the posterior sulci.

3. Patient position plays a crucial role in diagnosing pleural effusion. For example, in the supine patient fluid layers posterior to the lung in the pleural space; if the effusion is unilateral, this results in asymmetric increased opacity of the affected hemithorax. The underlying pulmonary vessels in this case are still surrounded by aerated lung and are well visualized, whereas in diffuse lung disease such as pneumonia the vessels cannot be seen.

B. Imaging Modalities

1. Plain chest radiograph
   a. Good first step.
   b. Upright, frontal and lateral preferred.
2. Lateral decubitus radiography
   a. Side of suspected effusion down.
   b. Improves detection of fluid and assessment of effusion size and mobility.
3. Ultrasonography
   a. Especially helpful with loculated effusion.
   b. A good tool for guidance of thoracentesis.
4. CT
   a. Good demonstration of pleural effusion.
   b. But so what?
   c. Rarely explains the etiology of an isolated effusion.
   d. Seldom needed.
5. MRI: Does not provide incremental information to justify added time and expense.

C. Recommended Imaging Approach

1. Chest radiography with or without lateral decubitus radiography.
2. Thoracentesis is the key tool in understanding the etiology of pleural effusion.
3. If thoracentesis is unsuccessful based on radiography, percussion, and standard techniques, ultrasonographic guidance is recommended.

D. Differential Diagnostic Considerations

1. Most pleural effusions result from CHF; these effusions are usually bilateral and symmetric, or the right pleural effusion may be somewhat larger.
2. Systemic lupus erythematosis (SLE) and rheumatoid arthritis are collagen vascular diseases that often result in pleural effusion; with SLE, there may also be a pericardial effusion.

3. Pancreatitis generally causes a left pleural effusion, while ascites and Meig's syndrome tend to result in right pleural effusion.

4. Subpulmonic pleural effusion displaces the apparent dome of the hemidiaphragm laterally (usually medial to midhemidiaphragm) and results in diffuse increased opacity of the hemidiaphragm because of displaced posterior costophrenic sulcus lung.

5. Fluid may accumulate in a fissure, usually assuming a biconvex (cigar-shaped), tapering configuration.

6. Differential diagnoses.
   a. Malignancy.
      - Pleural metastases.
      - Lymphoma.
      - Malignant mesothelioma.
      - Meig's syndrome (benign or malignant ovarian mass).
   b. Infection.
      - Pneumonia with sympathetic effusion.
      - Empyema.
   c. Inflammation.
      - Collagen vascular disease.
      - Postmyocardial infarction (Dressler's syndrome) or postcardiotomy.
      - Subdiaphragmatic (e.g., subphrenic abscess or pancreatitis).
   d. Trauma.
      - Community-acquired.
      - Iatrogenic.
   e. Vascular.
      - Congestive heart failure (CHF)—right more often than left ventricular failure, but usually biventricular.
      - Pulmonary emboli, bland or septic.
   f. Miscellaneous.
      - Hypoproteinemia.
      - Nephrotic syndrome.
      - Ascites with transdiaphragmatic migration.

References

Bartter T, Santarelli R, Akers SM, Pratter MR (1994). The evaluation of pleural effusion. Chest 106:1209–1214.

Ruskin JA, Gurney JW, Thorsen MK, Goodman LR (1987). Detection of pleural effusions on supine chest radiographs. AJR 148:681–683.

Vix VA (1974). Roentgenographic recognition of pleural effusion. JAMA 22:695–698.

OPPORTUNISTIC INFECTION

A. Clinical Findings

1. In the past, "rule out opportunistic infection" was an occasional indication for radiographic evaluation, usually in patients receiving chemotherapy.

2. Opportunistic infections have unfortunately become more common in the AIDS era, and the number of potential infecting agents has increased almost exponentially.

3. Radiologists spend years learning to apply Osler's rule ("No matter how you pinch and squeeze, it's got to fit just one disease") by sifting through a patient's radiologic and clinical findings and discovering the one underlying disease that explains them all. For an AIDS patient, however, Osler's rule is invalidated; if there's one radiographic pattern it's probably due to three concurrent organisms (Hictum's dictum: "A patient can have as many diseases as he damn well pleases").

B. Imaging Modalities

1. Plain chest radiograph
   a. A good screening tool.
   b. May miss subtle or early disease.
   c. High index of suspicion required in this setting.
2. CT
   a. Standard scanning of minimal value unless mediastinal abnormality is suspected.

   b. High-resolution CT (HRCT) using thin sections, bone recon-
      struction algorithm, and targeted images is a new modality for
      lung parenchymal disease.
   c. HRCT more sensitive than chest radiography, but current role
      unknown.
   d. Abdominal and pelvic CT may also be needed to exclude ab-
      dominal abscess.
3. Nuclear medicine scanning
   a. Gallium and indium-labeled white cell scanning are options for
      detecting inflammatory disease.
   b. High sensitivity, low specificity.
   c. Total body imaged, but anatomic resolution poor.

C. Recommended Imaging Approach

1. Chest radiograph is a first step.
2. If negative with persistent symptoms, consider HRCT.
3. Gallium and indium studies are alternative possibilities, but they
   take longer to complete.
4. Bronchoscopy with lavage is another alternative.

D. Differential Diagnostic Considerations

1. Typical features
   a. Pneumocystis: Diffuse radiographic abnormality, first intersti-
      tial and then alveolar; typically not associated with lymph node
      enlargement or pleural effusion.
   b. Aspergillus: Multiple cavitary nodules with central nondepen-
      dent debris.
   c. Other fungi: Multiple nodules, lymph nodes, multifocal air-
      space disease.
   d. Bacteria: Air-space disease, often more focal.
   e. Viruses: Similar to pneumocystis.
   f. TB: Not a common opportunistic organism except in AIDS,
      where lymph node enlargement predominates (on CT, nodes
      may have enhancing rims with low attenuation centers); cavi-

tation occurs more often than with primary TB in normal hosts.

2. HRCT findings
   a. Ground-glass opacity: Early air-space disease, often in pneumocystis or cytomegalovirus.
   b. "CT halo sign": A nodule surrounded by edema, usually indicating a hemorrhagic nodule. First described in invasive aspergillosis, but now with a long differential.

3. Remember malignancy (e.g., AIDS-related Kaposi sarcoma, lymphoma, or lung cancer or pulmonary involvement by leukemia or lymphoma).

4. Think before ordering: Most febrile immunocompromised patients are pancultured and pantreated. If that's the plan, why order HRCT?

5. Differential diagnoses: Any immunocompromised host can get any opportunistic infection; the following are common.
   a. Acute leukemia.
      - Gram-negative bacteria.
      - Fungi—especially *Aspergillus* and *Candida*.
   b. Chronic Leukemia: Multiple organisms.
   c. Hodgkin's Disease.
      - *Toxoplasma*
      - *Cryptococcus*
      - Other fungi
   d. Non-Hodgkin's Lymphoma.
      - Gram-negative bacteria.
      - Encapsulated bacteria.
   e. Transplant patients.
      - Cytomegalovirus—especially 1–6 months after surgery.
      - *Nocardia*.
      - Mycobacteria.
      - *Histoplasma*.
      - Herpes.
      - Pneumocystis.
      - *Strongyloides*.
   f. Cushing syndrome (endogenous or exogenous).

- *Cryptococcus.*
- *Aspergillus.*
- *Nocardia.*
- Pneumocystis.
- *Strongyloides.*

g. AIDS.
  - Any infection.
  - Especially pneumocystis and cytomegalovirus.

References

Morrison DL, Granton JT, Kesten S, Balter MS (1993). Cavitary aspergillosis as a complication of AIDS. Can Assoc Radiol J 44:35–38.

Naidich DO, Garay SM, Leitman BS, McCauley DI (1987). Radiographic manifestations of pulmonary disease in the acquired immunodeficiency syndrome (AIDS). Semin Roentgenol 22:14–30.

Wasserman K, Pithoff G, Kim E et al (1993). Chronic pneumocystic pneumonia in AIDS. Chest 104:667–672.

STAGING LUNG CANCER

A. Clinical Findings

1. Bronchogenic carcinoma is now the leading cause of cancer deaths in both American men and American women.

2. At the present time complete surgical resection is the only therapy that offers a significant likelihood of cure. Surgical resection is reserved for patients without distant spread of disease.

3. Determining whether there is distant spread requires a complex interplay of clinical, laboratory, radiologic, endoscopic, and surgical procedures. For example, signs or symptoms may point to the presence of distant metastases, or laboratory findings (elevation of enzymes) may suggest hepatic (or skeletal or other) spread. In most patients, there is no definite evidence of unresectability based on history, physical examination, and laboratory studies.

4. At this point there are three ways to proceed: directly to surgery, to preoperative mediastinoscopy, or to radiologic testing. If the patient

goes directly to surgery there will be a large number of unnecessary "exploratory thoracotomies," so the real question is whether preoperative testing should be radiologic or mediastinoscopic.

5. Proponents of radiologic staging point to the significant morbidity (and even mortality) of the surgical procedure and to its blind spots; certain lymph node groups (such as aortopulmonary window nodes) cannot be visualized or sampled, and the upper abdomen is obviously not evaluated. Furthermore, the sensitivity of radiologic staging has usually been reported in the 85%–90% range. If it looks like there is clear consensus in favor of radiologic staging, do not worry—things are never as obvious as they seem. Recent reports suggest that the sensitivity of radiologic staging for mediastinal lymph node metastases in lung cancer patients is closer to 50%.

Theory of Noninvasive Staging: When a therapeutic procedure is costly and invasive (such as lobectomy), the goal of noninvasive staging should be to prevent unnecessary intervention. Noninvasive staging should detect almost every example of unresectability. However, not every patient thus detected must be unresectable. Imaging is not the sole arbiter of unresectability; patients can be triaged so that only some patients require more invasive staging. The key is that negative imaging should almost always mean that the patient is resectable.

Findings of Unresectable Lung Cancer

1. Contralateral mediastinal or hilar lymph node metastases.
2. Distant metastases, such as
   - Liver: Many liver lesions in lung cancer patients are cysts or hemangiomas.
   - Adrenal glands: Two-thirds of adrenal masses in lung cancer patients are benign.
3. Malignant pleural effusion: Requires thoracentesis for definitive diagnosis.
4. Mediastinal invasion.
5. Cell type: Small cell unresectable.
6. Inoperability: Regardless of resectability, some patients cannot tolerate the proposed surgery because of insufficient pulmonary reserve or concurrent disease (e.g., cardiac disease).

B. Imaging Modalities

1. Plain chest radiograph
   a. The first step in diagnosis and staging.
   b. Good for pleural effusion (especially when supplemented by lateral decubitus radiography) and for parenchymal lung metastases.
   c. Poor for mediastinal lymph node spread until late in the course of disease; very poor for extrathoracic spread.

2. CT
   a. The best single noninvasive modality available.
   b. In most reports, very sensitive for mediastinal spread, parenchymal metastases, pleural disease, and upper abdominal spread.
   c. Not *specific*; positive CT does not prove disease.

3. MRI
   a. More expensive, slower, and less readily available than CT.
   b. Otherwise very similar in capability to CT.
   c. Especially helpful for patients with allergies to iodinated contrast and occasionally used to evaluate hepatic or adrenal masses.
   d. Better than CT at detecting local chest wall invasion, but this is not a determinant of resectability.

4. Ultrasound
   a. Occasionally helpful as an ancillary tool to characterize a liver lesion.
   b. Otherwise not helpful.

5. Nuclear medicine scanning
   a. NP-59 adrenal scanning very helpful for characterizing unilateral adrenal masses.
   b. Bone scans very sensitive for skeletal lesions in patients with signs, symptoms, or laboratory findings that point to bone metastases.

C. Recommended Imaging Approach

1. History, physical examination, and routine laboratory studies guide the workup. For example, focal CNS signs and symptoms can indicate the need for head CT.
2. Chest radiography to exclude obvious metastases (rib or spine

metastases, massive mediastinal lymph node enlargement, multiple lung nodules, or pleural effusion).

3. CT of the chest and upper abdomen as a triaging tool.
4. CT positive for apparent unresectable disease: Sample the CT abnormality via CT-guided, transbronchoscopic, mediastinoscopic, thoracoscopic, or open biopsy.
5. CT negative: Proceed directly to thoracotomy.
6. CT equivocal (e.g., small liver or adrenal lesions): Alternative imaging (MRI, nuclear medicine scanning) may be helpful. Otherwise, thoracotomy with follow-up CT.

D. Differential Diagnostic Considerations

1. Mediastinal and abdominal lymph nodes are considered abnormal if they exceed 1 cm in short-axis diameter (short-axis diameter is the axis perpendicular to the largest nodal dimension in a given image).
2. Adrenal masses are more worrisome for metastases if they are bilateral or larger than 3 cm.
3. Hepatic metastases from non-small lung cancer are rare until disease is widespread.
4. Think before you order—if the patient has squamous cell carcinoma in the sputum, a lung mass, and brain metastases, why order chest CT? The patient is already unresectable!

References

Glazer GM, Orrigner MG, Gross BH, Quint LE (1984). The mediastinum in non-small cell lung cancer: CT-surgical correlation. AJR 142:1101–1105.

McLoud TC, Bourgouin PM, Greenberg RW et al (1992). Bronchogenic carcinoma: Analysis of staging in the mediastinum with CT by correlative lymph node mapping and sampling. Radiology 182:319–323.

Quint LE, Francis IR, Wahl RL et al (1995). Pre-operative staging of non-small cell carcinoma of the lung: Imaging methods. AJR 164:1349–1359.

BLUNT THORACIC TRAUMA

A. Clinical Findings

1. Trauma is the third most common cause of death irrespective of age and the leading cause of death for people under the age of 40 years. Chest injury alone or in combination with other injuries accounts for more than half of all trauma-related deaths.

2. The overall death rate is 2%–12% for isolated chest injuries and 35% for chest injuries in patients with multiple trauma.

B. Imaging Modalities

1. Suspected aortic rupture: Approximately 80%–85% die at scene of injury, with a mortality rate of 1%–2% per hour in the first 24 hours if untreated. Most common site of rupture is the aortic root (most of these patients exsanguinate immediately), just distal to the ligamentum arteriosum (most common location for patients reaching the hospital), and less commonly the aortic hiatus of the diaphragm. At these three points the aorta is fixed in position.

   a. Plain chest radiograph
      - Screening tool with low specificity; often suboptimal technique in trauma patients on trauma boards (supine position and low lung volumes exaggerate width of mediastinum).
      - Findings suggestive of aortic rupture are all indirect findings of mediastinal blood or hematoma and include an indistinct aortic knob, wide superior mediastinum, left apical cap, deviation of the nasogastric tube or trachea to the right, depression of the left main bronchus deviated inferiorly.
      - Aortic and great vessel rupture are often associated with fractures of ribs 1–3, the clavicle, and/or sternum.

   b. Aortography
      - The gold standard for diagnosis of traumatic aortic injury.
      - There should be a low threshold for requesting aortography in patients with an abnormal chest film because of the mas-

sive early mortality associated with missed aortic laceration; at many institutions the positive aortic rupture rate for aortography is 1%–5%.

c. CT
- Role is controversial.
- CT more accurate than chest radiography in determining presence of a mediastinal hematoma and therefore could be used as a tool to screen patients before proceeding to aortography. A suggested algorithm is that if CT reveals mediastinal blood/hematoma then an aortogram should be performed, and if CT is negative no aortogram is necessary. However, little is yet known about the false-negative rate of CT. Is there ever aortic injury without mediastinal blood? Anecdotally, yes. More investigation is needed to assess the role of CT, particularly using the newer helical CT scanners that allow 2D and 3D reconstructions of the aorta and look similar to aortography, and to allow assessment of the aorta itself, not just indirect evidence of injury in the form of a hematoma.

2. Tracheobronchial tear: Seen in 1.5% of major blunt trauma; carries a high mortality rate (30%); diagnosis frequently delayed and confirmed with bronchoscopy. Approximately 80% occur within 2 cm of carina in either the distal trachea or mainstem bronchi.

   a. Plain chest radiograph
   - Should suspect when pneumothorax and/or pneumomediastinum persists or increases despite the placement of a chest tube or chest tubes.
   - Often associated with other signs of thoracic trauma; 90% have associated fractures of ribs 1–3; look for flail chest, lung contusion or laceration, and the classic "fallen-lung" sign of a collapsed lung dangling from the hilum surrounded by a large pneumothorax.

3. Diaphragmatic rupture: Approximately 90% related to motor vehicle accident; with blunt abdominal trauma the force of the trauma is transmitted up through the diaphragm. From 75% to 90% occur on

the left side; the right hemidiaphragm is protected by the shock-absorbing liver. Usually associated with other significant chest (45%) and abdominal (60%–80%) injuries.

a. Plain chest radiograph

- Invisible radiologically in up to 50% of cases initially; may be identified on radiographs weeks or months later as the tear enlarges; often discovered unexpectedly at laparotomy for abdominal trauma.
- Look for an elevated hemidiaphragm, bubble-like lucencies, or air–fluid levels (representing bowel) in lower chest, an unusual course of nasogastric tube down into the abdomen and then back up into the chest.

b. CT: Signs on CT are nonspecific and lack sensitivity and specificity; axial CT images are not in the ideal plane (coronal or sagittal would be better), and it is difficult to follow the shape of the entire diaphragm.

4. Lung injury

a. Plain chest radiograph

- Pulmonary contusion/laceration occurs in 30%–70% of cases and is of variable severity, from asymptomatic to severe respiratory failure.
- Blood accumulates in the first 6–8 hours; therefore, the initial chest film taken in the ER may demonstrate normal lungs. The lungs begins to clear within 48–72 hours; films demonstrate peripheral nonsegmental air-space opacities with or without air-bronchograms. May see associated rib fractures.
- Aspiration usually involves the basal segments of the lower lobes, as patients are typically upright during a motor vehicle accident. Aspiration related to intubation when patients are in the supine position typically occurs in the superior segments of the lower lobes.
- The course of aspiration depends on the aspirated material; gastric contents incite a chemical pneumonitis, oral flora may lead to aspiration pneumonia with air-space opacity that

persists and increases over 3–7 days, whereas water is quickly cleared from the lungs.

C. Recommended Imaging Approach

1. While the specifics depend on the type of trauma sustained and the clinical suspicion of injury, portable supine trauma board plain chest radiography is the initial screening study.
2. Aortography is the gold standard for aortic injury.
3. Echocardiography for suspected cardiac contusion or pericardial hematoma.
4. Barium swallow for suspected esophageal rupture, usually with penetrating trauma.

D. Differential Diagnostic Considerations

1. Fractures, especially of ribs, are common. Upper rib, clavicle, and sternal fractures are associated with injury to the great vessels/aorta, airway, and brachial plexus. Lower rib fractures are associated with injury to the liver, spleen, and kidneys.
2. Overall cardiac contusion is rare; it is associated with anterior rib and sternal fractures.
3. Esophageal perforation is uncommon with blunt trauma; consider if there is a left pleural effusion or pneumothorax and mediastinitis or penetrating mediastinal trauma.
4. Pneumomediastinum is most often "benign," seen in many patients with direct compression of chest, but do not forget ruptured airways (pneumothorax unresponsive to tube drainage) and esophageal rupture.

References

Mirvis SE, Bidwell JK, Buddmeyer EU et al (1987). Value of chest radiology in excluding traumatic aortic rupture. Radiology 163:487–493.

Mirvis SE, Templeton P (1992). Imaging in acute thoracic trauma. Semin Roentgenol 27;(3):184–210.

Raptopoulos V (1994). Chest CT for aortic injury: Maybe not for everyone. AJR 162:1053–1055.

SUSPECTED BRONCHIECTASIS (ABNORMAL PERSISTENT AND IRREVERSIBLE DILATATION OF THE BRONCHI)

A. Clinical Findings

1. Typically chronic cough producing copious amounts of purulent/mucopurulent secretions with frequent febrile exacerbations. May have a dry cough, intermittent hemoptysis, pleuritic chest pain related to infective episodes, wheezing, and shortness of breath. Sinusitis occurs in nearly half of patients.

2. Predisposing factors

   a. Bronchial obstruction (foreign body, tumor, inspissated secretions).

   b. Pneumonia (measles, pertussis, *Klebsiella*, *Staphylococcus*, *Pseudomonas*).

   c. Granulomatous diseases (tuberculosis, histoplasmosis, sarcoidosis).

   d. Immune disorders (X-linked agammaglobulinaemia, etc.).

   e. Hypersensitivity disorders (allergic bronchopulmonary aspergillosis type III immune complex reaction).

   f. Genetic disorders (cystic fibrosis, Kartagener's syndrome, Mounier-Kuhn syndrome [with tracheobronchomegaly], Williams-Campbell syndrome, yellow-nail syndrome, Young's syndrome).

B. Imaging Modalities

1. Plain chest radiograph

   a. Normal in one-fifth to one-fourth of cases.

   b. Look for increased size of bronchi and cystic spaces with air–fluid levels. Ill-defined bronchovascular bundles due to peribronchial fibrosis and retained secretions is more difficult to appreciate.

   c. Other findings include the "gloved-hand" or "finger-in-glove" appearance of dilated mucous-filled bronchi, atelectasis and crowding of vessels due to volume loss, oligemia of affected segments due to reflex vasoconstriction, and compensatory overinflation of normal lung.

2. Bronchography: Investigation of choice in the past, now superseded by CT.

3. CT
   a. Study of choice for suspected bronchiectasis.
   b. Requires minimum possible slice thickness (high resolution technique; 1–1.5 mm).
   c. Definition of bronchiectasis on CT is bronchial diameter greater than that of the accompanying pulmonary artery branch.
   d. If bronchi are mucous filled, they appear as branching tubular structures.

C. Recommended Imaging Approach

1. Chest radiograph as first step—many other diseases have similar clinical manifestations.

2. CT may be used for diagnosis when bronchiectasis cannot be identified by chest radiography and for assessment of the location and severity of bronchiectasis when surgery is planned.

D. Differential Diagnostic Considerations

1. Localized bronchiectasis is frequently related to recurrent infections in one lobe, possible due to partial bronchial obstruction.

2. Generalized bronchiectasis is usually part of a systemic process (e.g., agammaglobulinemia, Kartagener's syndrome or cystic fibrosis).

References

Fraser RG, Pare JAP (1989). Diagnosis of Diseases of the Chest. 3rd Ed. Philadelphia: WB Saunders.

Grenier P, Maurice F, Musset D, Menu Y, Nahum H (1986). Bronchiectasis: Assessment by thin-section CT. Radiology 161:95–99.

Lichter JP (1996). Hemoptysis. In Bordow RA, Moser KM (eds): Manual of Clinical Problems in Clinical Medicine. Boston: Little Brown.

► CHAPTER **8**

Central Nervous System and Head and Neck Disease

Douglas J. Quint, MD
University of Michigan Medical Center

With Contributions by

Katrina Gwinn, MD
Mayo Clinic

Mohamed Mohamed Amin, MD
Wayne Cornblath, MD
O. Petter Eldevik, MD
Stephen S. Gebarski, MD
David Jamadar, MB, BS, FRCS, FRCR
Thomas Kim, MD
Duc Tran, MD
University of Michigan Medical Center

Marie D. Acierno, MD
University of Mississippi Medical Center

Laurie Loevner, MD
University of Pennsylvania Medical Center

Harry Cloft, MD
University of Virginia Medical Center

Imaging Handbook for House Officers, Edited by Paul M. Silverman and Douglas J. Quint.
ISBN 0-471-13767-7 © 1997 Wiley-Liss, Inc.

ACUTE MENTAL STATUS CHANGES

Acute altered mental status (reduced consciousness, confusion, delirium, stupor, coma) are alarming neurologic emergencies. If persistent, the underlying conditions can be fatal or leave the patient in an irreparably damaged condition both physically and mentally. Normal mental status (awareness) is dependent on a normal interaction between the reticular activating substance of the brain stem, the thalami, and the cerebral cortex. Even small lesions in the upper brain stem reticular activating substance can deactivate the cerebral cortex.

A. Clinical Findings

1. Impairment of reticular activation of the cerebral cortex—mechanisms

   a. Intoxication (medications, drugs, poison): Chronic poisoning can also present as acute altered mental status.

   b. Head trauma: Cerebral concussion with torque on the upper brain stem impairs function of the reticular activating substance.

   c. Seizures: Sudden excessive neuronal discharge temporarily paralyzes the brain and can give a postictal period with confusion and somnolence.

   d. Metabolic derangements: Uremia, diabetic ketoacidosis, hepatic failure, hypoglycemia, hypercapnia.

   e. Destructive lesions involving upper brain stem or thalamus: Tumor, infarction, hemorrhage.

   f. Mass lesions of one cerebral hemisphere

      • Tumor, hemorrhage, contusion, subdural/epidural hematoma.

      • Mass effect on and compression of the midbrain, often with associated transtentorial temporal lobe herniation.

      • Can also be seen with posterior fossa mass lesions with upward herniation of brain stem structures.

   g. Hypotension (decline in blood pressure below 70 mm systolic): Blood loss, myocardial infarction.

2. Subarachnoid hemorrhage due to acutely ruptured aneurysm

3. Coma of unknown etiology: When mental status changes have no obvious cause (see above), the following diagnoses are most frequently encountered:

   a. Drug poisoning (30%).

   b. Metabolic causes (30%).

   c. Cerebrovascular disease (30%).

   d. Other (encephalitis, brain abscess).

4. "Beclouded" dementia: Most common mental disorder seen on the wards of a general hospital. It refers to the acute confusional states of elderly people in whom a preexisting brain disease is present, most often Alzheimer's disease, but is complicated by some more

acute medical or surgical illness. In such a person, almost any complicating illness may precipitate such confusion:

   a. Infections (lung, bladder).
   b. Head trauma.
   c. Heart failure.
   d. Anemia.
   e. Fever.
   f. Drug/alcohol intoxication.
   g. Dehydration.
   h. Electrolyte imbalance.

5. Potentially treatable causes of dementia:

   a. Neurosyphilis, cryptococcosis.
   b. Subdural hematoma, brain tumor.
   c. Chronic drug or poison intoxication.
   d. Normal-pressure hydrocephalus.
   e. Pellagra, vitamin B_{12} deficiency, hypothyroidism.
   f. Metabolic or electrolyte disorders.

B. Imaging Modalities

1. Plain radiographs: No role in the evaluation of acute mental status changes with the possible exception of documenting nondisplaced fractures of the skull in suspected child abuse cases.

2. CT: Advantages include direct visualization of the brain parenchyma, ventricular system and subarachnoid spaces, best demonstration of acute intracranial hemorrhage, ability to image sick, uncooperative patients, and more available and less expensive than MRI.

   Disadvantages include poor evaluation of the posterior fossa (including the brain stem), relatively insensitive to subacute or chronic hemorrhage (unless associated with mass effect), significantly less accurate than MRI with respect to identifying small strokes (particularly in the brain stem), other vascular processes, meningeal pathology, and some smaller tumors.

3. MRI: Advantages include that it is more sensitive than CT for

metabolic disease, ischemic changes, meningeal processes, posterior fossa lesions, and most small intracranial pathologic processes. MR angiography can also be performed in the setting of subarachnoid hemorrhage to screen for an aneurysm. Multiplanar scanning capabilities and lack of ionizing radiation are additional advantages. MRI is particularly useful for evaluation of the medulla, pons, midbrain, basal ganglia, and deep white matter.

Disadvantages include poor evaluation of bony structures, need for patient cooperation (which may not be possible in patients with acute mental status changes), the relative expense of the examination, and the inability to scan some patients with MRI-incompatible implants or life-support equipment.

Both CT and MRI are good (though MRI is better) for searching for treatable causes of acute mental status changes such as subdural or epidural hematomas, encephalitis, brain abscess, mass lesions, or hydrocephalus. Several additional processes that are not readily treatable at the present time but may also be diagnosed include brain infarctions, parenchymal hemorrhages, contusions, many primary and secondary brain neoplasms, and cerebral atrophy.

C. Recommended Imaging Approach

In the setting of a patient with acute altered mental status, establishing life support (e.g., securing the airway, monitoring of blood pressure) is the first concern. In some cases (e.g., drug overdose, intoxication, some metabolic derangements), clinical history, physical examination, and appropriate laboratory studies can obviate the need for imaging. EEG can be useful to differentiate between various degrees of altered consciousness.

When imaging is indicated, a head CT should be the first imaging examination performed to rule out a subarachnoid hemorrhage, hydrocephalus, or mass effect for any reason. If the CT is negative and the cause of the altered mental status remains unknown, or if the CT is positive but the abnormality requires additional characterization or delineation, a head MRI scan should be performed. In the setting of an acute nontraumatic subarachnoid hemorrhage, cerebral angiography to evaluate for an aneurysm should be performed.

D. Differential Diagnostic Considerations

1. Encephalitis: Herpes simplex encephalitis can be detected with MRI as early as 24 hours after onset of symptoms (usually altered mental status). It usually takes 2–3 days before a CT scan is positive. Look for edema, hemorrhage, and broken blood–brain barrier in the temporal lobes with sparing of the basal ganglia. Early treatment with anti-viral agents is essential. EEG is often diagnostic early on. Brain biopsy is required for definitive diagnosis.

2. Meningitis: Usually normal on noncontrast CT and MRI scans. Can see abnormal meningeal enhancement after intravenous contrast administration on MRI (and rarely CT).

3. Dementia: MRI and CT often do not demonstrate any specific focal abnormalities. Mild to moderate brain volume loss and small scattered high T2 signal lesions in the deep white matter (on MRI scans) are considered normal findings in patients over 60 years of age. Alzheimer's disease can result in volume loss of the temporal and parietal lobes, but this is not a specific or diagnostic finding.

4. Liver failure: May result in areas of high MRI signal on T1 images in the globus pallidus.

5. Intoxication: CT and MR scans are usually normal in acute alcohol, barbiturate, or cocaine poisoning. Carbon monoxide encephalopathy can give symmetric hypodense foci on CT and hyperintense T2 lesions on MRI scans in the globus pallidus and cerebral white matter.

6. Chronic subdural hematomas: Can be overlooked on CT scans if the hematomas are small or bilateral and symmetric, particularly if the lesions are several weeks old ("isodense" subdural hematomas). Administration of intravenous contrast material usually outlines the cortex and hematoma capsule and facilitates the diagnosis. MRI is exquisitely sensitive to small extraaxial fluid collections.

7. Increased intracranial pressure: Cannot always be diagnosed on CT or MRI scans. Imaging findings suggestive of increased intracranial pressure include presence of an intracranial mass, obliteration of the basal cisterns, subfalcine or transtentorial herniation, trans-

foramen magnum cerebellar tonsillar herniation, periventricular cerebrospinal fluid "migration," and hydrocephalus. Fundoscopy may reveal papilledema. Neck stiffness may be present. To avoid the possibility of cerebellar herniation, do not perform lumbar puncture.

APHASIA

A. Clinical Findings

Aphasia refers to a language disorder that may manifest as abnormal comprehension, decreased language output, and/or incorrect usage of words. Aphasia usually localizes the abnormality to the left cerebral hemisphere, and more specifically, the cortex supplied by the left middle cerebral artery. Exceptions to this include (1) a small percentage of left-handed people use the right cerebral hemisphere for language; (2) anomic aphasias secondary to toxic encephalopathies, metabolic disorders, or mass lesions that cause increased intracranial pressure; and (3) a small number of thalamic lesions leading to aphasia.

Aphasia in most cases is secondary to stroke (cerebral ischemia/infarction) and is frequently accompanied by a right hemiparesis. While the clinical diagnosis of stroke is usually evident based on history and physical examination, imaging plays an important role in excluding less common causes of aphasia such as intracranial hemorrhage or a structural abnormality.

B. Imaging Modalities

1. CT

Advantages

- Quick scanning time, especially with new rapid techniques.
- Readily identifies acute intracranial hemorrhage and mass lesions.

Disadvantages
- Radiation exposure.
- Scanning artifact, especially at the skull base and in the posterior fossa.

2. MRI

Advantages
- No ionizing radiation.
- Multiplanar capabilities.
- Ischemia/infarct demonstrated sooner (within minutes–hours) than with CT due to earlier detection of brain abnormalities as well as identification of intraarterial enhancement on contrast-enhanced scans in the affected vascular distribution (left MCA) due to slow flow.
- Better for evaluating vascular malformations, complicated hemorrhagic lesions, and underlying mass lesions.
- MR angiography can identify some vascular occlusions.

3. Cerebral Angiography

Advantages
- Gold standard for evaluating the cerebral vessels, especially the smaller distal branches (as is necessary to rule out vasculitis). Best for defining vascular abnormalities.
- Potential for endovascular treatment (lytic therapy) by the neuroradiologist following diagnostic cerebral angiography.

Disadvantages
- Interventional procedure with inherent risks including stroke, hemorrhage, and death.
- Thrombosed vascular malformations/aneurysms may not be identified and may be better seen on conventional spin-echo MR images.

C. Recommended Imaging Approach

Although aphasia associated with hemiparesis is most often secondary to stroke and is usually a clinical diagnosis, neuroimaging is important in excluding other less common etiologies that may mimic infarction. In the acute setting, CT is the imaging modality of choice. Its primary roles are to (1) exclude intracranial hemorrhage, (2) exclude an underlying mass lesion, and (3) identify, if present, changes associated with infarction. A normal CT scan in the setting of an acute stroke, especially within the first 24 hours of symptom onset, is common. If clinically indicated, follow-up CT scan to confirm the diagnosis may be warranted.

MRI is usually not necessary in the acute setting. In patients with atypical presentations (e.g., young patients, drug abusers, patients with unclear clinical histories), MRI because of its superior soft tissue resolution may be indicated following CT to help localize and better characterize cerebral abnormalities. MRI may also be helpful in further evaluating complicated hemorrhagic lesions/masses identified on CT.

Expedient evaluation of otherwise healthy patients presenting with symptoms of left MCA ischemia (aphasia, right hemiparesis) is vital. Specifically, a critical "window of opportunity" (usually patients must be evaluated with initiation of therapy within 4–6 hours of symptom onset) may allow for management with endovascular lytic therapy (e.g., urokinase) in some patients. These patients should have prompt CT evaluation (that will usually not reveal any areas of infarction or hemorrhage; however, a hyperdense acute intraluminal thrombus may be noted in the MCA or distal ICA). Diagnostic (endovascular) cerebral angiography confirming a thrombus with immediate initiation of endovascular lytic therapy instituted by the neuroradiologist may then be performed in patients meeting specific criteria.

D. Differential Diagnostic Considerations

1. Cerebral ischemia/infarction
   a. Vascular occlusion (internal carotid artery [ICA]/middle cerebral artery [MCA]) secondary to atheromatous disease.
   b. Embolic disease originating from

- Ulcerated plaque in the ICA.
- Cardiac source: Valvular disease, atrial fibrillation, mural thrombus following myocardial infarction, atrial myxoma.
- Underlying vascular injury (e.g., intimal tear [traumatic dissection] of ICA).

   c. Vasculitis, vasculopathy.

   d. Drugs, e.g., cocaine.

   e. Blood disorders: Hypercoagulable states.

2. Intracranial hemorrhage
   a. Brain neoplasm associated with acute hemorrhage within or around the tumor, e.g., primary glioblastoma multiforme, metastatic disease (i.e., melanoma).
   b. Hypertensive bleed.
   c. Vascular malformation.
   d. Amyloid angiopathy (elderly).
   e. Anticoagulation (heparin, coumadin).
   f. Bleeding diathesis.
   g. Posttraumatic (e.g., large subdural hematoma).

3. Complicated migraine: Frequently young adults. Transient neurologic deficits may precede headache. Neuroimaging (CT/MR) can be normal.

4. Postictal state: In unwitnessed seizure.

5. Anomic aphasia: Secondary to toxic/metabolic encephalopathies; often no associated hemiplegia.

ATAXIA/ABNORMAL GAIT

A. Clinical Findings

Stance and gait difficulties are often suggestive of specific disorders of motor or sensory function. Cerebellar disease is classically associated with ataxia. The patient will have a wide-based stance, often with associated titubation (tremor) of the head or trunk, nystagmus, and/or tremor of the extremities. A hemiparetic patient will flex the arm and extend the leg on the affected side. In Parkinsonism, the stance will be rigid and stooped, and the patient will have a Romberg sign. When lower motor neuron disease is the cause of gait disturbance, a foot drop is a common manifestation of distal weakness. Diseases of the muscles will cause proximal greater than distal weakness of the extremities and also a "waddling" gait. Hysterical gait disorders will often be associated with a hysterical paralysis, but standard reflexes and the Babinski reflex will be normal.

B. Imaging Modalities

1. Plain radiographs: The advantages of plain radiographs of the skull and cervical spine are cost, ease of obtaining them, and their ability to screen for certain types of pathology, most notably posttraumatic changes of the cervical spine.

    Disadvantages of plain radiographs are nonvisualization of intracranial and intraspinal structures. Therefore, while plain radiographs are acceptable as a first step for evaluating the cervical spine (for posttraumatic changes or spinal stenosis of any etiology), they are completely inappropriate for evaluation of the brain and are not enough to "rule out" spinal canal (spinal cord) abnormality.

2. CT: A CT scan is the imaging examination of choice for identifying acute posterior fossa hemorrhage. It is also best for identifying intracranial mineralization that might suggest an underlying vascular malformation. Bony abnormalities are best evaluated with CT; either posttraumatic changes of the intracranial compartment or the spinal canal (e.g., displaced bone fragments). CT after myelography can be used to assess compromise of the spinal cord by a spinal canal process, though MRI remains the best imaging modality for such evaluation.

    The main disadvantage of CT scanning is that it is less sensitive to abnormalities of the brain than MRI. This is particularly true in the posterior fossa, where extensive artifacts from the temporal bones severely limit evaluation of the brain stem and cerebellum such that they are not as well evaluated as even the supratentorial brain on CT scans. Such artifacts are not present on MRI scans. CT scanning is also limited with respect to scan planes. Sagittal scans cannot be obtained with CT.

3. MRI: MRI is the most sensitive imaging modality for the detection of intracranial pathology. It also provides some specificity with respect to diagnosis (e.g., subacute/chronic hematomas, some cystic processes). Delineation of anatomy is far superior to that achieved on CT (e.g., delineating brain stem/cerebellar atrophy in olivopontocerebellar atrophy, mammillary body changes in Wernicke-Korsakoff syndrome, demyelinating lesions in multiple sclerosis, etc.) An MRI examination can be tailored to evaluate some vascular lesions such as aneurysms, atherosclerotic vessel narrowing, and major dural venous occlusion by utilizing (noninvasive) MR angiography.

Disadvantages of MRI include poor evaluation of bone and mineralization (e.g., within lesions), need for greater patient cooperation than CT scanning (minutes vs. seconds), MRI-incompatible implants or foreign bodies, nondiagnostic examinations in claustrophobic patients who are unable to remain within the MRI scanner, and inability to image some patients with movement disorders without general anaesthesia. Also, while some intrinsic vascular pathology can be delineated on MR angiography, conventional endovascular angiography remains a better test.

4. Angiography: Catheter angiography is an invasive procedure with a risk of between 1:200 and 1:1,000 of *causing* a stroke. It is never the initial imaging modality for evaluating ataxia. However, it remains the gold standard for demonstrating intrinsic vascular abnormalities such as aneurysms, vascular malformations, and vasculitis. It also remains the best test for demonstrating vessel narrowing by atherosclerosis, fibromuscular dysplasia, etc., though MR angiography and ultrasound also have important roles in the evaluation of these processes. The chance of a serious reaction to injected contrast material is about 1:50,000.

C. Recommended Imaging Approach

1. Determine if the process is acute or chronic. If the process is acute and there is no history of trauma, an underlying vascular process should be considered first. An emergent head CT scan should be done to rule out an acute intracranial hemorrhage or mass effect on posterior fossa structures.

2. A thorough family history with an appropriate laboratory evaluation (including screening for toxins and/or anticonvulsant levels, as appropriate) should be performed.

3. Determine with a physical examination if the gait disturbance is truly ataxia or due to another problem such as weakness, bradykinesis, normal pressure hydrocephalus (in which the patient might have a "magnetic" gait), or psychogenic.

4. An emergent angiogram (either MR angiography or conventional endovascular angiography) may be necessary if there is concern (clinically, or on a CT or MRI scan) with respect to a vertebrobasilar dissection or acute arterial or dural venous sinus thrombosis.

5. If the problem is chronic, progressive, or suggestive of posterior fossa pathology, the imaging work-up should include an MRI scan to evaluate for masses or other intrinsic abnormalities of the posterior fossa (ischemic, inflammatory, neoplastic, etc.).

6. In addition to gait disturbances, posterior fossa processes often manifest with nystagmus, gaze palsies, or other cranial nerve abnormalities. In addition, posterior fossa disease is often accompanied by nausea, emesis, vertigo, and headache.

7. Acute stroke may not be visualized on CT or even MRI in the first 24 hours after an event.

8. Faster growing tumors can present relatively acutely in the posterior fossa, sometimes mimicking a stroke because the space in this compartment is limited. Similarly, an abscess can present acutely or subacutely in this region, also mimicking a stroke or other mass lesion.

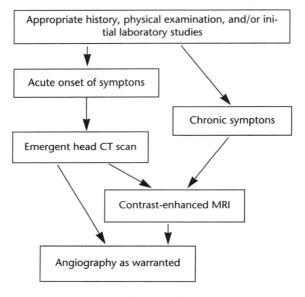

Imaging Algorithm

D. Differential Diagnostic Considerations

1. Vascular (stroke, migraine, cerebellar hemorrhage of any etiology).
2. Structural (tumor, vascular malformation, abscess, cyst, Chiari malformation, basilar invagination).
3. Myelin dysfunction (multiple sclerosis).
4. Inherited metabolic disease.
5. Acquired metabolic diseases (toxins such as alcohol and anticonvulsants, Wernicke-Korsakoff syndrome, hypothyroidism, renal/hepatic disease, vitamin E deficiency).
6. Infectious (viral/postinfectious, Creutzfeld-Jacob disease).

7. Degenerative (olivopontocerebellar atrophy, Frederich's ataxia, ataxia-telangectasia).

8. Paraneoplastic (subacute cerebellar degeneration, opsoclonus-myoclonus).

9. Other
   a. Normal pressure hydrocephalus.
   b. Sensory neuropathy.
   c. Weakness due to myopathy.
   d. Myelopathy.
   e. Polyneuropathy.
   f. Movement disorders.

10. Hysterical, malingering.

COMA

A. Clinical Findings

Coma is a pathologic state in which neither "arousal" nor "awareness" is present. Associated nonpurposeful reflex movements (decorticate/decerebrate posturing) may be present. Coma needs to be differentiated from a "vegetative state" in which there is severe bihemispheric cerebral dysfunction, particularly following an anoxic-ischemic injury or severe head trauma. Differentiation is important, as the prognosis for a vegetative state is usually significantly worse than for coma.

B. Imaging Modalities

1. Plain radiographs: There is no role for plain radiographs in the evaluation of coma.

2. Ultrasound: Due to the calvaria, with the exception of neonates, ultrasound is not feasible to evaluate the brain. However, with the advent of "power" Doppler techniques and the utilization of ultrasound intravascular contrast agents, the circle of Willis region and some of the other larger intracranial blood vessels can be evaluated with ultrasound (e.g., evaluate for vascular spasm, etc.).

3. CT: Advantages include optimal demonstration of acute intracra-

nial hemorrhage (including the ability to distinguish between bland and hemorrhagic strokes), demonstration of supratentorial mass effect and hydrocephalus equal to that of MRI, rapid acquisition of images so that the degree of patient cooperation required for CT scanning is minimal, the ability to monitor extremely sick patients in the CT scanner, excellent delineation of bony abnormalities (e.g., maxillofacial fractures) and (intracranial) foreign bodies.

Disadvantages include the risks of ionizing radiation, limited scan planes (particularly in sick patients), inferior ability to demonstrate some intracranial intraaxial pathology (in particular, the inability to evaluate adequately the posterior fossa, including the brain stem, which is an important structure to evaluate in coma patients), and the inability to evaluate blood vessels (e.g., to rule out vascular spasm, vasculitis, etc.).

4. Magnetic Resonance (MR) Imaging: Advantages include superior contrast resolution, permitting optimal evaluation of the intracranial compartment including more subtle areas of ischemic change (e.g., "shearing" injuries in the setting of trauma or small brain stem strokes that can be totally missed on CT scans), unlimited scan planes, the lack of ionizing radiation, and the potential use of MR angiography to evaluate for vascular spasm that may obviate the need for conventional angiography.

Disadvantages include motion artifacts in unstable/uncooperative patients who cannot remain motionless for the minutes required to obtain a series of MR images, inferior evaluation of bony structures, limited availability, high cost, and inability to evaluate some patients with MRI-incompatible implants (e.g., pacemakers, aneurysm clips, cochlear implants, etc.) or life-support equipment (e.g., some ventilators).

5. Angiography: Advantages of conventional endovascular catheter angiography include superior (clearly superior to MR angiography) delineation of arterial and venous anatomy, intrinsic vascular lesions (e.g., aneurysms and/or vascular spasm in the setting of subarachnoid hemorrhage) and vascular neoplasms, and the potential for interventional therapy of some vascular lesions (e.g., dural arteriovenous malformations, meningiomas, aneurysms, and lytic therapy of basilar artery thrombosis).

Disadvantages include the intrinsic risk of catheter angiography (between a 1:200 and 1:1,000 risk of *causing* a stroke), the relatively high dose of radiation, the risks of intravascular contrast material, and the relatively high cost of the examination.

In the setting of acute (<4–6 hours) symptoms that are believed to be secondary to a thrombus of the basilar artery, emergent angiography with the possibility of intraarterial lytic (urokinase) therapy should be considered.

C. Recommended Imaging Approach

The causes of coma are extremely varied. A careful history and physical examination and selected laboratory studies can eliminate the need for imaging in many patients. These include psychiatric disorders, hypothermia, and some of the exogenous/endogenous toxins outlined below.

In neonates, any neurologic symptoms should initially be evaluated with ultrasound. CT scanning should be considered if acute hemorrhage is of concern. MRI should be reserved to rule out structural (congenital) abnormalities, evaluate the brain stem for subtle lesions that can be missed on ultrasound or CT, or further delineate or characterize abnormalities seen on ultrasound or CT.

In the setting of acute onset of coma (either "spontaneous" or associated with trauma), the intracranial compartment should first be evaluated with a head CT to rule out acute intracerebral or subarachnoid hemorrhage, mass effect, or hydrocephalus. If negative, an MRI should be considered to search for more subtle (particularly brain stem) lesions.

In the setting of suspected basilar artery thrombosis (e.g., "locked-in syndrome"), CT should be performed to rule out associated hemorrhage. If the patient is being evaluated within the first 4–6 hours after their event, emergent angiography should be considered as intraarterial lytic therapy can be initiated in some patients.

In most cases of (nonacute, nontraumatic) coma, if clinical evaluation results in the need for imaging, MRI should be performed. CT scanning should also be performed only if evaluation of bony structures or possible lesion mineralization is of concern.

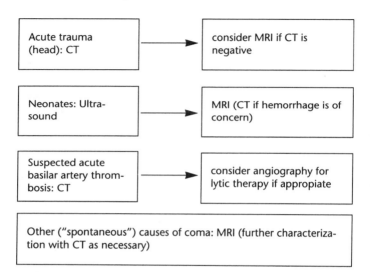

Acute trauma (head): CT	→	consider MRI if CT is negative
Neonates: Ultrasound	→	MRI (CT if hemorrhage is of concern)
Suspected acute basilar artery thrombosis: CT	→	consider angiography for lytic therapy if appropiate

Other ("spontaneous") causes of coma: MRI (further characterization with CT as necessary)

Imaging Algorithm

D. Differential Diagnostic Considerations

1. Supratentorial mass lesions with mass effect (usually with associated transtentorial temporal lobe herniation with compression of the brain stem (reticular activating system)

   a. Extracerebral fluid collections (epidural hematoma, subdural hematoma).

   b. Large intracerebral hemorrhage for any reason.

   c. Large stroke (associated mass effect can be significant several days after the stroke).

   d. Tumor (any neoplasm can have associated mass effect on the brain stem).

   e. Abscess (mass effect).

   f. Radiation necrosis (mass effect 6–24 months after radiation therapy).

2. Infratentorial mass lesions can directly invade and/or compress the brain stem
   a. Tumor.
   b. Hemorrhage.
   c. Stroke (e.g., basilar artery thrombosis).
3. Trauma or toxic/metabolic processes affecting the brain
   a. Trauma (concussion, contusion, laceration, "shear" hemorrhages).
   b. Subarachnoid hemorrhage (trauma, ruptured aneurysm).
   c. Epilepsy (status epilepticus, postictal state).
   d. Hypoxia/anoxia or ischemia
      • Carbon monoxide poisoning.
      • Pulmonary infarction, pulmonary insufficiency.
      • Cardiac arrhythmia, syncope of any etiology.
      • Collagen vascular disease.
   e. Endogenous toxins and deficiency states
      • Hypoglycemia, diabetic ketoacidosis.
      • Uremic or hepatic encephalopathy.
      • Hyponatremia.
      • Myxedema.
   f. Exogenous toxins
      • Ethyl alcohol, methyl alcohol.
      • Drugs (glutethimide, barbiturates, morphine, heroin).
4. Hypothermia
5. Psychiatric disorders
   a. Hysteria.
   b. Catatonia.
   c. Malingering.

DEMENTIA

A. Clinical Findings

Dementia refers to a clinical condition in which cognitive/intellectual deterioration is severe enough to interfere with social and/or occupational functioning. Memory impairment is the cardinal feature of dementia, though other cognitive functions (e.g., poor abstract thinking and/or judgement, aphasia, apraxia, agnosia) and personality disturbances are present to varying degrees.

B. Imaging Modalities

1. Plain radiographs: There is no role for plain radiographs in the evaluation of dementia.

2. CT: Advantages of CT include (1) rapid acquisition time, which therefore requires less patient cooperation than MRI (which can be important when evaluating dementia patients), (2) better delineation of bony abnormalities and mineralization, and (3) less expensive than MRI or nuclear medicine studies.

    Disadvantages include (1) poor evaluation of posterior fossa structures due to extensive artifacts; (2) provides only anatomic information (and not as well as MRI), i.e., does not provide functional information such as regional blood flow; and (3) utilizes ionizing radiation.

3. MRI: Advantages of MR include (1) best delineation of anatomy, (2) multiplanar capabilities, (3) lack of ionizing radiation, (4) ability to perform "functional" imaging (regional cerebral blood flow, diffusion imaging, etc.), and (5) possible lesion characterization in the future (e.g., spectroscopy).

    Disadvantages include (1) many dementia patients cannot stay motionless for the minutes currently required to acquire a series of MR images; (2) contraindications such as pacemakers, non-MRI-compatible life-support equipment, some cochlear implants, aneurysm clips, etc.; and (3) more expensive than CT.

4. Angiography: Advantages: Conventional endovascular angiography is superior to but more invasive than MR angiography as it gives unsurpassed depiction of intracranial vasculature, which is extremely useful when diagnosing some processes such as vasculitis.

    Disadvantages are that endovascular angiography is an invasive procedure that carries a risk of between 1:200 and 1:1,000 of *causing* a stroke, its uses ionizing radiation and is an expensive procedure, and it is somewhat nonspecific as vasculitis and atherosclerotic changes (and other processes) can be indistinguishable on angiograms.

Note: While MR angiography is noninvasive and does not have a risk of stroke, the spatial resolution of MR angiography is so inferior to "conventional" catheter angiography that small vessel vasculitis currently cannot be ruled out on such studies.

5. Single photon emission computed tomography (SPECT): The main advantage of SPECT is that it provides physiologic data (e.g., cerebral perfusion).

   Disadvantages of SPECT include problems with specificity (the appearance of many of the dementias can be similar), its expense (sometimes not covered by third party payers) and significantly inferior delineation of anatomic detail with respect to MRI and CT.

6. Positron emission tomography (PET): PET scanning also provides physiologic data (e.g., regional metabolism and perfusion). PET is only available at large institutions due to the need for an on-site cyclotron and is an expensive test that is rarely paid for by third party payers.

C. Recommended Imaging Approach

The workup of dementia starts with a comprehensive history and physical, neurologic, and psychiatric examinations in an attempt to identify potentially reversible conditions such as pseudodementia and drug toxicity.

Laboratory tests (including evaluation of cerebrospinal fluid) and neuroimaging are essential to evaluate for metabolic/infectious or structural abnormalities.

The National Institutes of Health Consensus Conference on Differential Diagnosis of Dementing diseases has recommended the following screening laboratory and imaging tests, which will identify the majority of reversible causes of dementia: CBC, electrolyte and metabolic screen, thyroid panel, vitamin B_{12}/folate levels, syphilis screening, urinalysis, EKG, chest radiographs, and a head CT.

Structural treatable causes of dementia such as NPH, intracranial neoplasms, and subdural hematomas can usually be diagnosed on CT scans. However, if further characterization or delineation of a lesion is necessary, MR imaging can be performed.

If the etiology of the dementia remains unclear, functional imaging (SPECT, PET, and/or newer MRI applications) can be helpful in demonstrating patterns of cerebral perfusion that have some specificity for certain dementias. For example, in Alzheimer's dementia, bilateral temporoparietal hypoperfusion is characteristic, and in multi-infarct dementia patchy periventricular areas of hypoperfusion are often seen. However, some overlap (e.g., Alzheimer's disease and multi-infarct dementia) can occur.

If structural studies (including MRI) are negative, cerebral angiography is the last test that should be considered (to rule out vasculitis as the cause of dementia).

D. Differential Diagnostic Considerations

1. CNS neuronal degeneration
   a. Alzheimer's disease: 50%–60% of all dementia patients.
   b. Parkinson's disease.
   c. Huntington's chorea.
   d. Pick's disease.
2. Multi-infarct dementia is the second most common cause of dementia (10%–15% of dementia patients). Vascular risk factors such as hypertension are almost always present. Abrupt onset of symptoms with a "stepwise" clinical decline are characteristic.
3. Pseudodementia should be considered when depressive symptoms precede cognitive decline.
4. Mass lesions
   a. Subdural hematomas.
   b. Primary or secondary neoplasms.
5. Cerebrospinal fluid circulation disorders
   a. Obstructive hydrocephalus (due to a process intrinsic to the ventricular system).
   b. Communicating hydrocephalus (due to a process extrinsic to the ventricular system).

    c. Normal pressure hydrocephalus (NPH) (classic triad: incontinence, ataxia, and dementia).

6. Drug toxicity (psychotrophic agents, anticholinergic agents, narcotics, anticonvulsants, etc.).
7. Intoxicants (alcohol, lead, mercury, organic solvents).
8. Infections (AIDS dementia complex, tuberculous/fungal/parasitic meningitis, Lyme disease, herpes encephalitis, neurosyphilis, Creutzfeldt-Jacob syndrome, Whipple's disease).
9. Endocrine disorders (hypoparathyroidism, hyperparathyroidism, hypothyroidism, hypopituitarism, Cushing's syndrome).
10. Metabolic disorders (hepatic and uremic encephalopathy, Wilson's disease).
11. Collagen-vascular disorders (systemic lupus erythematosis [SLE], temporal arteritis, primary CNS vasculitis).
12. Other: Radiation-induced dementia, postanoxic/posttraumatic dementia, sarcoidosis, dialysis encephalopathy.

DIPLOPIA

A. Clinical Findings

Diplopia is the perception of the same object in two different places ("double" vision). Diplopia can be either *monocular* (occurs with both eyes open and persists when one eye is closed) or *binocular* (occurs with both eyes open and disappears when one eye is closed). Monocular diplopia is either a refractive problem of an eye, psychogenic, or, rarely, cortical. Binocular diplopia may be *comitant* (the degree of visual misalignment is equal in all gaze directions) or *incomitant* (the degree of misalignment varies with the direction of gaze). The two images may be aligned horizontally, vertically, or obliquely.

The time course and age of a patient are important with respect to determining the etiology of diplopia. Binocular diplopia can be from orbital disease, neuromuscular junction disorders, cranial nerve palsies, or brain stem (fasicular, nuclear, internuclear) or supranuclear abnormality.

Diplopia from different causes will frequently have distinct patterns and associated features that can narrow the differential diagnosis.

B. Imaging Modalities

1. Plain radiographs: While plain radiographs can demonstrate orbital wall, lacrimal gland fossa, optic foramen, optic canal, sphenoid ridge, and paranasal sinus bony abnormalities, associated soft tissue (e.g., intraorbital) abnormalities cannot be assessed. Therefore, plain radiography, whether positive or negative, does not obviate the need for additional imaging (ultrasound, CT, or MRI) and is therefore of no value in evaluating diplopia.

2. Ultrasound (orbital echography): Inexpensive, safe (no ionizing radiation), reproducible method of evaluating orbital lesions. Does not permit visualization of the orbital apex or extraorbital spread of a process. May not be possible to use in severely traumatized or uncooperative patients.

   a. A-mode ultrasound: One-dimensional view of a lesion; can show lesion's "reflectivity," sound attenuation, and internal structure.

   b. B-mode ultrasound: Can demonstrate lesion's location, size, shape, and orientation to other structures.

   c. Color-Doppler ultrasound: Can show changes of blood flow direction and velocity.

3. CT: Superb delineation of the bones of the face, which is crucial when evaluating fractures or bony erosion/expansion/destruction by orbital neoplasms or infectious/inflammatory processes. Normal intraorbital fat provides excellent contrast to both normal and abnormal orbital soft tissue structures. CT is the examination of choice for ruling out foreign bodies. Can also scan in the direct coronal plane to better localize pathologic processes and detect orbital roof/floor fractures or extension of other pathologic processes. CT is also best for detecting acute hemorrhage and requires less patient cooperation than MRI.

4. MRI: Best delineation of soft tissue structures of the orbit. Contrast-enhanced imaging (with fat suppression technique) is ex-

tremely sensitive to pathologic processes (in particular, intrinsic optic nerve processes such as optic neuritis and glioma and perioptic nerve processes such as meningioma). The orbital apex is best seen on MRI as is extension of a cavernous sinus process or any intracranial process due to the lack of bone artifacts.

Disadvantages of MRI include lack of delineation of bony structures and mineralization in a lesion (which can help characterize lesions such as retinoblastoma). Even with MR angiography, most orbital vascular processes (most aneurysms, some varices, some fistulas) are inadequately evaluated and require dedicated endovascular angiography for diagnosis (and treatment).

5. Angiography: Formal catheter angiography is still considered the gold standard for evaluation of most intraorbital vascular processes. However, such processes are rarely the cause of diplopia. Cerebral angiography is the examination of choice for intracranial aneurysm and allows the neurosurgeon to plan a surgical approach.

Disadvantages of cerebral angiography include ionizing radiation, cost, and the 1:200 to 1:1,000 risk of *causing* a stroke during the examination.

C. Recommended Imaging Approach

Many causes of diplopia can be determined with a careful history and physical examination (by an ophthalmologist), which can obviate the need for imaging in some patients.

Monocular diplopia with a visual field defect should be evaluated with MRI to evaluate the occipital lobe region. Monocular diplopia without a field defect rarely requires imaging evaluation.

Binocular comitant diplopia is usually due to strabismus and rarely requires imaging.

Binocular incomitant diplopia (isolated or associated with other findings, acute or chronic) in a patient less than 50 years old requires imaging. MRI is the single best test, though CT should also be considered if a primarily bony process is of concern.

Acute binocular incomitant diplopia involving a single cranial nerve in a patient more than 50 years old is probably ischemic (the most common cause of diplopia) and does not require immediate imaging evaluation;

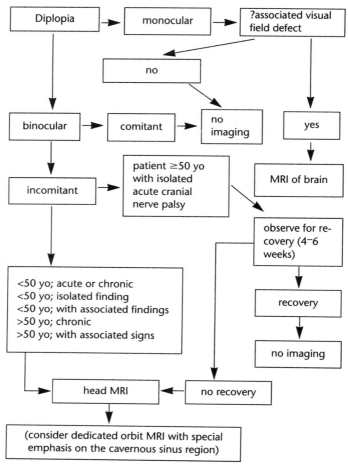

Imaging Algorithm

however, these patients should be followed for recovery. If no recovery is seen in 4–6 weeks, imaging should be performed. Again, MRI is the examination of choice.

Binocular incomitant diplopia that is chronic or associated with other orbital or brain stem signs/symptoms should be evaluated with MRI.

D. Differential Diagnostic Considerations

1. Monocular diplopia
   a. Refractive error (cornea, cataract, macula): Will resolve with pinhole testing.
   b. Cortical diplopia (rare): Will have associated visual field defect.
   c. Psychogenic.
2. Binocular diplopia
   a. Comitant: Usually a congenital problem (e.g., strabismus).
   b. Incomitant.
      - Orbital lesion.
         Inflammatory (thyroid eye disease, myositis).
         Traumatic.
         Neoplastic (primary, metastatic).
         Inherited (myopathy; e.g., chronic progressive external ophthalmoplegia).
      - Neuromuscular junction.
         Myasthenia gravis.
         Eaton-Lambert syndrome (can rarely affect eyes).
      - Cranial nerve palsy.
         Third nerve palsy (ischemia, trauma, aneurysm).
         Fourth nerve palsy (ischemia, trauma).
         Sixth nerve palsy (ischemia, trauma).
      - Central (brain stem) disorder.
         Fasicular.
         Nuclear.
         Internuclear ophthalmoplegia.
      - Supranuclear gaze palsy.

EAR PAIN

A. Clinical Findings

Ear pain, also known as otalgia, may be caused directly by ear pathology or referred from another location in the head, neck, or chest.

B. Imaging Modalities

1. Plain radiographs: Plain radiographs are rarely useful. Chest radiographs can occasionally demonstrate a thoracic aneurysm or other thoracic mass. Skull radiographs may demonstrate the elongated styloid process of Eagle syndrome. However, CT scanning better demonstrates thoracic and skull base processes and multiple other processes that cannot be seen on plain radiographs. Dental radiographs (Panorex) can be used to demonstrate alveolar/dental pathology.

2. CT: CT is best for evaluating intrinsic temporal bone pathology such as congenital abnormalities, neoplasm, and complications of otitis. CT is also useful for evaluating involvement of the skull base by head and neck neoplasms.

3. MRI: MRI is the most sensitive imaging modality for evaluating the extent of a soft tissue abnormality. Intracranial or extracranial extension of an intrinsic temporal bone process (neoplasm, infection, etc.) is best demonstrated with MRI. Therefore, in many cases, imaging evaluation of otalgia requires both CT and MRI. MRI is the examination of choice for evaluating the temporomandibular joint.

   Disadvantages of MRI include poor evaluation of bones and mineralization (e.g., within lesions), need for greater patient cooperation than with CT scanning (minutes vs. seconds), some MRI-incompatible implants or foreign bodies, nondiagnostic examinations of claustrophobic patients who cannot remain within the MRI scanner for imaging, and the limited availability of MRI scanners in many parts of the world.

C. Recommended Imaging Approach

Careful attention to the history and physical examination is the first step in the evaluation of ear pain. As most ear pain is due to uncomplicated otitis or mastoiditis, no imaging evaluation is necessary in the majority of patients. Imaging for patients with temporal bone infections is only considered when complications such as cholesteatoma or osteomyelitis is of clinical concern. CT scanning is the imaging test of choice for evaluation of such inflammatory processes, though extension outside the temporal bone by these processes is probably best evaluated with MRI.

If dental or temporomandibular joint pathology is suspected, referral to an oral surgeon is suggested. Dedicated dental radiographs [Panorex] for the evaluation of the teeth and immediate peridontal areas and/or MRI for evaluation of temporomandibular joints may then be ordered by them.

In adults, especially those with a history of tobacco and/or alcohol use, head and neck squamous cell carcinoma needs to be ruled out if no other causes of ear pain are identified. These patients should be referred to an otorhinolaryngologist for further evaluation. The otorhinolaryngologist may then order a CT or MRI scan of the head, skull base, and/or neck regions to evaluate areas of clinical concern identified on physical examination or to search for occult lesions.

D. Differential Diagnostic Considerations

1. Local causes.
   a. Otitis media.
   b. Otitis externa.
   c. Mastoiditis.
   d. Trauma.
   e. Foreign body.
   f. Impacted cerumen.
   g. Herpes zoster.
   h. Tumor (benign or malignant).
2. Referred pain.
   a. Dental pathology.
   b. Temporomandibular joint disease.
   c. Myofascial pain syndrome.
   d. Benign/malignant tumors or infection (oral cavity, pharynx, larynx, thyroid, lung/bronchus, esophagus).

   e. Neuralgia (trigeminal, geniculate, sphenopalatine, glossopharyngeal).
   f. Temporal arteritis.
   g. Thoracic aneurysm.
   h. Angina pectoris.
   i. Cervical spinal arthritis.
   j. Carotodynia (a rare, self-limited, idiopathic condition causing tenderness at the carotid bifurcation).
   k. Eagle syndrome (pain on swallowing due to elongated styloid process; pain exacerbated by swallowing, yawning, or chewing).

References

Meyeroff WL, Pownell PH (1991). Otalgia. In Meyeroff WL, Rice DH (eds.): Otolaryngology: Head and Neck Surgery. Philadelphia: WB Saunders.

Thaller SR, De Silva A (1987). Otalgia with a normal ear. Am Fam Physician 36:129–136.

HEADACHE

A. Clinical Findings

Headache refers to any pain in or of the head, excluding the lower face and ears.

B. Imaging Modalities

   1. Plain radiographs: These have an extremely limited role in the evaluation of headache. While they can demonstrate some paranasal sinus and skull pathology, CT scanning is far better for demonstrating bony abnormalities. A "limited" screening paranasal sinus region CT has a cost similar to a plain radiographic sinus series of films. In patients with shunt catheters (e.g., for hydrocephalus), plain films are useful for demonstrating shunt tubing abnormalities. Finally, plain radiographs are probably the best imaging modality for demonstrating non-depressed skull fractures (e.g., evaluation of possible child abuse).

2. CT: A head CT without administration of intravenous contrast media (NCCT = noncontrast head CT) demonstrates acute hemorrhagic lesions (including subarachnoid hemorrhage) and bone lesions best. It is the imaging modality of choice in the evaluation of trauma and acute mental status changes ("rule out intracranial hemorrhage"). NCCT detects many intracranial masses, but is less sensitive than CT scanning obtained after intravenous administration of contract material (CECT = contrast-enhanced head CT) or MRI for the detection of small neoplastic, inflammatory, or vascular lesions. However, NCCT is essentially risk-free and requires significantly less patient cooperation than MRI.

While a CECT is more sensitive than NCCT for the detection of small intracranial abnormalities, calcifications and hemorrhage can be misinterpreted as areas of enhancement on a CECT if an NCCT is not obtained first. Disadvantages of CECT include the risk of a serious reaction to intravenous contrast material (1:50,000) and less sensitivity to an intracranial abnormality than MRI.

3. MRI: MRI is the most sensitive imaging modality for the detection of most types of intracranial pathology. It also provides some specificity with respect to some diagnoses (e.g., hematomas, some cystic processes). An MRI examination can be tailored to evaluate some vascular lesions such as aneurysms, atherosclerotic vessel narrowing and major dural venous occlusion by utilizing (noninvasive) MR angiography. While MRI does demonstrate most paranasal sinus pathology, evaluation of maxillofacial bony structures is required when evaluating the paranasal sinuses, so CT remains the imaging modality of choice (see Sinusitis/Nasal Congestion).

Disadvantages of MRI include poor evaluation of bones and mineralization (e.g., within lesions), need for greater patient cooperation than CT scanning (minutes vs. seconds), MRI-incompatible implants or foreign bodies, nondiagnostic examinations when claustrophobic patients are unable to remain within the MRI scanner, and limited availability of MRI scanners in many parts of the world.

4. Angiography: Catheter angiography is an invasive procedure with a risk of between 1:200 and 1:1,000 of *causing* a stroke. It is never the

initial imaging modality for evaluating headache. It remains the gold standard for demonstrating intrinsic vascular abnormalities such as aneurysms, vascular malformations, and vasculitis. It also remains the best test for demonstrating vessel narrowing by atherosclerosis, fibromuscular dysplasia, etc., though MR angiography and ultrasound also have some role in the evaluation of these processes.

C. Recommended Imaging Approach

Evaluation of a patient with headache depends primarily on clinical history. If the clinical history is typical of a tension, cluster, or migraine headache, no imaging evaluation is necessary. If the clinical history is atypical or the patient does not respond as expected to conventional therapy, additional causes of headache need to be considered. MRI is by far the most sensitive imaging modality for such evaluation and can be performed on an elective basis. An exception to this is acute headache or an acute change in mental status, which requires emergent NCCT scanning to rule out intracranial hemorrhage or increasing intracranial pressure.

Headache following trauma should prompt NCCT scanning to evaluate for intracranial hemorrhage and/or calvarial/skull base fracture.

If a patient complains of an acute, severe headache ("worst headache of my life"), an acute subarachnoid hemorrhage (from a ruptured aneurysm) needs to be ruled out with NCCT. If the NCCT is negative, lumbar puncture should be considered. If the CT scan or lumbar puncture is positive for an acute subarachnoid bleed, then angiography to search for a ruptured aneurysm is the next test that should be performed. Often exactly when that test is performed will depend on the clinical status of the patient.

If a headache is accompanied by a fever, infection needs to be considered. While CECT or contrast-enhanced MRI (better test) imaging may demonstrate meningeal enhancement in this setting, lumbar puncture is necessary to establish the diagnosis. NCCT scanning is sometimes performed before lumbar puncture to rule out increasing intracranial pressure that might contraindicate lumbar puncture. Contrast-enhanced MRI is best for evaluating for meningitis versus encephalitis versus intracerebral/extracerebral abscess, but CECT is also diagnostic in many cases (or for following known lesions).

No imaging is necessary if the clinical history is typical of acute sinusitis. If it is necessary to confirm that sinus inflammatory changes are present, a "limited" screening paranasal sinus NCCT scan can be performed. NCCT can detect underlying bony abnormalities that can predispose to sinusitis and can also demonstrate bony remodeling/destruction due to an inflammatory sinus process.

D. Differential Diagnostic Considerations

1. Migraine headache (simple, classic, or complex).
2. Tension headache.
3. Cluster headache.
4. Trauma (may include skull fracture, epidural/subdural hematoma).
5. Subarachnoid hemorrhage (classic history: "worst headache of my life").
6. Meningitis (infectious, neoplastic, chemical).
7. Obstructive hydrocephalus.
8. Intracranial mass (infectious, neoplastic, vascular).
9. Benign intracranial hypertension.
10. Paroxysmal hypertension ("malignant" hypertension, pheochromocytoma).
11. Dural venous sinus thrombosis.
12. Status post recent lumbar puncture.
13. Temporal arteritis.
14. Sinusitus.
15. Post-herpetic neuralgia.
16. Upper cervical spine injury.
17. Psychogenic.

MYELOPATHY

A. Clinical Findings

Myelopathy refers to symptoms due to dysfunction of the spinal cord. Such dysfunction can be due to an intrinsic spinal cord abnormality or to a process extrinsic to the spinal cord compressing and/or invading the spinal cord. Rarely, intracranial processes can cause myelopathic symptoms.

B. Imaging Modalities

1. Plain Radiographs

Advantages
- High spatial resolution.
- Low cost.

Disadvantages
- Do not directly image the spinal cord or most soft tissue pathology.
- Superimposition of shadows.
- Difficult to visualize upper thoracic region.
- Regardless of results, still need CT or MRI scan.

2. Myelography with Postmyelogram CT

Advangates
- Directly outlines the spinal cord.
- Demonstrates morphologic abnormalities of cord (e.g., enlarged, atrophied).
- Can show blockages to the flow of subarachnoid contrast material.
- Requires less patient cooperation than MRI (see below).
- Demonstrates bony abnormalities and mineralized pathology better than MRI.
- Can be performed on patients with MRI-incompatible implants, ventilators, etc.

Disadvantages
- Invasive, requiring spinal needle placement in either the cervical or lumbar subarachnoid space with the instillation of contrast material.
- Involves ionizing radiation.
- Can exacerbate symptoms of spinal cord compression.
- May not adequately demonstrate tandem lesions.

- Usually cannot differentiate cystic from solid causes of spinal cord enlargement.
- Can require extensive patient manipulation.

3. MRI

Advantages
- No ionizing radiation.
- Does not require needle placement into the subarachnoid space, avoiding the potential risks of infection, bleeding, contrast (dye), etc.
- Does not require any special patient positioning.
- Only imaging modality that allows *direct visualization* of the spinal cord.
- Can demonstrate intrinsic, noncontour deforming abnormalities of the spinal cord (inflammatory/ischemic processes).
- Can differentiate cystic (syrinx) from solid (tumor) spinal cord processes.
- Better demonstrates associated developmental abnormalities (e.g., Chiari malformations, diastematomyelia, etc.).
- Some specificity (hematoma).
- Often less expensive than a complete myelogram followed by a CT scan.

Disadvantages
- Limited availability in many parts of the United States (and the world).
- Need for patient cooperation—even minimal movement during the minutes required to perform each series of scans usually results in nondiagnostic images.
- Potential complications of MRI-incompatible implants or life-support equipment.

C. Recommended Imaging Approach

In the setting of acute trauma, patient with myelopathic symptoms should initially be evaluated with plain radiographs and/or CT to best evaluate for bony abnormalities such as displaced or nondisplaced vertebral fractures or the location of fracture fragments or foreign bodies.

However, in most patients, once it has been decided that imaging is required, MRI is the examination of choice. For patients with both upper and lower body symptoms, cervical imaging is probably adequate. In the setting of only lower extremity and/or bowel/bladder problems, the entire spinal cord should be imaged. In the setting of myelopathy, contrast-enhanced scans must also be obtained to evaluate for noncontour deforming lesions that have resulted in breakdown of the blood–brain barrier.

In some patients with extrinsic impingement on the spinal cord (usually spondylosis or degenerative disc disease, but occasionally also primary and secondary bone neoplasms), plain radiographs and/or CT scans through the areas of abnormality may be necessary for further characterization of a lesion.

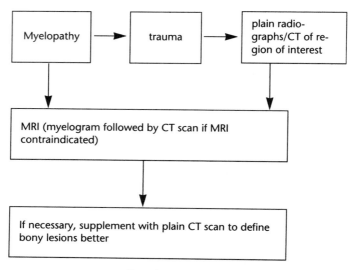

Imaging Algorithm

In patients unable to undergo MRI (machine unavailable, patient cannot lie still, patient with MRI-incompatible implants, etc.), myelography with postmyelogram CT is the examination of choice and will adequately demonstrate most surgical lesions.

D. Differential Diagnostic Considerations

1. Extrinsic spinal cord disease (compressing/invading cord)
    a. Extradural
        - Neoplasm (1°/2° benign/malignant tumor of spine/paraspinal regions invading canal).
        - Traumatic (fracture/dislocation, postoperative scar).
        - Inflammatory/infection (rheumatoid arthritis, abscess).
        - Vascular (hematoma).
        - Degenerative (spondylolisthesis, herniated discs, spondylosis).
        - Congenital (spinal stenosis, spinal dysraphic processes).
    b. Intradural/extramedullary
        - Neoplasm (neurofibroma, meningioma, metastases, dermoid, epidermoid, lipoma).
        - Inflammation (arachnoiditis).
        - Congenital (arachnoid cyst).
        - Vascular (vascular malformation, dural fistula, hematoma).
2. Intrinsic spinal cord disease (intramedullary; expanding and replacing normal cord)
    a. Neoplasm (astrocytoma, ependymoma, metastases).
    b. Syrinx (may be secondary to Chiari malformation, tumor, infection, trauma).
    c. Inflammatory/infection (myelitis, demyelinating disease, tuberculosis, radiation).
    d. Vascular (infarction, vascular malformation, posttraumatic hematoma/contusion).
    e. Degenerative.
    f. Metabolic (vitamin B_{12} deficiency).
    g. Congenital (diastematomyelia, neurenteric cyst).

NEONATAL SEIZURES

A. Clinical Findings

Seizures are a frequent problem encountered in neonatal nurseries. Seizures are defined clinically as a paroxysmal alteration in neurologic function with or without associated EEG seizure activity. There are four types of seizures:

1. Subtle or fragmentary: Episodes of apnea, abnormal facial or ocular movements, abnormal extremity movements such as "bicycling."
2. Clonic: Focal or multifocal rhythmic movements at a slow rate.
3. Tonic: Focal or generalized sustained posturing of axial or appendicular musculature.
4. Myoclonic: Generalized or focal/multifocal with rapid jerking movements with a predilection for flexor muscle groups.

B. Imaging Modalities

1. Plain radiographs: only potential use is in the setting of suspected child abuse to document skull fractures.
2. Ultrasound: Advantages include being able to perform the study at the patient's bedside (patient does not have to be transported to the CT or MRI scanner), no ionizing radiation, relatively little patient cooperation required, can document some intracranial hemorrhages (particularly subependymal/intraventricular bleeds), can delineate periventricular leukomalacia (which is often seen in premature infants), can demonstrate most major CNS malformations, and can differentiate a solid from a cystic mass.

   Disadvantages include extremely operator dependent, requires the presence of an open fontanelle, can miss some of the less extensive CNS malformations (e.g., focal heterotopias) and calcification, and posterior fossa processes can be difficult to appreciate.
2. CT: Mineralization (such as in infections) and acute hemorrhage are better seen with CT than with ultrasound or MRI.

   Disadvantages include that only axial images can be obtained in the vast majority of neonates, ionizing radiation is used, and it is not available at the bedside. Detail of intracranial structures is inferior to MRI.

3. MRI: Advantages include the absence of ionizing radiation; superior contrast resolution for delineation of intracranial abnormalities such as congenital malformations, strokes, infectious processes, etc.; hemorrhagic and vascular lesions better characterized; availability of MR angiography; multiplanar capabilities, only imaging modality that permits evaluation of meninges.

   Disadvantages include the requirement that the patient be transported to the MRI scanner for imaging, necessity of MRI-compatible life-support equipment, poor visualization of bone detail and mineralization, and need for heavy sedation or general anesthesia to avoid motion artifacts during the minutes required to acquire each set of images.

C. Recommended Imaging Approach

1. History and physical examination should provide most of the diagnostic clues
   a. Blood pressure should be measured because hypertensive encephalopathy may be the cause of seizures.
   b. A family history of neonatal seizures points to either an inborn error of metabolism or a benign neonatal seizure.
   c. Maternal rash, lymphadenopathy, and arthralgia suggest an intrauterine infection.
   d. Maternal labor history is important in establishing hypoxic, ischemic, or traumatic causes.
2. Laboratory studies should be tailored to rule out metabolic and electrolyte imbalances, inborn errors of metabolism, and infections.
3. Imaging workup
   a. *Ultrasound* is the initial imaging examination of choice, particularly because its portability allows quick access to the neonatal intracranial compartment and quick diagnosis of the majority of demonstrable intracranial causes of neonatal seizures. Ultrasound easily demonstrates the most common causes of neonatal

hypoxic seizures—subependymal/intraventricular hemorrhage, periventricular leukomalacia, and/or infarction. Large pathologic extracerebral fluid collections (associated with trauma or infection), many congenital CNS malformations (e.g., holoprosencephaly, lissencephaly), and the sequelae of in utero vascular insults (e.g., hydranencephaly) can be diagnosed with ultrasound.

b. If an abnormality needs further characterization, either *CT* or *MRI* can be used to better delineate the pertinent anatomy. While CT is better for demonstrating mineralization or bony ab-

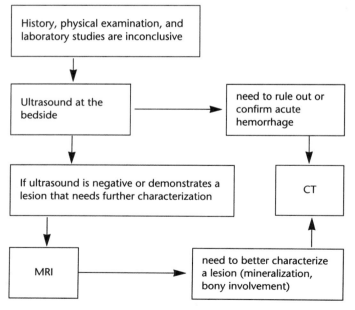

Imaging Algorithm

normalities (e.g., tumors or infections), MRI is far superior for demonstrating the vast majority of abnormalities (congenital malformations, tumors, meningeal processes, infections) that affect the intracranial compartment. *MR angiography* can also be used to visualize the dural venous sinuses in a noninvasive manner to rule out dural venous sinus thrombosis. As either CT or MRI will require general anesthesia in most neonates, MRI should be the examination of choice following ultrasound unless acute intracranial hemorrhage is of clinical concern (then CT should be performed).

D. Differential Diagnostic Considerations

1. Hypoxic-ischemic encephalopathy: Most common cause of neonatal seizure. Sequelae include subependymal/intraventricular hemorrhage, leukomalacia, and infarction. Ultrasound is the initial imaging examination of choice.
2. Trauma: Subdural hematoma, intraparenchymal hemorrhage, cortical vein thrombosis.
3. Hypertension.
4. Electrolyte disturbances: Hypoglycemia, hypocalcemia, hyponatremia, hypernatremia.
5. Infections: Congenital infections in the TORCH group; bacterial meningitis (group B *Streptococcus*); cerebral abscess.
6. Drug withdrawal: Methadone, heroin, barbiturate, alcohol.
7. Congenital malformations: Polymicrogyria, heterotopias, holoprosencephaly, hydranencephaly, lissencephaly, neurocutaneous syndromes (tuberous sclerosis, incontinentia pigmenti). MRI the best modality for evaluating these entities.
8. Inborn errors of metabolism: Amino acid disturbances (e.g., maple syrup urine disease), vitamin B_6 deficiency, pyridoxine deficiency.
9. Benign neonatal seizures ("fifth day convulsions"): Diagnosis of exclusion, which usually occur in previously healthy neonates; can be familial (autosomal dominant, localized to chromosome 20) or nonfamilial.

ORBITAL PAIN

A. Clinical Findings

Ocular pain is the result of stimulation of the trigeminal nerve fibers anywhere within the eye, the surrounding periorbital tissues, the deep (intraconal, retro-ocular) orbit, or the floor of the anterior or middle cranial fossae.

Ocular pathology may or may not result in eye pain. In addition, eye pain is often nonspecific with respect to underlying pathology.

Ocular pain may be described as a foreign body sensation, periocular in location, a throbbing pain, or as a retro-ocular dull ache. Clinical history with respect to the nature, frequency, and duration of the pain can be helpful. If ocular pain is associated with visual loss, diplopia, ptosis, or proptosis, further evaluation with imaging is almost always warranted.

B. Imaging Modalities

1. Plain radiographs: While plain radiographs can demonstrate orbital wall, lacrimal gland fossa, optic foramen, optic canal, sphenoid ridge, and paranasal sinus bony abnormalities, associated soft tissue (i.e., intraorbital, facial, etc.) abnormalities cannot be assessed. Therefore, plain radiography, whether positive or negative, does not obviate the need for additional imaging (ultrasound, CT or MRI) and is therefore of no value in evaluating orbital pain.

2. Ultrasound (orbital echography): Inexpensive, safe (no ionizing radiation), reproducible method of evaluating orbital lesions. Does not permit visualization of the orbital apex or extraorbital spread of a process. May not be possible to use in severely traumatized or uncooperative patients.

   a. A-mode ultrasound: One-dimensional view of a lesion; can show lesion's "reflectivity," sound attenuation, and internal structure.

   b. B-mode ultrasound: Can demonstrate lesion's location, size, shape, and orientation to other structures.

3. CT: Superb delineation of the bones of the face, which is crucial when evaluating fractures or bony erosion/expansion/destruction

by orbital neoplasms or infectious/inflammatory processes. Native intraorbital fat provides excellent contrast to both normal and abnormal orbital soft tissue structures. Examination of choice for ruling out foreign bodies. Can also scan in the direct coronal plane to better localize pathologic processes and detect orbital roof/floor fractures. CT is also best for detecting acute hemorrhage and requires less patient cooperation than MRI.

4. MRI: Best delineation of soft tissue structures of the orbit. Contrast-enhanced imaging (with fat suppression technique) is extremely sensitive to pathologic processes (in particular, intrinsic optic nerve processes such as optic neuritis and glioma and perioptic nerve processes such as meningioma). The orbital apex is best seen on MRI as is extension of a cavernous sinus process or any intracranial process due to the lack of bone artifacts.

Disadvantages of MRI include lack of delineation of bony structures and mineralization in a lesion (which can help characterize lesions such as retinoblastoma). Even with MR angiography, most orbital vascular processes (most aneurysms, some varices, some fistulas) are inadequately evaluated and require dedicated endovascular angiography for diagnosis (and treatment).

5. Angiography: Formal catheter angiography is still considered the gold standard for evaluation of most intraorbital vascular processes. Cerebral angiography is the examination of choice for carotid cavernous fistulas, as definitive endovascular therapy can be performed at the time of the diagnostic evaluation.

Disadvantages of cerebral angiography include ionizing radiation, cost, and the 1:200 to 1:1,000 risk of *causing* a stroke during the examination.

C. Recommended Imaging Approach

Orbital pain is often a nonspecific, nonlocalizing symptom that spontaneously resolves. However, the clinical presentation of orbital pain, associated visual complaints, and associated external ocular findings can narrow a differential diagnosis. Therefore, a careful history and physical examination can obviate the need for imaging in many patients.

In the setting of trauma including blunt or lacerating injury to the eye, a painful red eye may reflect an intraocular and/or retro-ocular intraorbital foreign body. The eye should be manipulated as little as possible and an emergent CT scan obtained to search for a foreign body, evaluate surrounding bony structures, rule out retro-ocular hematoma, etc.

Acute ocular pain with eye movements in the setting of visual loss in a young adult strongly suggests optic neuritis (suggesting underlying multiple sclerosis). The Optic Neuritis Treatment Trial Study has concluded that the extent of abnormalities consistent with demyelination on an MRI scan in a patient with optic neuritis is a strong predictor of a patient's future clinical course.

Conjunctival chemosis, eyelid edema, limited ocular motility, and visual compromise may reflect an underlying infectious or inflammatory orbital process. Imaging is required to evaluate the extent of disease so that appropriate medical or surgical management can be initiated. CT scanning is the examination of choice so that both intraorbital structures and surrounding bony structures (including nearby paranasal sinuses that can be a source of infection) are fully evaluated. If orbital apex or frank intracranial extension of a process is suspected, then MRI should also be performed.

In patients older than 10 years who have orbit pain and a third nerve palsy (with abnormal pupillary reflexes), an intracranial aneurysm (posterior communicating artery) should be ruled out. Aneurysms greater than 4–5 mm can comfortably be ruled out on a high-quality MR angiogram. However, if the MR angiogram is negative, then formal endovascular catheter angiography to rule out a smaller aneurysm remains the examination of choice.

Conjunctival hyperemia in the setting of periocular pain, diplopia, elevated intraocular pressure, and visual loss may suggest an arteriovenous malformation (i.e., carotid-cavernous fistula). Sometimes, the patient will describe a "whooshing" sound (subjective bruit) that may or may not be audible to the examining physician. A dilated (usually superior) ophthalmic vein on an imaging study is suggestive of drainage from a carotid-cavernous fistula. This finding is equally well evaluated on CT and MRI, and, while the draining vein can be seen on MR angiography, the actual fistula is difficult to delineate on MR angiography. Endovascular angiography is the examination of choice for both diagnosing and *treating* such a fistula.

In summary, when imaging is considered necessary in the setting of orbital pain, a CT scan is the examination of choice particularly if symptoms are acute or an infectious process is of concern. MRI can be used to characterize and delineate a lesion more fully and is the examination of choice for intrinsic optic nerve, orbital apex, or intracranial processes. Angiography should be reserved for suspected aneurysms or vascular malformations.

D. Differential Diagnostic Considerations

1. Ocular pain *without extraocular findings.*
   a. Deep orbital/retro-orbital process.
      * Benign/malignant orbital mass.
      * Orbital infiltrative process (neoplasm, infection).
   b. Inflammatory
      * Demyelination (optic neuritis).
2. Ocular pain with *extraocular findings.*
   a. Infectious—orbital cellulitis.
   b. Inflammatory.
      * Idiopathic orbital inflammatory disease or orbital pseudotumor.

         Diffuse (anterior globe, posterior globe, orbital apex).

         Local (myositis, dacryoadenitis, periscleritis, perineuritis).
      * Tolosa-Hunt syndrome (idiopathic inflammation restricted to the superior orbital fissure, optic canal or the cavernous sinus).
   c. Orbital mass.
   d. Systemic disease (e.g., thyroid ophthalmopathy [Graves' disease]).
   e. Arteriovenous malformation—carotid-cavernous fistula (traumatic or spontaneous).
   f. Trauma.
      * Blunt or penetrating eye injury.
      * Retro-ocular hemorrhage.
3. Ocular pain *with cranial motor/sensory neuropathy.*

a. Vascular lesions.
   - Arteriovenous malformations.
   - Intracranial aneurysms (anterior circle of Willis).
   - Carotid-cavernous fistulas.
b. Masses

PARALYSIS

A. Clinical Findings

Paralysis refers to complete loss of movement (paresis = partial paralysis). Paralysis may be due to a lesion of the brain, spinal cord or peripheral nerve(s). It may present as a "spastic" (upper motor neuron: spinal cord or brain) or "flaccid" (lower motor neuron) process. It can present as a monoplegia, hemiplegia (most common), paraplegia (most commonly due to spinal cord abnormality), quadraplegia or may involve only a single nerve.

B. Imaging Modalities

1. Plain radiographs: Advantages include low cost and ability to acquire them at the bedside or in the Emergency Room. Useful to evaluate the cervical spine in the setting of trauma.

   Disadvantages include lack of cross-sectional imaging capabilities, "superimposition of shadows," and low contrast resolution; soft tissue injuries/pathology in the head and spinal canal cannot be delineated. Therefore, plain radiographs are not indicated in the evaluation of paralysis except in the setting of spinal trauma to assess the status of the spinal column before CT or MRI.

2. Ultrasound: Advantages include portability, low cost, absence of ionizing radiation, and universal availability. Newer transcranial Doppler applications (particularly in conjunction with intravascular ultrasound contrast agents) allow some evaluation of intracranial vasculature.

   Disadvantages include the need for an "acoustic window." Specifically, an open fontanelle is necessary to evaluate the intracranial compartment. Also, the resolution of intracranial and spinal canal structures is inferior to MRI, and any ultrasound examination is dependent on the skill of the sonologist performing the study. Therefore, ultrasound is essentially limited to evaluation of neonates, the lumbosacral spine to evaluate dysraphism in younger patients, and intraoperatively when a craniotomy or laminectomy has already been performed.

3. Myelography (with postmyelogram CT): In the era of MRI, myelography with postmyelogram CT should rarely be the imaging examination of choice to evaluate the spinal canal.

   Advantages of this procedure include excellent delineation of bony abnormalities and their relationship to the spinal canal and exiting nerve roots. In addition, patients with implants that are MRI-incompatible or internal fixation hardware that obscures the spine on MRI can still be evaluated.

   Disadvantages of this procedure include inferior evaluation of the spinal cord compared with MRI, the risks of ionizing radiation and intrathecal contrast, and the risk of placing a spinal needle below the level of a lesion that compresses the spinal cord.

4. CT: Advantages include optimal demonstration of intracranial hemorrhage, rapid acquisition of images so that the degree of patient cooperation required is minimal, ability to monitor sick patients in the CT scanner, excellent delineation of bony abnormalities (e.g., spinal fractures), and ability to distinguish between bland and hemorrhagic strokes.

   Disadvantages include the risks of ionizing radiation, limited scan planes (particularly in sick patients), inferior ability to demonstrate intracranial intraaxial pathology, inability to demonstrate intrinsic spinal cord pathology, and the possibility of missing *nondisplaced* lesions (e.g., spinal and skull fractures).

5. MRI: Advantages include superior contrast resolution permitting optimal evaluation of the intracranial and spinal compartments, unlimited scan planes, and the lack of ionizing radiation.

   Disadvantages include motion artifacts in unstable/uncooperative patients who cannot remain motionless for the minutes required to obtain a series of MR images, inferior evaluation of bony structures, limited availability of the technology, high cost, and inability to evaluate some patients with MRI-incompatible implants (e.g., pacemakers, aneurysm clips, cochlear implants) or life-support equipment (e.g., ventilators).

6. Angiography: Advantages of conventional endovascular catheter angiography include superior delineation of arterial and venous anatomy (clearly superior to MR angiography) and vascular neoplasms and the potential for interventional therapy of some vascular lesions (e.g., dural arteriovenous malformations, meningiomas, aneurysms).

Disadvantages include the intrinsic risk of catheter angiography (between a 1:200 and 1:1,000 risk of *causing* a stroke), the relatively high dose of radiation, the risks of intravascular contrast material, and the relatively high cost of the examination.

In the setting of acute (<4–6 hours) paralysis (hemiparesis) believed to be secondary to an occluding thrombus, emergent angiography with the possibility of intraarterial lytic (urokinase) therapy should be considered.

C. Recommended Imaging Approach

The causes of the different types of paralysis are extremely varied. A careful history and physical examination and selected laboratory studies can eliminate the need for imaging in many patients. These include hysterical paralysis and many types of toxic/metabolic insults.

In neonates, any neurologic symptoms should initially be evaluated with ultrasound. CT scanning should be considered if acute hemorrhage is of concern. MRI should be reserved to rule out structural (congenital) abnormalities or to further delineate or characterize abnormalities seen on ultrasound or CT.

In the setting of acute trauma, the intracranial compartment should be evaluated with a head CT to rule out acute hemorrhage, mass effect, or hydrocephalus. The spine should initially be evaluated with plain radiographs to look for areas of gross abnormality. Even if plain radiographs are negative, any region of clinical concern should be evaluated with dedicated CT scanning through that region. If the patient has any myelopathic symptoms or signs, MRI to further evaluate the spinal canal and spinal cord should then be performed.

In the setting of a stroke, CT should be performed to rule out associated hemorrhage. If the patient is being evaluated within the first 4–6 hours after the event, emergent angiography should be considered as intraarterial lytic therapy can be initiated in some patients.

In most cases of (nonacute, nontraumatic) paralysis, clinical evaluation can localize a region of the central nervous system for dedicated imaging evaluation that should begin with MRI. CT scanning should also be performed only if evaluation of bony structures is of concern. Peripheral nervous system etiologies of focal paralysis rarely require imaging. If so, dedicated CT or MRI is suggested, depending on the region.

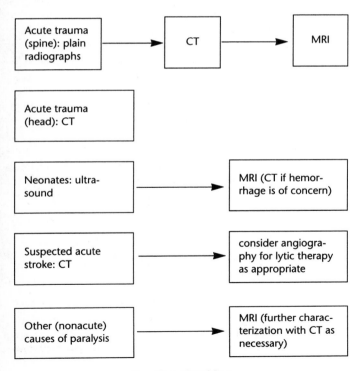

Imaging Algorithm

D. Differential Diagnostic Considerations

1. Vascular.
   a. Infarction (hemorrhagic, embolic, ischemic, hypoxic): Brain, spinal cord.
   b. Vascular malformation: Brain, spinal cord.
   c. Aneurysm: Brain.
   d. Hematoma (hypertensive, amyloid, trauma, etc.): Brain, spinal cord.
   e. Postoperative (e.g., spinal cord infarction).
2. Trauma.
   a. Intracranial hemorrhage, mass effect, etc.
   b. Spinal canal compromise due to vertebral fracture, epidural hematoma, frank cord injury, etc.
   c. Blunt/lacerating injury to extraspinal nerves, root avulsions.
   d. Birth injury (Klumpke, Erb palsies).
3. Neoplasm.
   a. Space-occupying benign or malignant mass in the head or spinal canal; mass compromising extraspinal nerve or nerve plexus.
4. Degenerative.
   a. Spinal canal compromise by herniated disc, spondylosis, spondylolisthesis.
   b. Craniovertebral junction compromise by rheumatoid arthritis, etc.
5. Infections/inflammatory.
   a. Frank abscess within the head or spinal cord/canal.
   b. Tuberculosis/granulomatous/fungal disease.
   c. Syphilitic meningomyelitis.
   d. Encephalitis, myelitis (e.g., poliomyelitis).
   e. Demyelinating disease (acute disseminated encephalomyelitis, multiple sclerosis).
6. Syrinx/syringobulbia.
   a. Associated with congenital malformation (Chiari malformations).

    b. Tumor.

    c. Postinfectious.

    d. Posttraumatic.

7. Congenital.

    a. Brain and/or spinal malformations (Chiari malformation, holoprosencephaly, dysraphism, neurenteric cyst, tethered cord, etc.).

    b. Dysmyelinating processes.

8. Metabolic.

    a. Hypokalemia, vitamin B_{12} deficiency, "familial periodic paralysis."

9. Hysterical (need to be distinguished from organic pathology).

10. Iatrogenic.

    a. Anesthesia (general, regional, local).

    b. Curarization (induced paralysis with curare: flail chest, tetanus).

11. Other (myasthenia gravis, tetanus, tetany, botulism, lead poisoning, thyroid myopathy).

PITUITARY DYSFUNCTION

A. Clinical Findings

Sellar region lesions present with either clinical signs or symptoms of pituitary hormone overproduction or underproduction due to an intrinsic or extrinsic pituitary process or by local mass effect on, or invasion of, nearby structures by a "nonfunctioning" pituitary region lesion. Once intrinsic pituitary dysfunction has been confirmed biochemically, imaging is usually performed. Imaging is usually also performed if the patient has signs or symptoms referable to the peri-sellar region (e.g., cavernous sinus cranial nerve [3, 4, 6] findings, bitemporal field cut, hypothalamic symptoms) even if biochemical studies are normal.

B. Imaging Modalities

1. Plain radiographs: These can show bony changes of the sella turci-

ca and surrounding structures, but cannot directly image the pituitary gland or the vast majority of pathologic processes. Therefore, they are of no value (do not replace or add information to the other imaging modalities described below) and should not be performed as part of the evaluation of these patients.

2. CT: Directly visualizes sellar region structures. Direct coronal imaging can be performed. Demonstrates acute hemorrhage, mineralization (within a lesion), and erosion/destruction of nearby bony structures better than MRI. However, direct coronal CT scanning requires positioning that many patients cannot tolerate, and coronal scans are often severely limited by artifacts from dental amalgam.

3. MRI: Like CT, this modality allows direct visualization of the pituitary gland. Advantages of this technique include no use of ionizing radiation, does not require any special patient positioning, can demonstrate intrinsic abnormalities of the pituitary gland better than CT (better contrast resolution), allows sagittal imaging, is somewhat more specific than CT (better defines subacute/chronic hemorrhage and highly proteinaceous material which might be found in craniopharyngiomas), shows only minimal artifact from dental amalgam, and includes the ability to perform MR angiography, which can define aneurysms, some fistulas, and anomalous vessels.

   Disadvantages of this technique include the requirement of patient cooperation—even minimal movement during the minutes required to perform each series of scans usually results in nondiagnostic images; the potential complications of MRI-incompatible implants or life-support equipment; and poor visualization of mineralization, which can limit evaluation of craniopharyngiomas, aneurysm walls, and erosion of nearby bony structures (e.g., sellar floor, dorsum sella).

4. Angiography: This technique remains the gold standard for evaluating blood vessels. Advantages of this technique include best definition (spatial resolution) of aneurysms (necks, etc.), fistulas, and anomalous vessels; and the potential for endovascular therapy by an interventional neuroradiologist at the time of angiography to

treat an abnormality (occlude a carotid-cavernous fistula, balloon/coil an aneurysm, etc.), avoiding more costly and potentially more dangerous surgery.

Disadvantages of endovascular angiography include poor evaluation of nonvascular lesions (mass effect on vessels is often a late finding; therefore most mass lesions are missed at angiography); cannot evaluate thrombosed portions of vascular abnormalities (e.g., partially thrombosed aneurysms) which are better seen with MRI; and the increased risks of cerebral arteriography, including stroke and death.

C. Recommended Imaging Approach

Imaging of suspected sellar region pathology should begin with multiplanar contrast-enhanced MRI. CT scanning should be performed only to rule out acute hemorrhage, further characterize a mass (e.g., calcification), or assess nearby associated bony changes or suspected intrinsic bony processes that have spread to the sella turcica region. If a vascular abnormality such as a carotid-cavernous fistula or aneurysm is identified or suspected either on a clinical basis or from MRI/CT scanning, endovascular cerebral angiography should be performed for diagnostic (and possibly therapeutic) purposes. In most cases, MRI scanning will be the only imaging test required.

D. Differential Diagnostic Considerations

1. Primary pituitary fossa process
   a. Neoplasm (pituitary adenoma [functioning, nonfunctioning], craniopharyngioma, metastases).
   b. Developmental (Rathke cleft cysts).
   c. Infection (hypophysitis, abscess).
   d. Vascular (infarction, hemorrhage [pituitary apoplexy]).
2. Process secondarily involving pituitary fossa or hypothalamic/pituitary axis
   a. Neoplasm (meningioma, chiasmal and hypothalamic gliomas, metastases, skull base tumors [chordomas, sarcomas, myeloma, metastases], germ cell tumors).

    b. Developmental (arachnoid cysts, epidermoid, dermoid, hamartoma).

    c. Infection/inflammation (abscess, granulomatous disease, Langerhans histiocytosis).

    d. Vascular (extension of parasellar or suprasellar aneurysms, carotid-cavernous fistulas, anomalous vessels).

PROPTOSIS

A. Clinical Findings

Proptosis or exophthalmos refers to abnormal anterior displacement of the eye (axial protrusion). There may be simultaneous transverse (medial or lateral) and/or vertical (superior or inferior) displacement of the globe. Proptosis is more commonly unilateral, but may be bilateral. It may be acute (developing over a few days), subacute, or more insidious (developing over weeks to months) in onset.

B. Imaging Modalities

1. Ultrasound: Usually Performed by an Ophthalmologist

Advantages

- No ionizing radiation.
- Relatively inexpensive.
- Obtain dynamic (real-time) information.
- As an initial exam, can quickly establish the presence of a lesion in many cases. However, further evaluation with CT or MRI to determine lesion morphology, extension, and its relationship to adjacent anatomic structures is usually necessary.
- Doppler capabilities allow evaluation of some vascular abnormalities (e.g., varix, carotid-cavernous fistula).

Disadvantages

- Operator dependent.

- Lesions in the posterior orbit and orbital apex and those with intracranial or maxillofacial extension may be missed.

2. CT

Advantages
- Relatively quick scanning time with new rapid techniques.
- Provides excellent bone detail.
- Direct axial and coronal imaging.
- Coronal, sagittal, and oblique CT sections may be obtained by reformation of information obtained in the axial plane. These reformations do not require additional imaging time and may be performed after the patient has left the scanner.

Disadvantages
- Radiation exposure.
- Artifact from dental hardware may degrade coronal images.

3. MRI

Advantages
- No ionizing radiation.
- Multiplanar capabilities (coronal, axial, and sagittal images may be obtained without changing the patient's position on the MRI table).
- Improved soft tissue contrast resolution.
- Better for evaluating vascular and hemorrhagic lesions; MR angiography may also be performed as needed to evaluate vascular abnormalities.

Disadvantages
- Contraindicated in certain circumstances, including patients with cardiac pacemakers, some metallic foreign bodies in or around the orbits, some aneurysm clips, and certain prosthetic devices.
- Poor visualization of bone detail.
- Requires strict patient cooperation—patient motion results in artifact that degrades images, limiting interpretation.

- Mascara and other eye make-up may result in significant "susceptibility" artifacts and should be removed prior to imaging.

C. Recommended Imaging Approach

In the setting of acute trauma, proptosis should initially be evaluated with CT, which allows excellent evaluation of both the soft tissues and the bones. Retrobulbar hematomas, associated abnormalities of the globe, fractures, and radiopaque foreign bodies are readily detected. In select circumstances, patients may require additional imaging for unexplained symptoms (such as MRI to evaluate optic neuropathy or cerebral angiography to evaluate suspected posttraumatic carotid-cavernous fistulas).

The diagnosis of thyroid ophthalmopathy is often obvious due to associated clinical findings and coexisting abnormal thyroid function tests (however, thyroid ophthalmopathy may occur in euthyroid patients). In thyroid ophthalmopathy, imaging may be necessary for those patients with secondary symptoms, in particular, optic neuropathy due to compression of the optic nerve by enlarged extraocular muscles at the orbital apex. While CT and MRI nicely delineate soft tissue abnormalities, in this instance CT may be preferred as it better depicts bone detail that may be important in preparing for decompressive surgery.

In the remaining patients, proptosis frequently implies an intraorbital lesion. It is important that a complete imaging evaluation be obtained to evaluate not only the lesion location but also its extent both within and beyond the orbit. Selection of CT or MRI in evaluating exophthalmos depends on several factors, including the clinical setting and the availability of these imaging modalities. CT will adequately demonstrate a variety of lesions and is sufficient in many cases. Because of improved soft tissue contrast resolution with MRI as well as its ability to evaluate subacute/chronic hemorrhage, MRI can be helpful in characterizing lesions that remain confusing on CT. When there is concern for intracranial extension of an orbital abnormality or when a vascular etiology such as a carotid-cavernous fistula is suspected. MRI should be performed rather than CT. If a vascular abnormality is identified on an MRI scan, or if a vascular abnormality remains suspected in the setting of a normal MRI study, endovascular cerebral angiography should be performed.

D. Differential Diagnostic Considerations

1. Graves' disease: Most common cause of unilateral or bilateral proptosis in adults.

2. Orbital cellulitis: Usually acute in onset in patients with a known inflammatory process of adjacent structures (periorbital cellulitis, sinusitis, dental abscess).

3. Neoplasms: Proptosis usually more insidious in onset
   a. Children
      - Rhabdomyosarcoma: Most common primary orbital malignancy.
      - Dermoid.
      - Optic nerve glioma.
      - Hemangioma, lymphangioma.
      - Lymphoma/leukemia.
      - Metastatic disease: Sarcoma, neuroblastoma (often bilateral).
   b. Adults
      - Cavernous hemangioma.
      - Lymphoma.
      - Metastatic disease: Especially breast, lung, extension of nasopharyngeal carcinoma.
      - Meningioma.
      - Lacrimal gland tumors.

4. Hemorrhage: Acute proptosis
   a. Posttraumatic.
   b. Spontaneous: Frequently secondary to underlying lesion (tumor, hemangioma, varix). While ultrasound or CT may confirm the presence of a hematoma, MRI is frequently necessary to identify and characterize an associated underlying lesion.

5. Orbital pseudotumor (idiopathic inflammation).

6. Carotid-cavernous fistula (CCF): Posttraumatic or spontaneous. May present with pulsatile exophthalmos, chemosis, papilledema.

7. Encephaloceles: May have pulsatile exophthalmos.

    a. Posttraumatic orbital roof defect.

    b. Congenital skull defect such as dysplasia of the sphenoid wing in neurofibromatosis.

8. Mucoceles.

9. Pseudoproptosis: Large eye, giving appearance of proptosis.

    a. Myopic eye.

    b. Unilateral congenital glaucoma.

10. Contralateral enophthalmos: Normal eye appears proptotic.

RADICULOPATHY

A. Clinical Findings

Radicular pain, particularly if accompanied by paresthesia and loss of sensation, suggests mechanical compression of the nerve root supplying that dermatome possibly due to a structural process, like a herniated disc. *Low back pain* is not a diagnosis, but a symptom complex with many potential etiologies. *Discogenic pain* is characteristically aggravated by cough or sneeze. Usually, onset of acute symptoms of lumbar radiculopathy are preceded by chronic intermittent low back pain.

A patient with a clinical history of neoplasm, infection, or vascular disease who presents with radicular pain of the upper or lower extremity should be imaged without delay. Similarly, if, in addition to radiculopathy, *weakness* is present, imaging should be performed without delay. However, if radiculopathy is a new or isolated symptom, conservative management with bedrest, warmth, pain medication, and muscle relaxants is recommended for several weeks before imaging studies are considered.

B. Imaging Modalities

1. Plain films: Radiographs of the spine rarely reveal clinically unsuspected findings. Frontal, lateral, and oblique views of the cervical or lumbosacral spine can demonstrate intervertebral foraminal encroachment by vertebral endplate and facet degenerative changes, compression fractures, and subluxations (spondylolistheses). In conjunction with an MRI scan, they can be useful for distinguish-

ing between a hypertrophic spur and a herniated disc.

Plain radiographs do not demonstrate intracanalicular structures.

2. Plain (without intrathecal contrast) CT: Can directly visualize abnormalities such as herniated discs in asymptomatic as well as symptomatic patients. CT gives good delineation of the discs, vertebral bodies, spinal canal dimensions, and facet joints. CT is almost as accurate as MRI in unoperated patients with lumbar radiculopathy and is used in many institutions as the primary imaging modality in patients with lumbar radiculopathy. CT is less expensive than MRI and requires less patient cooperation.

Plain CT is rarely useful in patients with cervical radiculopathy even with high-resolution and thin-slice technique. Artifacts from the shoulders (and the iliac bones in the lumbar region) limits evaluation of the spinal canal and its contents at those levels. Without intrathecal contrast, spinal cord morphology/compression cannot be assessed. Even with intrathecal contrast, intrinsic, noncontour deforming spinal cord processes cannot be ruled out.

3. Myelography with postmyelogram CT: Now primarily used as a preoperative study when the surgeon is not comfortable with the other imaging studies and/or needs more information (such as the appearance of the bones). Patients with radiculopathy but who either cannot tolerate MRI or who have contraindications to MRI are well-evaluated with this procedure.

As this procedure is an invasive study involving lumbar puncture and injection of contrast material into the subarachnoid space, there are risks of postprocedure headache (15%–20%), ionizing radiation, and injected contrast material. Again, noncontour deforming intrinsic spinal cord lesions will be missed with this technique.

4. MRI: The study of choice for radiculopathy (probably superior to cervical myelography with postmyelogram CT and equivalent to lumbar myelography with postmyelogram CT). Superior contrast resolution, the lack of ionizing radiation, the absence of the risks of a lumbar puncture and instillation of subarachnoid contrast material, and the ability to image in any scan plane are all advantages of MRI with respect to myelography with postmyelogram CT.

Disadvantages of MRI include that the patient must be able to lie motionless for minutes at a time as even minor movement can degrade images significantly. Also, bony lesions and lesion mineralization are poorly seen on MR. An additional process not easily identified by MR imaging are subluxations of vertebral bodies that are only seen with movement (i.e., flexion/extension). However, limited flexion/extension MR imaging is possible.

C. Recommended Imaging Approach

If history and physical examination suggest radiculopathy due to a process involving the neck or back (such as degenerative disease or a herniated disc) and if pain does not respond to a several week course of conservative management, imaging workup should begin with MRI. CT is an acceptable alternative for patients with *lumbar* radiculopathy. Myelography with postmyelogram CT of the appropriate spinal region should be reserved for cases where MRI is nondiagnostic or if an MR lesion needs further characterization or delineation.

Patients with radiculopathy and a known neoplasm or other clinical findings of neoplasm or infection should undergo MRI immediately.

D. Differential Diagnostic Considerations

1. Disc herniation
   a. Cervical
      - C5/6 (20%)–C6 nerve root compression causes radiating pain to the lateral forearm and thumb and index finger with biceps motor deficit.
      - C6/7 (70%)–C7 nerve root compression causes radiating pain to the lateral hand with triceps, wrist flexor, and wrist extensor motor deficits.
   b. Lumbar
      - 90% of lumbar disc herniations are at the L4–5 and L5–S1 levels; 5% at the L3/4 level.
      - L3/4–L4 nerve root compression causes pain referred along the course of the femoral nerve. Knee extension may be weak and the patellar reflex reduced or absent.

- L4/5–L5 nerve root compression causes radiating pain to the posterior thigh and the anteromedial leg and foot with weakness of the toe extensors.
- L5/S1–S1 nerve root compression is associated with pain over the posterior thigh, calf, and heel, weakness of the ankle and toe flexors, and reduced or absent Achilles tendon reflex.

c. Thoracic
  - Less than 1% of herniated discs are in the thoracic region.
  - Thoracic herniated discs are often calcified and can be mistaken for neoplasm (e.g., meningioma) at imaging.

2. Spondylosis: Cervical or lumbar, rarely thoracic; often asymptomatic. However, when reactive tissue compresses a nerve root or the spinal cord, the symptoms are similar to those of a herniated disc with a less abrupt onset of symptoms. More likely to be symptomatic if the sagittal diameter of the spinal canal is congenitally narrow (congenital spinal stenosis).

3. Spinal stenosis
   a. Most common etiologies include spondylosis, large disc herniation, or tumor.
   b. In the cervical region, radicular and/or myelopathic symptoms may be present.
   c. In the lumbar region, radicular or polyradicular symptoms may be present.
   d. At the thoracolumbar junction, a cauda equina syndrome may result that is characterized by severe bilateral leg pain, urinary retention, weakness of the anal sphincter, and bilateral nerve root abnormalities.
   e. Conservative treatment usually fails with spinal stenosis, and surgery is the treatment of choice.

4. Neoplasms
   a. Can cause nerve root or spinal cord compression.
   b. Can be paravertebral, extradural, intradural, or intramedullary.
   c. Most of the neoplasms causing spinal cord compression are extradural metastases that extend into the spinal canal from the

vertebral body and compress spinal nerve roots and/or the spinal cord without frank invasion of those structures.

5. Paravertebral tumors: Can cause confusing/ambiguous neurologic signs and symptoms as the tumor extends longitudinally within the paravertebral space and invades one or more intervertebral foramina; may compress both the spinal cord and one or more nerve roots.

6. Myofascial pain syndromes
   a. Can cause paravertebral neck pain or low back pain, often with marked tenderness and "trigger" points, but no radiculopathy.
   b. Imaging studies are not useful.

7. Entrapment neuropathies: Can mimic paravertebral tumor.

8. Arachnoiditis
   a. Due to inflammatory, infectious, or hemorrhagic subarachnoid space process. Can be seen in the setting of previous spinal trauma (including surgery and myelography).
   b. Characterized by neck or back pain and/or by radicular pain in the distribution of the nerve roots involved by the process. Dysfunction of several roots, particularly in the lumbosacral region, is common.
   c. Can progress to spinal "block" (equivalent to thecal sac compression) with obliteration of the spinal canal and resultant paraplegia.
   d. No definite treatment (if no specific infectious organism is identified, which is usually the case).

RED EYE

A. Clinical Findings

The term "red-eye" includes a spectrum of eye conditions. A red eye represents conjunctival vascular congestion. It is important to decide if the red eye condition is vision-threatening or not.

A red eye may be the result of infection, inflammation, degeneration, trauma, glaucoma or vascular malformation. Clinical history with respect to the chronicity of redness, visual loss, pain, trauma, chemical exposure and photophobia can help determine the cause of the red eye.

If the etiology of the red eye is not straightforward after initial history and physical examination, a thorough evaluation of the patient should be performed by an ophthalmologist. Such an examination will include formal assessment of visual acuity, ocular adnexal structures, direct pupillary response to light, extraocular motility, evaluation of the anterior segment of the eye with fluorescein instillation, a cobalt light examination to evaluate the corneal epithelium, measurement of intraocular pressure and funduscopic evaluation.

Signs/symptoms that suggest that vision may be threatened include severe ocular pain, persistent blurred vision, proptosis, reduced ocular motility, an unreactive pupil, worsening of the red eye with pharmacologic treatment and/or a history of immunosuppression.

Some ocular processes present with a red eye and require only clinical observation and/or medical management without imaging evaluation. Other ocular conditions associated with a red eye require an imaging study as part of the initial assessment.

B. Imaging Modalities

1. Plain radiographs: While plain radiographs can demonstrate orbital wall, lacrimal gland fossa, optic foramen, optic canal, sphenoid ridge, and paranasal sinus bony abnormalities, associated soft tissue (i.e., intraorbital, facial) abnormalities cannot be assessed. Therefore, plain radiography, whether positive or negative, does not obviate the need for additional imaging (ultrasound, CT, or MRI) and is therefore of no value in evaluating red eye.

2. Ultrasound (orbital echography): Inexpensive, safe (no ionizing radiation), reproducible method of evaluating orbital lesions. Does not permit visualization of the orbital apex or extraorbital spread of a process. May not be possible to use in severely traumatized or uncooperative patients.

   a. A-mode ultrasound: One-dimensional view of a lesion; can show lesion's "reflectivity," sound attenuation, and internal structure.

   b. B-mode ultrasound: Can demonstrate lesion's location, size, shape, and orientation to other structures.

3. CT: Superb delineation of the bones of the face, which is crucial when evaluating fractures or bony erosion/expansion/destruction by orbital neoplasms or infectious/inflammatory processes. Native intraorbital fat provides excellent contrast to both normal and abnormal orbital soft tissue structures. Examination of choice for ruling out foreign bodies. Can also scan in the direct coronal plane to better localize pathologic processes and detect orbital roof/floor fractures. CT is also best for detecting acute hemorrhage and requires less patient cooperation than MRI.

4. MRI: Best delineation of soft tissue structures of the orbit. Contrast-enhanced imaging (with fat suppression technique) is extremely sensitive to pathologic processes (in particular, intrinsic optic nerve processes such as optic neuritis and glioma and perioptic nerve processes such as meningioma). The orbital apex is best seen on MRI as is extension of a cavernous sinus process or any intracranial process due to the lack of bone artifacts.

   Disadvantages of MRI include lack of delineation of bony structures and mineralization in a lesion (which can help characterize lesions such as retinoblastoma). Even with MR angiography, most orbital vascular processes (most aneurysms, some varices, some fistulas) are inadequately evaluated and still require dedicated endovascular angiography for diagnosis (and treatment).

4. Angiography: Formal catheter angiography is still considered the gold standard for evaluation of most intraorbital vascular lesions. Cerebral angiography is the examination of choice for a carotid-cavernous fistula, as definitive endovascular therapy can be performed at the time of the diagnostic evaluation.

   Disadvantages of cerebral angiography include ionizing radiation, cost, and the 1:200 to 1:1,000 risk of *causing* a stroke during the examination.

C. Recommended Imaging Approach

Red eye conditions associated with either periocular or retro-ocular pain, fever, edematous or ecchymotic eyelids, tenderness of the lids and/or globe, reduced ocular motility, proptosis, and/or enophthalmos or visual loss require an imaging study to help differentiate between an infectious, inflammatory, neoplastic, or vascular process involving the orbit. Similarly, any traumatized orbit needs an imaging examination. Imaging examinations help narrow a differential diagnosis and also define the extent of an abnormality.

In the setting of trauma (blunt or lacerating trauma, concern about foreign body), a red eye needs to be evaluated by an ophthalmologist. The eye should be manipulated as little as possible and shielded for protection. A CT scan is the examination of choice to search for foreign material, bone fractures, intraorbital hematomata, mass effect, etc.

For children and adults, if symptoms and signs suggest a postseptal infection, a sinonasal imaging study should be done to rule out sinusitis, orbital subperiosteal abscess, or tumor. Immunocompromised patients are at risk for aggressive infectious processes such as mucormycosis and aspergillus. As the appearance of orbital bones is crucial in these patients, CT scanning is the imaging examination of choice.

Conjunctival hyperemia in the setting of diplopia, periocular pain, elevated intraocular pressure, and visual loss may suggest increased orbital venous pressure due to a posttraumatic or spontaneous carotid-cavernous fistula. Sometimes, the patient will hear a "whooshing" sound. The clinician may or may not be able to appreciate a cephalic bruit. A dilated ophthalmic vein (usually the superior ophthalmic vein) can be seen on imaging studies. Such a vein is equally well seen on MRI or direct coronal CT. However, as all CCF do not drain antegrade through the orbit, if clinical suspicion of a cavernous fistula persists in the setting of negative CT and MRI scans, angiography may still be necessary. As mentioned above, conventional endovascular catheter angiography is preferred over MR angiography, as definitive therapy ("ballooning" or embolization) of a fistula can be performed at the time of the angiography.

In summary, when imaging is required, in the setting of acute signs and symptoms (which is the case with most patients), CT is the examination of choice. MRI can add complementary information particularly with respect to an extraorbital component of an orbital process. If a CCF is of concern, the next study considered should be angiography which may have to be performed emergently to preserve visual function.

D. Differential Diagnostic Considerations

1. Imaging studies required (to evaluate extent of the disease process that can be occult to the examining ophthalmologist)

   a. Orbital infection/cellulitis (bacterial or fungal infection posterior to the orbital septum).

   b. Orbital inflammation (idiopathic orbital inflammation, pseudotumor).
      - Diffuse (anterior globe, posterior globe, orbital apex).
      - Local (myositis, dacryoadenitis, periscleritis, perineuritis).

   c. Orbital mass (may involve the orbit primarily via direct extension from the paranasal sinuses or secondarily from metastases).

   d. Orbital vascular malformation: Cavernous sinus arteriovenous malformation.
      - Direct, high-flow fistula.
      - Indirect, low-flow fistula.

   e. Orbital trauma.
      - Retrobulbar hemorrhage.
      - Orbital fracture (direct or indirect "blow-out" fracture).
      - Ruptured globe.
      - Intraocular foreign body.

2. Imaging studies not required

   a. Infections
      - Viral

         Adenoviral keratoconjunctivitis (adenovirus types 3 and 7).

         Epidemic keratoconjunctivitis (adenovirus types 8 and 19).

         Acute hemorrhagic conjunctivitis (enterovirus 70 or coxsackievirus A24).

         Molluscum contagiosum.

         Herpes simplex conjunctivitis/keratitis.

      - Bacterial.

         Gonococcal conjunctivitis (*Neisseria gonorrhoeae*).

         Chlamydial inclusion conjunctivitis (neonatal inclusion conjunctivitis acquired from an infected cervix and adult inclusion conjunctivitis acquired by sexual contact).

Corneal ulcers (secondary to contact lens wear, trauma, environmental exposure).

Blepharitis (most often due to *Staphylococcus* infection).

Hordeolum (acute *Staphylococcus* infection of the eyelid).

Dacryocystitis (inflammation of the lacrimal sac usually caused by bacterial infection in the setting of an obstructed nasolacrimal passage).

Preseptal cellulitis.

Endophthalmitis (infection of the intraocular tissues).

- Fungal: Keratitis (caused by filamentous species such as *Fusarium* and *Aspergillus*).

b. Inflammation.
- Hayfever conjunctivitis (allergic reaction to airborne allergens).
- Vernal keratoconjunctivitis (seasonally recurring; mediated by IgE antibodies).
- Atopic keratoconjunctivitis (IgE-mediated allergic reaction in patient with h/o atopy).
- Toxic conjunctivitis (exposure to topical ocular medications, cosmetics, contact lens solutions, etc.).
- Meibomitis (inflammation of meibomian glands secondary to secretory dysfunction).
- Chalazion or internal hordeolum (inflammation of the meibomian or Zeiss glands).
- Episcleritis (focal inflammation of the deep subconjunctival/episcleral tissue).
- Scleritis (focal or diffuse inflammation of the sclera).
- Anterior uveitis (iritis, iridocyclitis; inflammation of the iris and/or ciliary muscle).

c. Conjunctival degeneration.
- Inflamed pingueculum (yellowish elevation at the inner/outer corneal margins).
- Pterygium (focal thickened conjunctivum; can partially cover cornea).

d. Trauma.
- Subconjunctival hemorrhage.
- Chemical burn.
- Corneal abrasion (mechanical or foreign body irritation).
- Conjunctival laceration.
- Corneal laceration.
- Iritis.
- Hyphema (blood in the anterior chamber of the eye).

e. Glaucoma: Acute angle-closure glaucoma.

SALIVARY GLAND SWELLING

A. Clinical Findings

The major salivary glands (parotid, submandibular, and sublingual) typically become enlarged when affected by disease, usually due to the retention of secretions that cannot flow normally into the oral cavity. Intermittent swelling related to eating suggests intermittent obstruction (usually by a stone). Persistent or progressive swelling of a salivary gland suggests tumor.

Salivary calculi most commonly arise in the submandibular gland or duct.

All parotid region masses should be considered parotid gland tumors until proven otherwise. Parotid gland swelling with facial nerve palsy is usually due to an underlying neoplasm.

In adults, pleomorphic adenoma and adenoid cystic carcinoma are the most common salivary gland tumors. In children, mucoepidermoid carcinoma is the most common tumor.

Salivary gland masses should not be subjected to incisional biopsy, as there is a 90% chance that a solitary parotid gland mass is a pleomorphic adenoma; incising such a lesion is not only unnecessary, but will almost certainly lead to lesion recurrence.

B. Imaging Modalities

1. Plain radiographs: Plain radiographs are of limited value except possibly in the assessment of submandibular calculi, most of which

are radio-opaque. However, noncontrast CT remains a more sensitive test for the detection of all types of calculi.

2. Sialography: Sialography (cannulation of the Stenson's duct [parotid] or Wharton's duct [sublingual] with injection of contrast followed by plain radiography (or preferably CT scanning; see below) can display the entire ductal system, delineating distortion of ducts by intrinsic or extrinsic neoplastic or inflammatory processes. It is a useful test for demonstrating radiolucent stones. It is more sensitive than CT or MRI for demonstrating the effects of inflammatory processes on the ductal system. For example, there are characteristic appearances of congenital saccular sialectasis and in advanced cystic sialectasis which are not well seen on plain CT or MRI scans.

   Disadvantages of sialography are that it must be performed by an experienced physician, since artifacts can be created by traumatic cannulation and/or overfilling the ductal system/gland; it cannot differentiate between benign and malignant tumors; tumors <1 cm are difficult to demonstrate; sialography does not give the final histologic diagnosis; and it involves ionizing radiation.

3. CT: CT scanning is the single most useful scanning technique for imaging assessment of salivary gland neoplasms. It can demonstrate erosion/destruction of bony structures adjacent to malignant lesions. It nicely outlines the deep face (parapharyngeal) extent of larger parotid tumors. CT after sialography can delineate whether a mass is intrinsic or extrinsic to the parotid gland, can localize a mass within the parotid gland with respect to the facial nerve, and is more sensitive than conventional sialography for identifying small or multiple lesions.

4. MRI: The advantages of MRI include greater contrast between the tumor and surrounding tissue, no ionizing radiation, and multiplanar capabilities.

   Disadvantages include insensitivity for detection of ductal calculi and requirements for patient cooperation during scanning.

5. Percutaneous fine-needle aspiration cytology: Cells can be obtained for cytologic analysis by fine-needle (22-gauge) aspiration on an outpatient basis from any portion of a major salivary gland

using CT guidance. However, interpretation of salivary cell smears is difficult and requires an exceptionally high level of expertise. Incisional biopsies are not necessary and carry the risk of late recurrence in 90% of neoplasms.

C. Recommended Imaging Approach

If a salivary gland mass is palpable, no imaging is required if biopsy proves the benign nature of the lesion. If a lesion is malignant or if the margin of the lesion cannot definitely be identified by palpation, CT or MRI to better define the extent of the lesion should be performed. Such scanning also permits evaluation of the neck for lymph nodes not detectable by physical examination.

For diffuse salivary gland swelling, often clinical history and physical examination is diagnostic and no imaging is necessary. However, when imaging is deemed appropriate, sialography is the initial imaging study of choice, especially when the swelling is bilateral. If the sialogram suggests a mass, CT or MRI should be performed.

If (less invasive) CT or MRI is performed as the first examination and is suggestive of ductal disease (calculi or stenosis), sialography to evaluate the ductal system more fully should be considered.

D. Differential Diagnostic Considerations

1. Congenital.
   a. Hemangioma (pediatric).
   b. Lymphangioma (pediatric).
   c. Branchial cleft cyst.
2. Inflammatory.
   a. Acute.
      - Viral (mumps) is the most common acute inflammatory condition.
      - Bacterial.
         Acute suppurative parotiditis.
         Acute sialadenitis (duct stone).
         Abscess.
   b. Chronic: Punctate sialadenitis, usually due to sialectasis.

3. Neoplastic.
    a. Benign tumors.
        - Pleomorphic adenoma (mixed salivary tumor)—most common benign tumor.
        - Adenolymphoma (Warthin's tumor).
    b. Malignant tumors.
        - Adenoid cystic carcinoma—most common malignant tumor.
        - Squamous cell carcinoma.
        - Malignant pleomorphic adenoma.
        - Mucoepidermoid tumors.
        - Acinic cell carcinoma.
        - Non-Hodgkin's lymphoma.
    c. Rare tumors.
        - Oncocytoma.
        - Lipoma.
        - Sarcoma.
        - Metastatic tumors.
            Melanoma of the facial skin.
            Adenocarcinoma of the GI tract or urogenital system.
4. Miscellaneous.
    a. Bilateral benign lymphoepithelial cysts in immunocompromised patients.
    b. Calculi (sialolithiasis).
    c. Sialectasis.
    d. Sjögren's syndrome.

SINUSITUS/NASAL CONGESTION

A. Clinical Findings

Nasal congestion and sinus complaints are the most common of all upper respiratory disorders. They are both usually due to allergic and/or viral processes and are almost always self-limited. However, both chronic and acute complaints of this type are also common causes for a person to seek medical attention. Though imaging is important in further evaluation, clinical history, patient symptoms and physical examination findings are critical for delineating significant disease (which, in some cases, may require immediate intervention) from a self-limited nuisance.

B. Imaging Modalities

1. Plain films of the sinuses: Common and usually least expensive. Water's view alone may be adequate, but addition of lateral very helpful.

   Very insensitive to distribution and detail, but *can* find large air–fluid levels that can assist the diagnosis of acute/subacute bacterial sinusitis (which history and physical examination have probably already made anyway).

   Can miss *huge* amounts of bone destruction, but *do* show some bone detail. Replaced at some medical centers with limited coronal CT scanning (see below), which provides much higher sensitivity at similar cost.

2. Focused paranasal sinus CT: Coronal images alone adequate, but axials add detail (e.g., of sinus backwalls). Intravenous contrast material almost never needed for routine allergic/chronic sinusitis evaluation. Contrast material is required if mass or associated intracranial/orbital infection is suspected.

   Overall, CT provides the best sensitivity and clinical utility because cortical bone is precisely defined, allowing a major differential diagnostic division to be made between aggressive and nonaggressive processes.

   Required for preoperative evaluation.

3. MRI: Usually more expensive, and less available, than CT. Can provide a superb evaluation of sinonasal disease. However, cannot precisely define cortical bone detail; therefore, early aggressive changes can be difficult to appreciate.

   Superior to CT for identifying spread of sinonasal disease intracranially, determining etiology of associated cranial neuropathies, demonstrating secondary venous or arterial occlusive disease and their sequelae, and characterizing some forms of fungal sinusitis.

C. Recommended Imaging Approach

1. No imaging: Most sinonasal disease.

    Plain films of the sinuses add very little to a good history and physical examination. They miss significant findings, which can result in a false sense of security. Because of established referral patterns, they are still used by some practitioners to find large air–fluid levels.

    Unilateral paranasal sinus air–fluid levels with ipsilateral signs and symptoms support the diagnosis of acute/subacute bacterial sinusitis.

    Bilateral sinus air–fluid levels are more nonspecific; they are common and are *not* predictors of superimposed infection in patients with allergic sinonasal disease, patients with an nasogastric or endotracheal tube in place, or in the setting of trauma (even without sinus wall fractures).

    Plain films, while insensitive to most sinonasal pathology, can show significant findings that history and physical examination have missed. These include occult fractures and bone destruction. If you cannot see a large bony structure, this may not be a "technical" limitation—bone may be *totally* destroyed. Bone destruction is critical. If it is present, it needs to be explained. Though this depends on the population being studied, lesions with bone destruction will usually turn out to be neoplasms.

2. Focused paranasal sinus CT: Should be performed when history and physical examination reveal allergic and/or inflammatory disease resistant to (antibiotic) therapy; immunocompromised state; disproportionate pain, anesthesia, anosmia; or findings suggestive of cranial neuropathy or maxillofacial mass.

3. MRI: Usually reserved to further classify and topographically define disease found on CT. Outstanding with respect to the depiction of spread of sinonasal disease to the intracranial compartment,

evaluation of cranial neuropathy, and evaluation of venous and arterial occlusive sequelae of sinonasal disease.

Though CT may show high attenuation in a sinus and MRI may show low signal in the same region, these findings *still* usually represent chronic allergic/bacterial sinusitis and not fungal infection. In fungal infections, the high attenuation on CT is usually calcification and may be in a striated pattern. The low signal on MRI represents minerals concentrated by the fungus in its growth. However, inspissated, desiccated mucus and chronic small-volume bleeding from "simple" chronic sinusitis can simulate these findings and are *far more common* than fungal sinusitis. In addition, the most common imaging appearance for early fungal sinusitis is nonspecific inflammatory change of the mucosa. Clinical history may help lead to aspiration and/or biopsy to make the correct diagnosis before bone destruction occurs.

D. Differential Diagnostic Considerations

In order of frequency for a Northern American practice:

1. Viral upper respiratory tract infection: Probably the most common cause of nasal congestion, "runny nose," etc. History critical.

2. Allergy: Patients almost always have a history of other allergies. May be the most common cause of chronic sinusitis.

    Hypertrophic lamina propria nasal polyps and *pan*sinusitis are common. Samter's triad (nasal polyps, asthma, hypersensitivity to nonsteroidal antiinflammatory agents, including aspirin) is rarely seen. Other causes of nasal polyps (trauma, cystic fibrosis) are less common.

    Complications of chronic sinusitis include mucous and serous retention cysts, polyps, and granulation tissue (more common) and mucocele and orbital/intracranial infection (less common).

3. Environment: Inhaled irritants/allergens. The clinical history of exposure is critical. Patients usually also have other allergies.

4. Bacterial infection: Usually preceded by an upper respiratory viral infection or allergic flare-up. Usually *focally* more painful than the disorder that led to it (i.e., patient may have pressure tenderness over a sinus). Usually isolated paranasal sinus infections result

from poor drainage of that sinus. Paranasal sinus infections can extend into the orbit, resulting in infection/abscess, and can also extend intracranially and cause dural venous sinus thromboses and/or meningoencephalitis if not treated.

These infections may be the result of an intranasal *foreign body* in children or the mentally impaired.

5. Neoplasm
   a. Squamous cell carcinoma: Usually older males with environmental exposure history (smoking, nickel and chromium production, woodworkers).
   b. Schneiderian papillomas: Most common is *inverted papilloma,* which grows from the lateral nasal wall under the middle turbinate, is locally aggressive, and may lead to development of an adjacent carcinoma.
   c. Angiofibroma: Teen-age male with chronic, recurrent nasal stuffiness and epistaxis. Posterior nasal cavity origin, locally very aggressive. *Angiomatous polyp* (probably posttraumatic) can mimic it on imaging, but usually enhances much less and is far less aggressive.
   d. Lymphoma: Including non-Hodgkin's, Hodgkin's and Burkitt-type non-Hodgkin's.
   e. Other neoplasms: Minor salivary gland neoplasms from the tiny mucosal glands. *Primary* melanoma. Neurogenic neoplasms, most often *Schwannoma* or *olfactory neuroblastoma* (esthesioneuroblastoma).

6. Autoimmune.
   a. Wegener's granulomatosis: Usually an adult with painful nasal ulcer and/or otitis who gradually develops bronchitis, pneumonia, and glomerulonephritis.
   b. Midline granuloma: Usually presents as nasal obstruction, pain, and ulcer.
   c. Sarcoidosis: Usually presents in blacks or Scandinavians as nasal obstruction.

7. Fungal infections: Still uncommon, but on the rise with the ever-increasing population of immunocompromised individuals.

    a. Allergies: More benign, noninvasive, environmental exposure-related.

    b. Aspergillosis: Can be chronic and relatively benign, but, in immunocompromised patients, may aggressively invade the maxillofacial and skull base regions and occlude arteries, infarcting portions of the CNS.

    c. Mucormycosis: *Diabetics* and immunocompromised. Aggressive and arteriopathic, just like aspergillosis. *Requires* urgent surgical treatment.

8. Less common etiologies.

    a. Tuberculosis.

    b. Syphilis.

    c. Cilia dysmotility: Smoking, Kartagener's syndrome.

    d. Cystic fibrosis: Consider in a child with polyps and chronic sinusitis.

TINNITUS

A. Clinical Findings

Tinnitus (from the Latin *tinnire* meaning "to jingle") may affect up to 37 million Americans, though only a minority of these patients seek medical attention. For any given patient, tinnitus may vary from a minor irritation to a major psychosocial upheaval resulting in depression and even suicide.

Patients will describe tinnitus as a "ringing," "rushing," "steam-escaping," "roaring," or "buzzing" sound in one or both ears and sometimes apparently originating from other regions of the head and neck. The intensity and character of the tinnitus can vary depending on the position of the head, exercise, and Valsalva and other maneuvers.

There is no consensus on a uniform classification system of the various types of tinnitus. Different classification systems include paraauditory versus sensorineural, vibratory versus nonvibratory, subjective versus objective, or by location (tympanic, cochlear, or central).

Many of the causes of sensorineural/nonvibratory tinnitus (see below) are not as well understood as the mechanical/vibratory causes. However, it is believed that the most common cause of sensorineural/nonvibratory tinnitus is intrinsic cochlear pathology.

B. Imaging Modalities

1. Plain radiographs: There is no role for plain radiographs in the evaluation of tinnitus.

2. CT: The main advantage of CT scanning is the excellent delineation of skull base (in particular temporal bone) anatomy when 1–2 mm sections are obtained in both the axial and coronal planes. In addition, contrast-enhanced images can demonstrate some vascular abnormalities and tumors.

    Disadvantages include limited evaluation of the intracranial compartment due to extensive artifact from the temporal bones and the intrinsic risks of ionizing radiation and intravenous contrast material.

3. MRI: The main advantage of MRI is the direct visualization of intracranial structures such as the brain stem, cerebellum, cerebellopontine angle cistern, the internal auditory canal, and any pathologic mass (tumor, infection). Also, extension of a temporal bone process either intracranially or extracranially is best delineated with MRI. MR angiography can be used to assess for anomalous vasculature and also invasion of intracranial vascular structures (e.g., transverse or sigmoid sinus involvement by a temporal bone inflammatory or neoplastic process). With MRI, there is no ionizing radiation, and the risk of contrast agents is less than that with CT.

    Disadvantages include poor delineation of bones, poor demonstration of mineralization of some pathologic processes, and the necessity for the patient to lie motionless for the 5–10 minutes required to obtain the MR images. MR angiography cannot demonstrate all vascular anomalies of the temporal bone (e.g., dural malformations can be occult on MR angiography).

4. Angiography: Advantages of conventional endovascular catheter angiography include superior delineation of arterial and venous anatomy (clearly superior to MR angiography) and vascular neo-

plasms and the potential for interventional therapy of some vascular lesions (e.g., dural arteriovenous malformations, meningiomas, aneurysms).

Disadvantages include the intrinsic risks of catheter angiography (between a 1:200 and 1:1,000 risk of *causing* a stroke), the relatively high dose of radiation, the risks of intravascular contrast material, and the relatively high cost of the examination.

C. Recommended Imaging Approach

The evaluation of tinnitus can be frustrating, as often the tinnitus is completely subjective (cannot be appreciated by the examining physician). Evaluation begins with a history and physical examination. As warranted by an otolaryngologist, audiometry, tympanometry, and possibly electromyography may be performed.

If imaging is required, either CT or MRI is the examination of choice. As these studies are often complimentary, depending on the clinical concerns, both studies may be necessary. Intrinsic temporal bone abnormalities such as a dehiscent jugular bulb, an anomalous vessel, congenital abnormalities, or postinflammatory changes of the otic capsule are best evaluated with CT. The relationship of any temporal bone process to nearby normal bony structures (e.g., as in the evaluation of a secondary cholesteatoma) is also better evaluated with CT. Masses of the temporal bone or the internal auditory canal or intracranial/extracranial masses with temporal bone invasion are best evaluated with MRI. Acute inflammatory processes that involve cranial nerves or the otic capsule are probably also better evaluated with MRI.

Angiography is reserved for the few cases in which a vascular malformation remains of clinical concern or if endovascular interventional therapy (either definitive or preoperative) is necessary.

D. Differential Diagnostic Considerations

1. Mechanical (vibratory).
   a. Vascular.
      - Normal variant (dehiscent jugular bulb, venous "hum," persistent stapedial artery).

- High flow state (hypertension, pregnancy, thyrotoxicosis, anemia, Paget's disease).
- Vascular neoplasms (e.g., paragangliomas).
- Arteriovenous malformations.
- Aneurysm.
- Fibromuscular dysplasia.

  b. Neuromuscular.
  - Temporomandibular joint dysfunction.
  - Stapedial muscle spasm.
  - Tensor tympani muscle spasm.
  - Palatal myoclonus (spasm of the tensor and levator veli palatani muscles).

2. Sensorineural (nonvibratory).
   a. Peripheral (intrinsic cochlear lesions).
   - Trauma.
   - Labyrinthitis: Allergies, bacterial, spirochetal, viral.
   - Meniere's disease.
   - Otosclerosis.

   b. Central
   - Auditory nerve (cranial nerve VIII) dysfunction (Schwannoma).
   - Any cerebellopontine angle mass (other cranial nerve lesions, meningioma).
   - Brain stem lesions.

   c. Other
   - Diabetes mellitus.
   - Hypothyroidism.
   - Drugs.
   - Trace metal deficiencies (zinc, copper, iron).

References

Lo WM (1991). Vascular tinnitus. In Som PM, Bergeron RT (eds.): Head and Neck Imaging, 2nd Ed. St. Louis: Mosby-Yearbook, pp. 1108–1115.

Meyerhoff WL, Cooper JC (1991). Tinnitus. In Paparella MM, Schumarik DA, Gluckman JL, Meyerhoff WL (eds): Otolaryngology, 3rd Ed. Philadelphia: WB Saunders, pp. 1169–1179.

Tyler RS, Babin RW (1986). Tinnitus. In Cummins CW, Frederickson JM et al (eds): Otolaryngology—Head and Neck Surgery, St. Louis: CV Mosby, pp. 3201–3217.

TRANSIENT VISUAL CHANGES

A. Clinical Findings

Transient (less than 24 hour) visual changes can be described as *negative phenomena* such as a curtain coming up or down, blurring, missing portions of a visual field, peripheral constriction, central scotoma, or fog. They can also be described as *positive phenomena* such as jagged lines, sparkles, or lightning bolts. Either description may be unilateral or bilateral.

B. Imaging Modalities

1. Plain radiographs: While plain radiographs can demonstrate orbital wall, lacrimal gland fossa, optic foramen, optic canal, sphenoid ridge, and paranasal sinus bony abnormalities, associated soft tissue (e.g., intraorbital) abnormalities cannot be assessed. Therefore, plain radiography, whether positive or negative, does not obviate the need for additional imaging (ultrasound, CT, or MRI) and is therefore of no value in evaluating transient visual changes.

2. Ultrasound: Inexpensive, safe (no ionizing radiation), reproducible method of evaluating orbital lesions. Does not permit visualization of the orbital apex or extraorbital spread of a process. May not be possible to use in severely traumatized or uncooperative patients. Very operator-dependent modality.

   a. A-mode orbital ultrasound (echography): One-dimensional view of an orbital lesion; can show lesion's "reflectivity," sound attenuation, and internal structure.

    b. B-mode orbital ultrasound (echography): Can demonstrate orbital lesion's location, size, shape, and orientation to other structures.

    c. Color Doppler ultrasound of the carotid arteries: Can accurately demonstrate carotid artery bifurcation region atherosclerotic changes, including vessel narrowing. Ultrasound can misinterpret a high-grade (but still patent) vessel narrowing for a completely occluded vessel.

    d. Transesophageal echogram (TEE): Can be used to evaluate the heart, valves, and aortic root for source of emboli.

3. CT: Superb delineation of the bones of the face, which is crucial when evaluating fractures or bony erosion/expansion/destruction by orbital neoplasms or infectious/inflammatory processes. Native intraorbital fat provides excellent contrast to both normal and abnormal orbital soft tissue structures. CT is the examination of choice for ruling out orbital foreign bodies. Can also scan in the direct coronal plane to better localize pathologic processes and detect orbital roof/floor fractures or extension of other pathologic processes. CT is also best for detecting acute hemorrhage and requires less patient cooperation than MRI.

4. MRI: Best delineation of soft tissue structures of the orbit. Contrast-enhanced imaging (with fat suppression technique) is extremely sensitive to pathologic processes (in particular, intrinsic optic nerve processes such as optic neuritis and glioma and perioptic nerve processes such as meningioma). The orbital apex is best seen on MRI as is extension of a cavernous sinus process or any intracranial process due to the lack of bone artifacts.

    Disadvantages of MRI include lack of delineation of bony structures and mineralization in a lesion (which can help characterize lesions such as retinoblastoma). Even with MR angiography most orbital vascular processes (most aneurysms, some varices, some fistulas) are inadequately evaluated and require dedicated endovascular angiography for diagnosis (and treatment).

    MR angiography can be used to evaluate the carotid artery bifurcations for atherosclerotic narrowing. High grade (99%)

(though still patent) vessel narrowing can be misinterpreted as a completely occluded vessel on MR angiography.

5. Angiography: Formal catheter angiography is still considered the gold standard for evaluation of the carotid arteries (or any arteries) for atherosclerotic narrowing. Similarly, most intraorbital vascular processes are best evaluated with angiography.

Disadvantages of cerebral angiography include ionizing radiation, cost, and the 1:200 to 1:1,000 risk of *causing* a stroke during the examination.

C. Recommended Imaging Approach

A major cause of transient visual changes is embolic phenomena from atherosclerotic changes of the carotid artery or, less commonly, from the ophthalmic artery itself or from intrinsic cardiac, heart valve, or aortic root embolic sources.

In patients with unilateral negative phenomena and no signs of optic neuropathy, a source of emboli should be ruled out with screening ultrasound (TEE) of the heart, valves, and aortic root and ultrasound or MR angiography of the carotid arteries. As a 70%-99% internal carotid arterial narrowing is best treated surgically, such narrowing is often confirmed with endovascular catheter angiography, which also permits evaluation of other areas of the internal carotid artery (including its intracranial portion), which are poorly evaluated by ultrasound or MR angiography.

If signs of optic neuropathy are present in the setting of unilateral negative phenomena, dedicated orbital imaging with MRI is suggested to rule out an intrinsic or extrinsic lesion compromising the optic nerve.

If unilateral or bilateral positive phenomena are present with associated features of a typical migraine headache in a patient <50 years old, no further evaluation is necessary and the patient may be treated for migraine headaches.

If unilateral positive phenomena are present in a patient >50 years old without a history of migraine headaches, MRI of the head and orbits and evaluation of the heart and neck with ultrasound and/or MR angiography should be performed.

If bilateral positive phenomena without a history of migraine

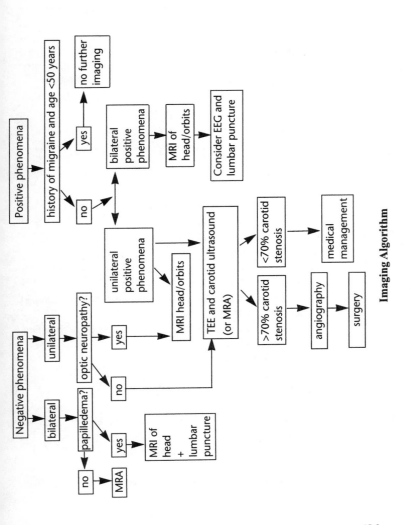

Imaging Algorithm

headache are present, head MRI and possibly EEG and lumbar puncture should be performed.

For bilateral negative phenomena without papilledema, MR angiography is recommended to rule out a posterior circulation stenosis; with evidence of papilledema, additional imaging (MRI of the head and orbits) should be performed to rule out an intraorbital or intracranial process.

D. Differential Diagnostic Considerations

1. Unilateral negative phenomena: Usually ischemic (1–5 minutes).
   a. Embolic (sources: heart, aortic root, carotid artery, ophthalmic artery).
   b. Thrombotic.
      - Low flow states.
      - Anticardiolipin antibody syndrome (age <50 years).
      - Giant cell arteritis (age >50 years).
   c. Recent eye surgery, angle closure glaucoma, hyphema.
   d. Compressive lesion (with signs of optic neuropathy).
2. Bilateral negative phenomena.
   a. Posterior circulation ischemia (<5 minutes).
   b. Papilledema: Multiple causes including increased intracranial pressure (<1 minute).
   c. Migraine (consider when other classic features of migraine headaches are present).
3. Unilateral positive phenomena.
   a. Retinal migraine.
   b. Retinal detachment (flashers and floaters).
4. Bilateral positive phenomena.
   a. Migraine: Reproducible pattern; spreading visual loss.
   b. Seizure.
   c. Vasculitis (e.g., systemic lupus erythematosis).
   d. Occipital tumor.
   e. Chronic meningitis (consider risk factors such as immunosuppression).

VERTIGO

A. Clinical Findings

Vertigo is the subjective sensation of rotary movement. Patients may describe the sensation that they are revolving in space, or they may feel that objects are moving around them. One of the keys to successfully treating vertigo is establishing its presence. Patients frequently find it difficult to describe what they are feeling and often use the term "dizziness" to describe vertigo. Therefore, it is important that patients describe their symptoms in detail to determine if they are experiencing "vertigo" or other symptoms. Nonvertiginous dizziness (sensation of light headedness, faintness, etc.) is frequently caused by processes that are easily identified by history and physical examination (e.g., medications, dehydration, anxiety, visual problems, heart disease, etc.) rather than by imaging.

B. Imaging Modalities

1. Plain radiographs: While skull films may identify temporal bone fractures in trauma patients or secondary osseous changes due to mass lesions (e.g., widening of the internal auditory canal with acoustic neuromas), they cannot directly evaluate the temporal bone or intracranial contents. When imaging is required in the workup of vertigo, one is typically looking for lesions of the brain stem, small structures contained within the temporal bone, or brain parenchyma. Therefore, plain films should not be used in the evaluation of these patients.

2. CT: Due to the excellent bone detail afforded by direct axial and coronal images, CT is better than MRI in the evaluation of many temporal bone abnormalities, especially those related to trauma. While CT is excellent for identifying many cerebral abnormalities, examination of the brain stem and posterior fossa contents by CT is inferior to MRI.

3. MRI: The major advantage of MRI over CT in the evaluation of vertigo is its superior visualization of the brain stem and posterior fossa contents due to its improved soft tissue contrast and mul-

tiplanar capabilities (coronal and sagittal images may be obtained without changes in patient position within the MRI scanner). In addition, unlike CT, MR images are not degraded by artifact from adjacent osseous structures. Noninvasive MR angiography may also be performed in select patients with suspected vascular abnormalities.

The major disadvantages of MRI are that it requires complete patient cooperation to prevent image degradation by motion artifact and that it is contraindicated in patients with cardiac pacemakers, some metallic aneurysm clips, some metallic orbital or periorbital foreign bodies, and certain prosthetic devices.

C. Recommended Imaging Approach

In the evaluation of vertigo, localization of the anatomic level of dysfunction based on clinical history and physical examination is most important in determining the need for imaging evaluation.

In most cases, labyrinthine vertigo may be diagnosed and treated based on history and physical examination alone. In cases of posttraumatic labyrinthitis, imaging is frequently necessary and CT is the modality of choice as it allows excellent evaluation of the temporal bone.

In patients with suspected acoustic Schwannomas and in patients with central vertigo (lesions localized to brain stem/brain), imaging evaluation should begin with MRI. In select cases when a vascular abnormality (such as vertebrobasilar ischemic disease) is suspected, MR angiography should be included as part of the MRI examination. If a vascular abnormality is identified or remains highly suspected in the setting of a normal MRI study, conventional endovascular cerebral angiography should be performed, as presently it remains the gold standard for evaluating blood vessels and cerebrovascular disease.

D. Differential Diagnostic Considerations

Vertigo may be secondary to dysfunction at multiple levels, including the labyrinth, eighth cranial nerve, brain stem, or the cerebral cortex. On occasion, vertigo may be secondary to systemic (extracranial) causes.

1. Labyrinthine vertigo most common.

    a. Acute: Viral or bacterial infections. Frequently accompanied by nausea and emesis, nystagmus, gait disturbance.

    b. Chronic labyrinthitis (Meniere's): Frequently accompanied by tinnitus and hearing loss.

    c. Benign positional vertigo.

    d. Ototoxic medications: Aspirin, lasix, streptomycin, etc.

    e. Posttraumatic: Sequela of temporal bone fracture.

    f. Cerebrovascular disease: Ischemia affecting the auditory artery.

2. Brain stem: Vertical nystagmus localizes lesion to the brain stem. Other findings that may localize to brain stem include cranial nerve symptoms and/or motor or sensory loss.

    a. Ischemia: Vertebrobasilar insufficiency.

    b. Inflammatory: Demyelinating disease, radiation, infection.

    c. Mass lesion: Neoplasm (astrocytoma, metastases), vascular malformation.

3. Acoustic nerve lesions: Uncommon cause of vertigo. Schwannoma of the vestibular portion of the cranial nerve VIII: Usually other signs of nerve VIII dysfunction are present (tinnitus, hearing loss). When the tumor extends into the cerebellopontine angle cistern, cranial nerve V and VII symptoms may be present.

4. Cerebral cortex: Temporal lobe seizure (rare).

5. Systemic (extracranial).

    a. Cardiovascular: Arrhythmias.

    b. Medications: Ototoxic drugs (antihypertensives, antibiotics).

    c. Metabolic: Hypoglycemia.

    d. Subclavian steal syndrome.

VOCAL CORD PARALYSIS

A. Clinical Findings

Depending on the cause, vocal cord paresis/paralysis may be unilateral or bilateral, complete or incomplete. In general, vocal cord paralysis arises from processes at some distance from the larynx.

All of the intrinsic muscles of the larynx, with the exception of the cricothyroid muscles, are supplied by the *recurrent* laryngeal branches of the tenth cranial nerves. The cricothyroid muscles, which act as tensors of the vocal cords, are supplied by an external branch of the *superior* laryngeal branch of the tenth cranial nerves. The courses of the right and left recurrent laryngeal nerves differ, and, as a result, the left recurrent laryngeal nerve is more vulnerable to acute and chronic injuries.

B. Imaging Modalities

1. Plain radiographs (i.e., chest radiography).
   a. Low cost and high-resolution screening examination.
   b. Will detect left bronchial carcinoma and left apical tuberculosis because these lesions are usually quite extensive before involving the left recurrent laryngeal nerve.
2. Barium swallow.
   a. Useful in identifying esophageal lesions such as esophageal carcinoma (best test for detecting intrinsic esophageal pathology), compression by a thyroid mass or an enlarged left atrium.
   b. Risk of aspiration of barium in the setting of laryngeal dysfunction.
3. Ultrasonography of the neck.
   a. Detect and differentiate between solid and cystic thyroid lesions.
   b. Limited value for detection of invasion of neck structures.
   c. No ionizing radiation.
4. CT.
   a. Superior to plain radiographs, barium swallow, or ultrasound for detection of structural abnormalities of the skull base, neck, or chest that can affect laryngeal nerves.
   b. Superior to MRI for the detection of pulmonary parenchymal processes (less motion artifact).
   c. Superior to MRI for the detection of skull base (e.g., petrous temporal bone) lesions.
   d. Inferior to MRI for the detection of intraaxial (e.g., brain stem) lesions.

5. MRI.
   a. Superior to CT for the detection of intracranial (in particular, intraaxial) pathology.
   b. Similar to CT for the detection of chest wall and/or mediastinal invasion.
   c. Coronal/sagittal capabilities make it superior to CT for the detection of apical thoracic lesions.
   d. High soft tissue discrimination for the evaluation of the neck (*probably* superior to CT).
   e. Inferior to CT for the detection and evaluation of bony lesions (e.g., skull base).

C. Recommended Imaging Approach

Clinical history and physical examination can often localize the region (brain stem, skull base, neck, or chest) of a lesion suspected to be causing a vocal cord paresis/paralysis. For example, an "intermediate" position of vocal cords (as determined by the otolaryngologist) indicates that an offending lesion is above the level of larynx.

Chest radiography is usually performed first to rule out lung carcinoma or apical thoracic tuberculosis. A barium swallow can also be performed if a primary esophageal etiology is of clinical concern. Neck and upper chest CT is the best test for ruling out mass lesions in these locations. MRI is probably as good, but is often degraded by respiratory motion artifacts and costs more without a proven superiority with respect to lesion detection. If a skull base (petrous temporal bone) lesion is of concern, CT evaluation should be performed. If an intracranial (i.e., brain stem) process is suspected, MRI is the examination of choice.

Conventional tomography and cinefluoroscopy are useful for evaluating vocal cord symmetry and mobility, but are of limited value for detecting the cause of the dysfunction.

D. Differential Diagnostic Considerations

1. Left recurrent laryngeal nerve paresis.
   a. In the chest.
      • Carcinoma of the bronchus.

- Carcinoma of the thoracic esophagus.
- Malignant mediastinal nodes and primary neoplasms.
- Pulmonary tuberculosis and/or associated surgery.
- Aortic (arch) aneurysm.
- Cardiac hypertrophy.
- Any cardiac surgery.
- Peripheral neuritis (idiopathic); often follows viral infection.

  b. In the neck.
  - Trauma during thyroid, cardiac, or esophageal surgery.
  - Penetrating wounds.
  - Malignant cervical lymph nodes.
  - Carcinoma of the hypopharynx, esophagus, or thyroid gland.

2. Right recurrent laryngeal nerve paresis: Much less common than left-sided recurrent laryngeal nerve paresis. While the causes are the same as for the left side, they are usually confined to the neck, with a thoracic etiology being extremely unusual.

3. Bilateral recurrent laryngeal nerve paresis: Thyroid (or any midline/paramidline neck) surgery is the most common cause; other lesions are the same as those listed for the left recurrent laryngeal nerve in the neck. A similar condition is sometimes seen in patients with rheumatoid arthritis, when there may be cricoarytenoid joint ankylosis.

4. Combined superior and recurrent laryngeal nerve paresis: Only can occur in lesions of the medulla oblongata or of the tenth cranial nerve above the level of the origin of the superior laryngeal nerve (which is approximately at the level of the skull base).

5. Tenth cranial nerve (vagus) lesion.
   - Carcinoma of the nasopharynx.
   - Tumors of the jugular foramen (e.g., glomus jugulare, Schwannoma, meningioma).

6. Brain stem (medullary) lesions.
   - Vascular (e.g., ischemic, vascular malformation).
   - Neoplastic (e.g., primary/secondary).
   - Inflammatory (e.g., demyelinating).

- Infectious (e.g., bulbar poliomyelitis).
- Congenital (e.g., syringobulbia).

7. Key points

   a. Left vocal cord paresis/paralysis is considered due to lung carcinoma until proven otherwise.

   b. Bilateral vocal cord palsies are uncommon and tend to occur after thyroid or chest surgery.

▶ Index

MRI Spine

CSF dark on T1
Bright on T2

Flair similar to T2 but
abnormalities bright +
normal CSF made dark